Imperial College London
2407854953

AF606506

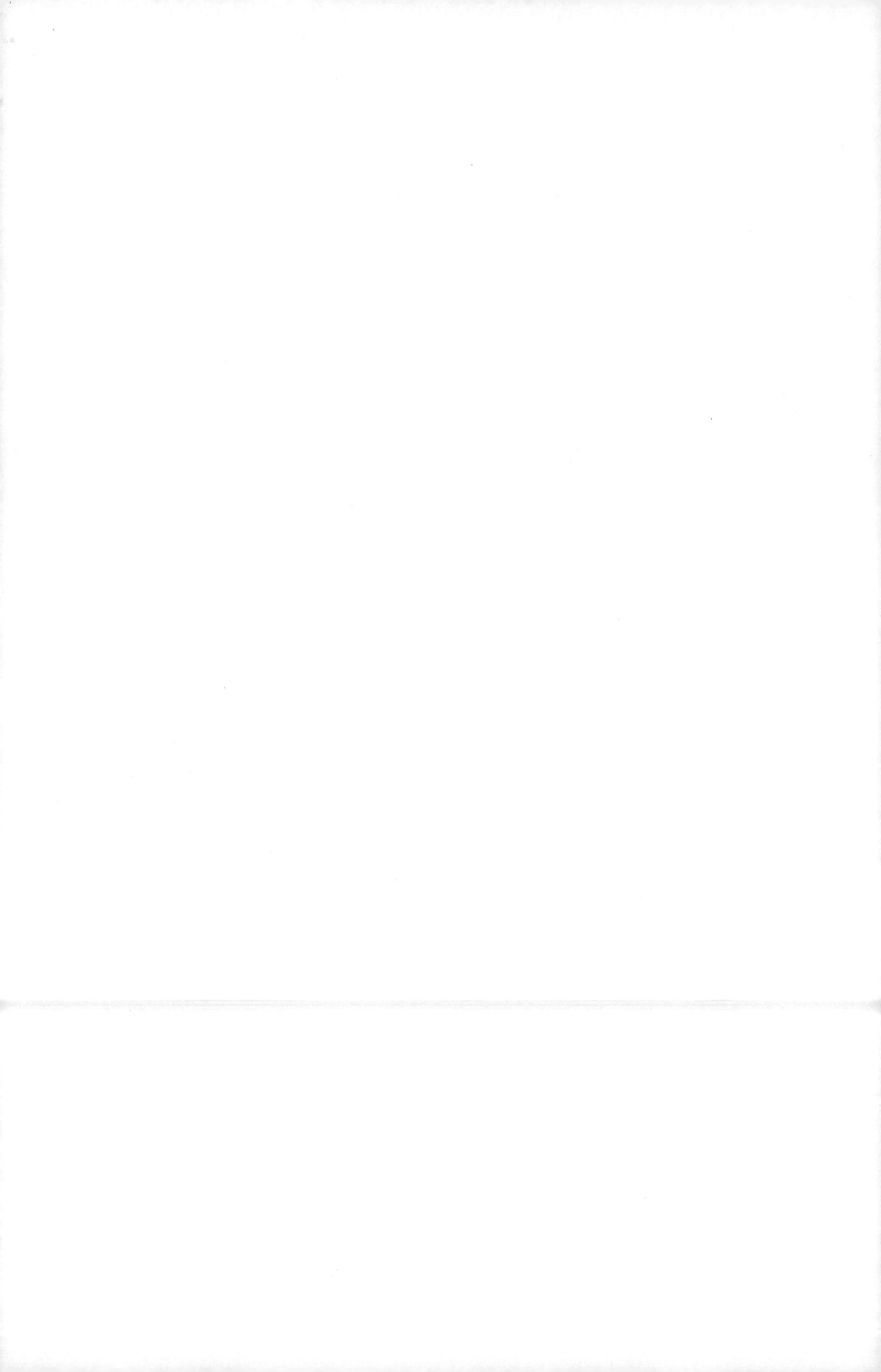

Functional Mitral and Tricuspid Regurgitation

Kok Meng John Chan
Editor

Functional Mitral and Tricuspid Regurgitation

Pathophysiology, Assessment and Treatment

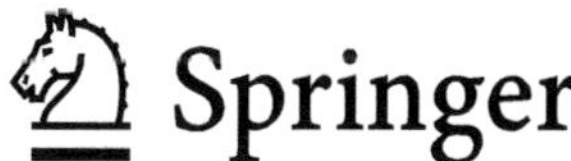

Editor
Kok Meng John Chan
Department of Cardiothoracic Surgery
Gleneagles Hospital
Kuala Lumpur
Malaysia

ISBN 978-3-319-43508-4 ISBN 978-3-319-43510-7 (eBook)
DOI 10.1007/978-3-319-43510-7

Library of Congress Control Number: 2016959032

Printed on acid-free paper

This Springer imprint is published by Springer Nature
The registered company is Springer International Publishing AG Switzerland
The registered company is Gewerbestrasse 11, 6330 Cham, Switzerland

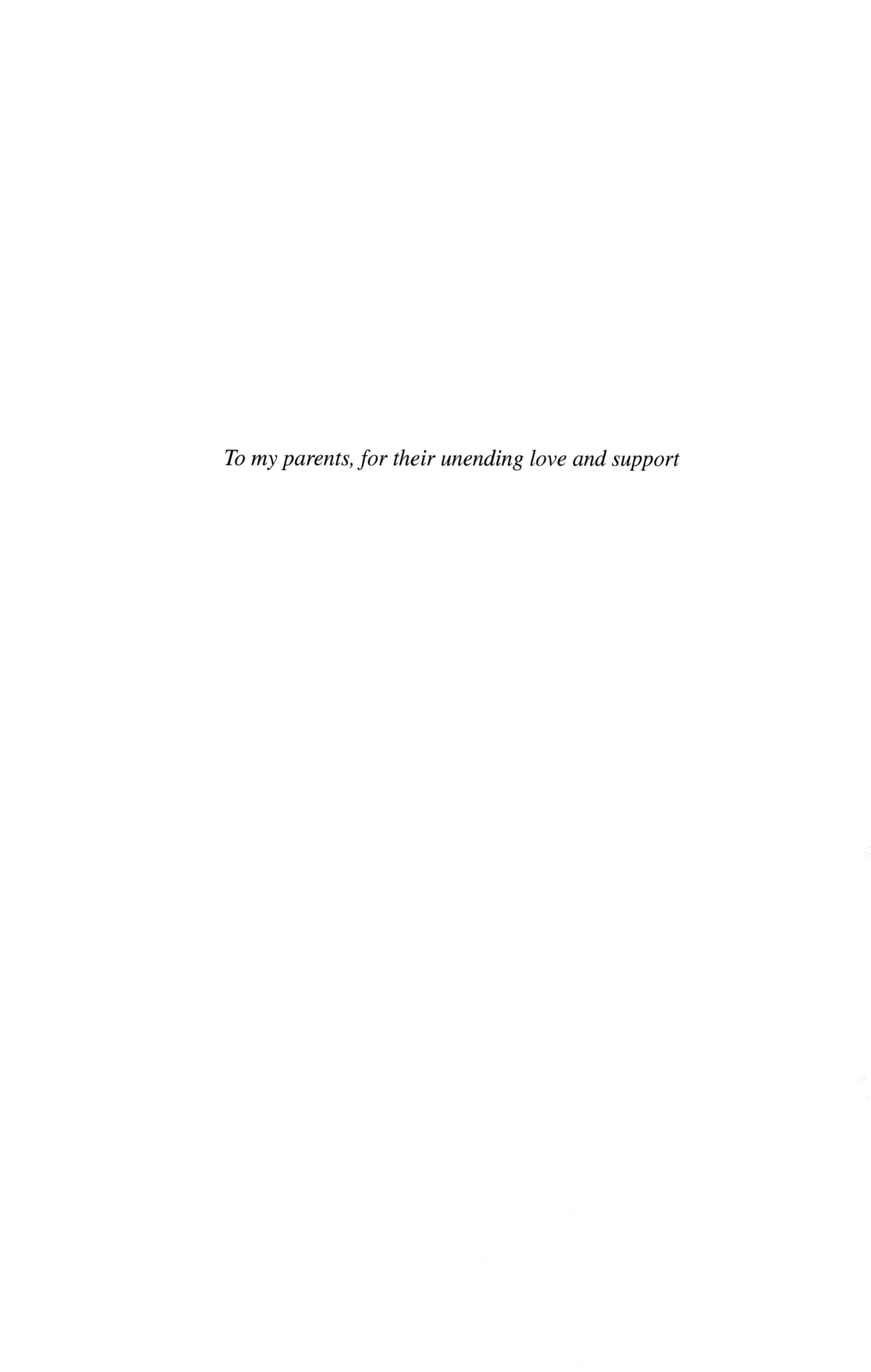

To my parents, for their unending love and support

Preface

Functional mitral and tricuspid regurgitation have proved challenging to clinicians and surgeons. Both conditions lead to adverse outcomes with reduced survival and functional capacity. Both share a common pathology in that they are diseases primarily of the ventricle, rather than of the valve itself. Hence the term "functional" as the function of the valve is impaired secondary to disease affecting the ventricle.

Our understanding of both conditions have increased substantially in recent years, and along with this better assessment and indications for surgery have been put into practice. Important operative surgical principles and techniques have also been learnt and taught over the years to ensure a successful long-term outcome with our operations. Newer surgical techniques and procedures have also been developed to treat the more advanced stages of the disease more effectively and durably. However, although we are able to restore the competency of the regurgitant valves and improve the symptoms, functional capacity and cardiac function of these patients, restoring their life expectancy back to that of a normal individual has proven challenging.

In functional mitral regurgitation, much new knowledge has emerged on the functional anatomy of the normal mitral valve and the pathophysiology of functional mitral regurgitation. This helps us better understand the importance of the surgical principles for performing a mitral annuloplasty for functional mitral regurgitation. In addition, new surgical techniques and procedures have been developed and used to address the lesions which limit the durability of a mitral annuloplasty. Surgical repair techniques now not only treat the lesion at the mitral annular level but address the subvalvular apparatus contributing to the leaflet restriction, and also the leaflet itself, as appropriate. Several randomised controlled trials comparing coronary artery bypass grafting (CABG) only against CABG plus concomitant mitral valve repair, and comparing mitral valve repair against mitral valve replacement, in the treatment of functional ischemic mitral regurgitation have been reported recently. These trials have provided important and useful insights on the best treatment for our patients depending on the severity of the mitral regurgitation and the stage of the disease process. A tailored approach for the treatment of functional ischaemic mitral regurgitation in different patients is now possible.

In functional tricuspid regurgitation, our knowledge and understanding of this condition is constantly advancing. Important concepts on the pathophysiology of functional tricuspid regurgitation with regards to annular dilatation have been emphasised in recent years. More recently, an appreciation of leaflet tethering and right ventricular dilatation and eccentricity contributing to functional tricuspid regurgitation is now known. Along with this, a better understanding of how to assess functional tricuspid regurgitation has emerged. New surgical procedures have also been developed to address these lesions at the leaflet level and are now in use. At the same time, recent studies have provided important insights into the long-term durability and complications with both bioprosthetic and mechanical valves in the tricuspid position, helping us select the right surgical procedure and choice of prosthesis if required.

With so many advances in functional mitral and tricuspid regurgitation in recent years, and so many emerging new concepts and principles to appreciate and understand, not only in the surgical treatment but also in the pathophysiology and the assessment of the conditions, the need to bring all of these together in a comprehensive book on the subject became apparent. This book will provide the reader with a comprehensive understanding and knowledge of all aspects of functional mitral and tricuspid regurgitation, from its natural history and pathophysiology, to its assessment, and treatment by various surgical techniques, procedures and devices. It will arm the reader with sufficient knowledge and understanding to select the most appropriate treatment option for the individual patient and tailor the management accordingly depending on patient characteristics and stage of the disease.

The contributors to this book are recognised international experts and leaders in functional mitral and tricuspid regurgitation, with a vast clinical, medical and surgical experience. All have done extensive research and published widely on the subject. Of note, the main authors of the recently reported randomised controlled trials on functional ischemic mitral regurgitation have each contributed chapters to the book on their respective research findings, providing unique insights and perspectives on the subject. The participation of authors from the United States, Europe and Asia has given the book an international perspective which is hoped will be applicable to your practice wherever you are working.

Kuala Lumpur, Malaysia K.M. John Chan

Contents

Contributors

Michael A. Acker, MD Division of Cardiovascular Surgery, Penn Medicine Heart and Vascular Center, Philadelphia, PA, USA

Hospital of the University of Pennsylvania, Perelman School of Medicine of the University of Pennsylvania, Philadelphia, PA, USA

Ottavio Alfieri, MD San Raffaele University Hospital, Milan, Italy

Manuel J. Antunes, MD, PhD, DSc University Hospital of Coimbra, Coimbra, Portugal

Rimantas Benetis Department of Cardiac Surgery, Hospital of Lithuanian University of Health Sciences, Kaunas Clinics, Kaunas, Lithuania

Serenella Castelvecchio, MD Department of Cardiac Surgery, IRCCS Policlinico San Donato, San Donato Milanese (MI), Italy

K.M. John Chan, BM BS, MSc, PhD, FRCS CTh Department of Cardiothoracic Surgery, Gleneagles Hospital, Kuala Lumpur, Malaysia

Antonio Colombo, MD Cardiac Cath Lab and Interventional Cardiology Unit, San Raffaele Hospital, Milan, Italy

Michele De Bonis, MD "Vita e Salute" San Raffaele University Medical School, San Raffaele University Hospital, Milan, Italy

Paolo Denti, MD Department of Heart Surgery, San Raffaele Hospital, Milan, Italy

Andrea Garatti, MD Cardiac Surgery Unit, IRCCS Policlinico San Donato, San Donato Milanese (Milan), Italy

Barbara Vidal I. Hagemeijer, MD, PhD Department of Cardiology, Hospital Clinic de Barcelona, Barcelona, Spain

Shelley L. Rahman Haley, MA (Cantab), MD, FRCP, FESC Harefield Echo Department, Royal Brompton & Harefield NHS Foundation Trust, Harefield, Middlesex, UK

Arminder S. Jassar, MBBS Division of Cardiovascular Surgery, Hospital of the University of Pennsylvania, Philadelphia, PA, USA

Afshin Khalatbari, MD, PhD, MRCP (UK) Liverpool Heart and Chest Hospital, Liverpool, UK

Philip Kilner, MD, PhD CMR Unit, Royal Brompton Hospital, London, UK

Irving Kron, MD Department of Surgery, University of Virginia Hospital, Charlottesville, VA, USA

Elisabetta Lapenna, MD "Vita e Salute" San Raffaele University Medical School, San Raffaele University Hospital, Milan, Italy

Azeem Latib, MB BCh, FCP, FESC, FACC Department of Interventional Cardiology, San Raffaele Scientific Institute and EMO-GVM Centro Cuore Columbus, Milan, Italy

Randolph P. Martin, MD, FACC, FASE, FESC Structural and Valvular Heart Disease and Principal Advisor, Education, Marcus Heart Valve Center, Piedmont Heart Institute, Piedmont Hospital, Atlanta, GA, USA

Lorenzo Menicanti, MD I.R.C.C.S. Policlinico San Donato, San Donato Milanese (MI), Italy

Daniel P. Mulloy, MD Division of Cardiothoracic Surgery, Department of Surgery, University of Virginia Medical Center, Charlottesville, VA, USA

Michael Sean Mulvihill, MD Department of Surgery, Duke University Medical Center, Durham, NC, USA

John R. Pepper, MChir, FRCS Royal Brompton Hospital, London, UK

Venkateshwar Polsani, MD Piedmont Heart Institute, Piedmont Atlanta Hospital, Atlanta, GA, USA

Alberto Pozzoli, MD Heart Surgery Unit, San Raffaele University Hospital, Milan, Italy

Marta Sitges, MD, PhD Hospital Clinic, Barcelona, Spain

Peter K. Smith, MD Department of Surgery, Duke University Medical Center, Durham, NC, USA

Amin Yehya, MD, MSc Samsky Heart Failure Center, Piedmont Heart Institute, Atlanta, GA, USA

Part I

Functional Ischaemic Mitral Regurgitation

The Mitral Valve and Mitral Regurgitation

1

K.M. John Chan

Abstract

An understanding of the normal anatomy, geometry and motion of the mitral valve is necessary to fully understand the pathophysiology of functional ischemic mitral regurgitation. The mitral valve apparatus is a dynamic structure with changes in its shape and geometry throughout the cardiac cycle. Six phases of the normal mitral valve motion and geometry can be identified.

Keywords

Mitral valve anatomy • Mitral valve motion • Mitral valve function • Mitral valve geometry • Mitral regurgitation

Structure of the Normal Mitral Valve

The mitral valve separates the left ventricle from the left atrium. It comprises two leaflets, the anterior and posterior leaflets, which are attached at their hinge ends to the mitral annulus, and at their free edge to chordae tendinae which in turn attach to papillary muscles [1] (Fig. 1.1). Some chordae tendinae, termed secondary chordae, attach to the body of the valve leaflets from papillary muscles, while others, termed tertiary chordae attach to the body of the valve leaflets directly from the mitral annulus and the left ventricle. The chordae tendinae at the free edge and body of the valve leaflets prevent excessive movement of the valve leaflets into the left atrium during left ventricular systole and are therefore essential for valve competency.

The papillary muscles are usually organized into two groups, the posteromedial and anterolateral papillary muscles, and are attached to the left ventricle wall approximately one third distance from the apex and two thirds from the annulus. The anterolateral papillary muscle usually attaches to the left ventricle at the junction between the septum and the posterior wall while the posteromedial papillary muscle usually attaches on the lateral wall of the left ventricle [1].

Each of the two mitral leaflets are further divided by two indentations at their free edges into

K.M.J. Chan, BM BS, MSc, PhD, FRCS CTh
Department of Cardiothoracic Surgery,
Gleneagles Hospital, Jalan Ampang,
Kuala Lumpur 50450, Malaysia
e-mail: kmjohnchan@yahoo.com

K.M.J. Chan (ed.), *Functional Mitral and Tricuspid Regurgitation*,
DOI 10.1007/978-3-319-43510-7_1

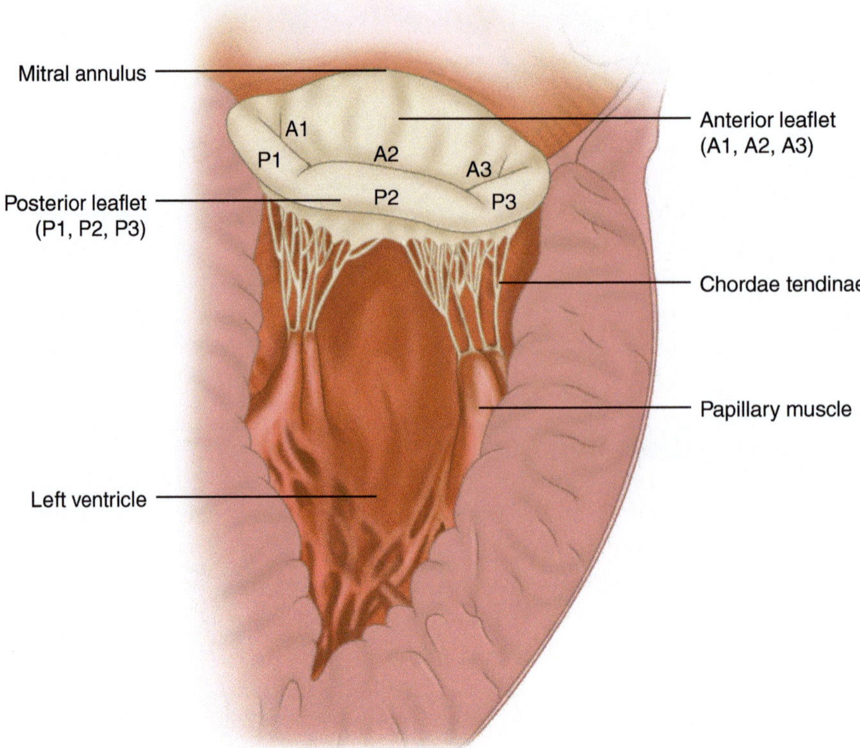

Fig. 1.1 The normal mitral valve (Adapted from Chan et al. [11]. With permission from Elsevier)

three scallops, termed A1, A2 and A3 in the anterior leaflet, and P1, P2 and P3 in the posterior leaflet (Fig. 1.1). The area between the two leaflets at the annulus is termed the commissures. A small commissural leaflet is present in this area which forms the continuity between the anterior and posterior leaflets. The anterior and posterior leaflets approximate and overlap each other at their free edges and commissures, forming a surface of coaptation of about 7–9 mm. This surface of coaptation between the free edges of the two leaflets is essential for valve competency. The normal coaptation line lies parallel to the posterior annulus [1].

Mitral Valve Motion and Geometry

The normal motion and geometry of the mitral valve has been previously studied mainly using radio-opaque markers in animals and also by echocardiography [2–5]. More recently, Chan, et al., used cardiovascular magnetic resonance to study the motion and geometry of the normal mitral valve apparatus in normal healthy volunteers; the results of this study are described here [6]. Six phases of mitral annular and leaflet motion can be identified during the normal cardiac cycle (Figs. 1.2 and 1.3):

Phase I: Ventricular systolic excursion
Phase II: Leaflet opening and annular recoil
Phase III: Leaflet approximation
Phase IV: Mid diastolic pause
Phase V: Atrial systolic excursion
Phase VI: Leaflet closure

Left ventricular systole starts in Phase VI with leaflet closure and occurs throughout Phase I. Left ventricular diastole starts in Phase II with leaflet opening, continues throughout Phases III to V, and ends in Phase VI with leaflet closure.

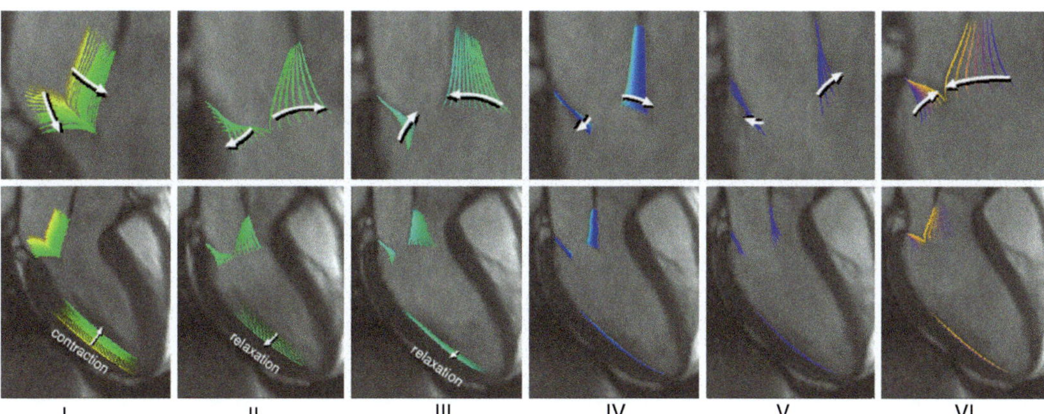

Fig. 1.2 The six phases of mitral annular and leaflet motion during the cardiac cycle in a normal individual. The motion of the mitral valve leaflets, annulus and left ventricle at its inferolateral wall were traced from individual cardiovascular magnetic resonance cine images and superimposed on each other to produce the image. Phase I represents left ventricular systole, Phases II–V represent left ventricular diastole, Phase VI represents the end of left ventricular diastole and the onset of left ventricular systole (Reprinted from Chan, et al. with permission. From Chan et al. [6])

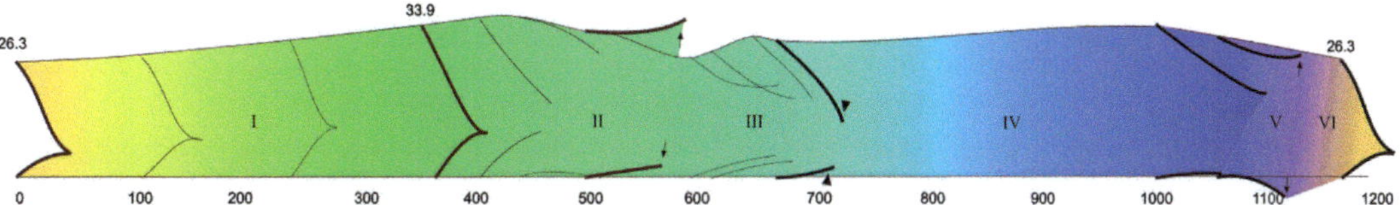

Fig. 1.3 "Two-dimensional M-Mode" display of mitral annular and leaflet motion during the cardiac cycle in a normal individual. The figure was produced by superimposing and tracing the images from individual cardiovascular magnetic resonance cine images. The view is that of the septo-lateral dimension of the mitral annulus. Phase I represents left ventricular systole, Phases II–V represent left ventricular diastole, Phase VI represents the end of left ventricular diastole and the onset of left ventricular systole. Arrows indicate maximal early and late diastolic opening of the leaflet tips, and arrow heads the diastolic leaflet approximation. Horizontal axis represents time in msec. Numbers at the top is the septo-lateral diameter in mm (From Chan et al. [6])

Phase I: Ventricular Systolic Excursion

Left ventricular systole occurs in this phase and as the left ventricle contracts, the mitral annulus moves towards the left ventricular apex. This excursion of the mitral annulus towards the left ventricular apex is asymmetrical with greater excursion of the posterior annulus and leaflets compared to the anterior annulus and leaflets (Fig. 1.2) [6]. The septo-lateral diameter of the mitral annulus increases in size during this phase but the commissure-commissure diameter remains relatively unchanged in size. The mitral leaflets remain approximated throughout this phase. During this phase of left ventricular systole, the papillary muscles contract, becoming shorter in length, and also approximate medially towards each other, towards the mitral annulus, and towards the left ventricular septum. The direction of greatest approximation is towards each other. Although both the papillary muscles and the mitral annulus move towards each other during this phase, contraction of the papillary muscles with corresponding reduction in their length means that the distance between the papillary muscle tips and the mitral annulus is relatively unchanged. Therefore, during this phase of left ventricular systole, both the anterolateral and posteromedial papillary muscles approximate towards each other and towards the long-axis midline of the left ventricle, and the anterolateral papillary muscle approximates towards the left ventricular septum. The distance between the tips of the papillary muscles and the mitral annulus remains relatively constant throughout this phase despite the mitral annulus and the left ventricular wall moving towards each other, accounted for by the 30–40 % contraction in its length.

Phase II: Leaflet Opening and Annular Recoil

This phase corresponds to the end of left ventricular systole and the start of left ventricular diastole. At the start of this phase, the mitral leaflets open and this is followed closely by recoil of the mitral annulus back towards the left atrium (Figs. 1.2 and 1.3). The septo-lateral diameter of the mitral annulus continues to increase in size reaching its maximal size in the middle of this phase, corresponding to maximal separation of the mitral leaflets. The left ventricle starts to relax and the papillary muscles move apart from each other, away from the long axis midline of the left ventricle and from the left ventricular septum.

Phase III: Leaflet Approximation

This phase occurs during left ventricular diastole. During this phase, the mitral leaflets move passively to a partially closed position (Figs. 1.2 and 1.3).

Phase IV: Mid Diastolic Pause

Left ventricular diastole continues throughout this phase. The mitral leaflets drift about in a neutral position during this phase. This represents the phase of diastolic inactivity and is the true neutral position of the heart.

Phase V: Atrial Systolic Excursion

Left ventricular diastole continues throughout this phase. Left atrial systole pulls the mitral annulus back towards the left atrium from its neutral position. The separation of the mitral leaflet edges increases (Figs. 1.2 and 1.3). The annulus begins to contract (pre-systolic contraction) and its septo-lateral diameter starts to decrease in size during this phase.

Phase VI: Leaflet Closure

This phase marks the end of left ventricular diastole and the onset of left ventricular systole. The leaflets close. The annulus continues to contract and reduce in size at its septo-lateral dimension.

The ability of cardiovascular magnetic resonance to image the entire mitral valve apparatus (mitral leaflets, annulus and papillary muscles) and the left ventricle, and to visualise these together in a single image, has given unique insights into the function, motion and geometry of the mitral valve apparatus. The entire mitral valve apparatus changes in size, shape and position during the cardiac cycle.

Mitral annular contraction begins as left atrial systole begins (in Phase V). As the annulus is pulled towards the left atrium with left atrial contraction, it also contracts and reduces in size in its septo-lateral dimension. It reaches its smallest size just before the onset of left ventricular systole when leaflet closure occurs (in phase VI and the beginning of phase I). At this stage, the annulus has reduced in size by about 15 % from its size in the middle of left ventricular diastole (Phase IV) [6]. This helps to increase the coaptation between the mitral leaflets as left ventricular systole begins. The annulus then starts to relax as left ventricular systole begins, and throughout left ventricular systole (Phase I), the annulus continues to increase in size in its septo-lateral dimension by about 15 %, so that its diameter is maximal during leaflet opening (Phase II) (Fig. 1.3). The annulus also moves longitudinally along the long axis of the heart. Throughout left ventricular systole (Phase I), the annulus moves towards the apex of the left ventricle (Fig. 1.2). At the end of left ventricular systole, the annulus recoils back towards the left atrium (Phase II), towards its neutral position. This movement actually helps to pull the mitral leaflets further apart so that it achieves its maximal separation distance at this time (Figs. 1.1 and 1.2). The annulus then stays in a relaxed state (Phase III and IV) until left atrial systole pulls it away from its neutral position towards the left atrium (Phase V). This movement helps to separate the mitral leaflets again. The annulus starts to contract again at this stage and its septo-lateral diameter reduces in size again until leaflet closure (Phase VI).

Several other studies have been done on mitral annular motion and function, mainly using radio-opaque markers in animal models and echocardiography. Most studies also report a pre-systolic mitral annular contraction, consistent with that reported by Chan et al. [2–5]. Ormiston et al. using transthoracic echocardiography, and Glasson et al. using radio-opaque markers in sheep hearts reported very similar results [2, 3]. There is, however, some variation in the precise changes in mitral annular size during the cardiac cycle in some studies, which may be related to differences in the imaging and analysis techniques used, and different definitions of the onset of systole and diastole. Many studies also did not analyse mitral annular size throughout the cardiac cycle, but only performed measurements at fixed time intervals, and some only measured the maximal and minimal size of the annulus. Transthoracic echocardiography, unlike cardiovascular magnetic resonance, is unable to precisely image the mitral annulus in the same position consistently between different patients, and does not always image the mitral annulus in a position which would enable accurate and reproducible measurements of its true dimensions, due to the orientation and direction of placement of the probe on the patient's chest.

The mitral leaflets show distinct motion throughout the cardiac cycle and its movement is influenced by the motion of the mitral annulus, and also by the flow of blood around it. The leaflets remain approximated throughout left ventricular systole (Phase I and VI) and separates during left ventricular diastole (Phases II–V) (Fig. 1.2). Separation of the leaflets is maximal at early diastole (Phase II) and occurs when the annulus recoils back towards the left atrium following apically directed systolic excursion in Phase I (Fig. 1.3). They then approximate to a partially closed position in the middle of diastole (Phase III) (Figs. 1.2 and 1.3). The leaflets then drift about the left ventricle in its neutral position during a period of diastolic inactivity (Phase IV). The leaflets open fully again towards the end of diastole when left atrial systole pulls the mitral annulus (and the base of the leaflets) towards the left atrium (Phase V) (Figs. 1.2 and 1.3). Finally, the leaflets close at the end of left ventricular diastole and the onset of systole (Phase VI) (Figs. 1.2 and 1.3).

The normal function of the papillary muscles is necessary to maintain mitral valve competency during left ventricular systole. The mitral annulus and the left ventricle supporting the papillary muscles move towards each other during left ventricular systole. To achieve mitral valve competency and prevent leaflet prolapse, it is necessary for the papillary muscles to contract and shorten in length so as to maintain an approximately constant distance between the tips of the papillary muscles and the mitral annulus during left ventricular systole. The papillary muscle length shortens by 30–40 % with maintenance of an approximately constant length between the tips of both papillary muscles and the mitral annulus.

The papillary muscles approximate towards each other and towards the long-axis midline of the left ventricular chamber during left ventricular systole. This realignment of the papillary muscles towards each other during left ventricular systole may be important to allow adequate coaptation between the mitral leaflets by avoiding excessive tension in the papillary muscles and chordae tendinae. In this regard, the position of the papillary muscles is dependent on both left ventricular size and function.

Mechanisms and Causes of Mitral Regurgitation

Mitral regurgitation refers to the backflow of blood from the left ventricle into the left atrium during left ventricular systole. It can occur with normal leaflet motion, so called Type I dysfunction, due to annular dilatation (e.g., due to atrial

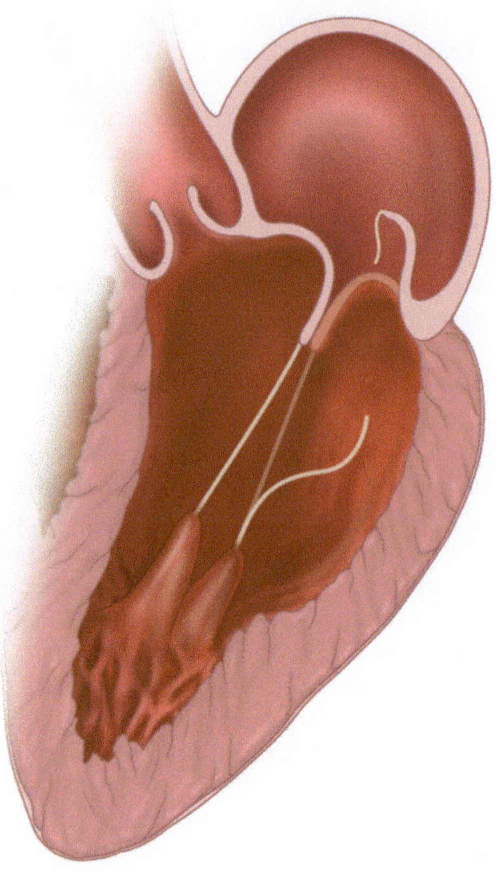

Fig. 1.4 Mitral regurgitation due to chordal rupture (Type II dysfunction) (Adapted from Amirak et al. [12]. With permission from Elsevier)

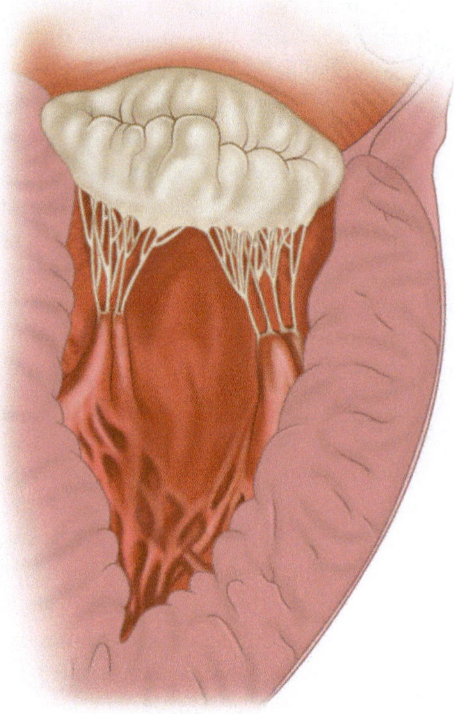

Fig. 1.5 Mitral regurgitation due to excessive leaflet tissue in Barlow's disease (Type II dysfunction) (Adapted from Amirak et al. [2]. With permission from Elsevier)

fibrillation) which pulls the leaflets apart preventing adequate leaflet coaptation during left ventricular systole and resulting in mitral regurgitation, or to leaflet tear or perforation (e.g., from endocarditis), or to vegetations from endocarditis preventing adequate leaflet coaptation [1].

More commonly, mitral regurgitation occurs due to excessive leaflet motion or leaflet prolapse into the left atrium during left ventricular systole, so called Type II dysfunction. The resulting lack of leaflet coaptation results in mitral regurgitation. This typically occurs due to chordal rupture or elongation from degenerative valve disease or endocarditis, excessive leaflet tissue from Barlow's or other connective tissue diseases, or papillary muscle rupture from myocardial infarction (Figs. 1.4 and 1.5) [1].

Mitral regurgitation can also occur due to restricted leaflet motion, so called Type III dysfunction. This is seen in rheumatic valve disease where thickened and fused leaflets limit leaflet motion and prevent adequate leaflet coaptation resulting in mitral regurgitation. It can also occur due to dilatation and dysfunction of the left ventricle following myocardial infarction or due to dilated cardiomyopathy. In these cases, the dilated or poorly contracting left ventricle pulls the mitral valve leaflets apart through their attachments to the chordae tendinae and papillary muscles, preventing adequate leaflet coaptation and resulting in mitral regurgitation (Figs. 1.6 and 1.7). This type of mitral regurgitation is also termed functional mitral regurgitation as the mitral valve apparatus is normal in structure but its function is abnormal secondary to the effects of a dilated or dysfunctional left ventricle. It will be discussed in more detail in Chap. 2.

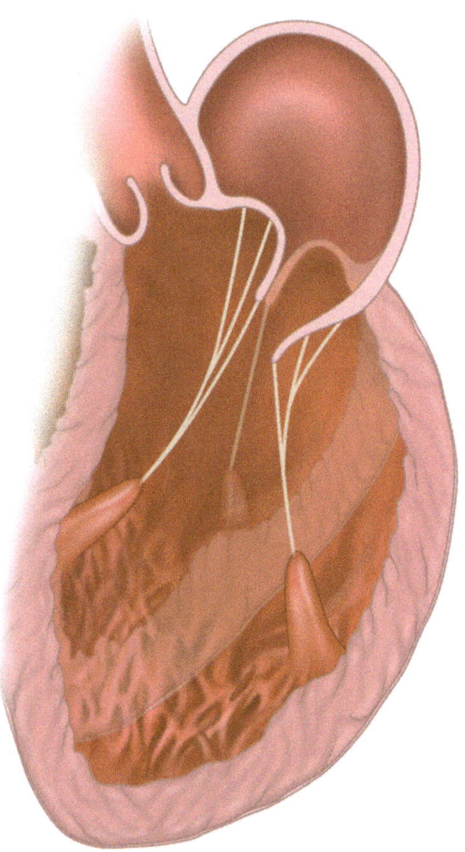

Fig. 1.6 Mitral regurgitation due to posterior leaflet restriction or tethering in functional ischaemic mitral regurgitation (Type III dysfunction). Left ventricular remodelling occurs following an inferior myocardial infarction. The resulting dilatation and displacement of the left ventricle wall tethers or restricts the posterior mitral valve leaflet during left ventricular systole preventing adequate leaflet coaptation and resulting in mitral regurgitation (Adapted from Chan et al. [11]. With permission from Elsevier)

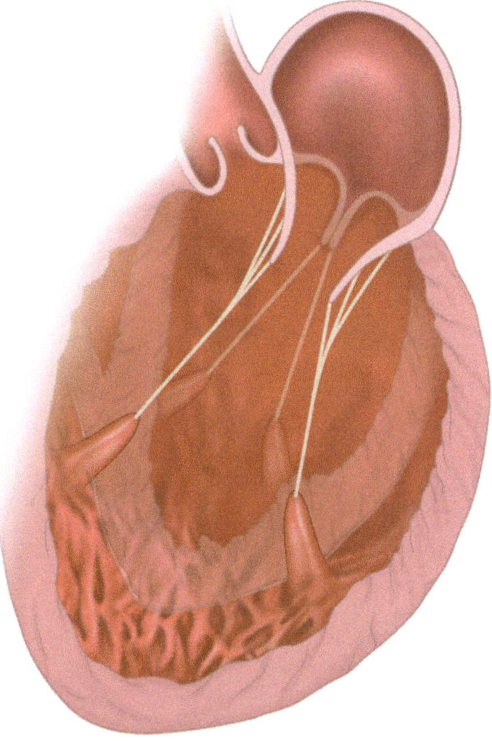

Fig. 1.7 Mitral regurgitation due to restriction or tethering of both anterior and posterior leaflets in functional mitral regurgitation due to dilated cardiomyopathy (Type III dysfunction). Global left ventricular dilatation and dysfunction tethers or restricts both mitral valve leaflets during left ventricular systole preventing adequate leaflet coaptation and resulting in mitral regurgitation (Adapted from Chan et al. [11]. With permission from Elsevier)

Consequences of Mitral Regurgitation

Mitral regurgitation results in an increase in preload and a decrease in afterload due to the backflow of blood into the left atrium. To maintain forward stroke volume, the left ventricle adapts by dilating in order to increase forward cardiac output with each systolic contraction; eccentric left ventricular hypertrophy occurs with the laying down of extra sarcomeres in series [7, 8]. This is also triggered as a result of increased left ventricular wall stress due to the increased preload. Geometrical changes also occur in the left ventricle which becomes more spherical. The left atrium enlarges as a result of the regurgitant flow into it. The enlargement of the left atrium results in left atrial pressures remaining normal or only being slightly elevated. As a result, pulmonary oedema is avoided and significant increases in pulmonary vascular resistance seldom occur. During this period of compensation, the patient may remain entirely asymptomatic but the heart is getting larger [9, 10].

After a period of compensation, with progressive left ventricular dilatation, contractile dysfunction occurs with increased myocyte length and decreased myofibril content. Consequently, left ventricular systolic contractility becomes progressively impaired as mitral regurgitation progresses. However, the calculated ejection fraction and stroke volume may still remain normal despite impaired left ventricular contractility, because the calculated ejection fraction and stroke volume includes the backflow of blood into the left atrium. The forward stroke volume will be decreased with progressive impairment of left ventricular contractility. Pulmonary congestion eventually ensues [9, 10].

References

1. Carpentier A, Adams DH, Filsoufi F. Carpentier's reconstructive valve surgery. From valve analysis to valve reconstruction. Maryland Heights: Saunders Elsevier; 2010.
2. Glasson JR, Komeda M, Daughters GT. Most ovine mitral annular size three-dimensional size reduction occurs before ventricular systole and is abolished with ventricular pacing. Circulation. 1997;96(9 Suppl):II-115–22.
3. Ormiston JA, Shah PM, Tei C, Wong M. Size and motion of the mitral valve annulus in man. A two dimensional echocardiographic method and findings in normal subjects. Circulation. 1981;64:113–20.
4. Saito S, Araki Y, Usui A, Akita T, Oshima H, Yokote J, Ueda Y. Mitral valve motion assessed by high speed video camera in isolated swine hearts. Eur J Cardiothorac Surg. 2006;30:584–91.
5. Flachskampf FA, Chandra S, Gaddipatti A. Analysis of shape and motion of the mitral annulus in subjects with and without cardiomyopathy by echocardiographic 3D reconstruction. J Am Soc Echocardiogr. 2000;13:277–87.
6. Chan KMJ, Merrifield R, Wage RR, Symmonds K, Cannell T, Firmin DN, Pepper JR, Pennell DJ, Kilner PJ. Two-dimensional M-mode display of the mitral valve from CMR cine acquisitions: insights into normal leaflet and annular motion. J Cardiovasc Magn Reson. 2008;10 Suppl 1:A351.
7. Zile MR, Gaasch WH, Carroll JD, Levine HJ. Chronic mitral regurgitation: predictive value of pre-operative echocardiographic indexes of left ventricular function and wall stress. J Am Coll Cardiol. 1984;3:235–42.
8. Carabello BA. Mitral regurgitation: basic pathophysiologic principles, part 1. Mod Concepts Cardiovasc Dis. 1988;57:53–8.
9. Bonow RO, Carabello BA, Kanu C, de Leon AC, Jr., Faxon DP, Freed MD, Gaasch WH, Lytle BW, Nishimura RA, O'Gara PT, O'Rourke RA, Otto CM, Shah PM, Shanewise JS, Smith SC, Jr., Jacobs AK, Adams CD, Anderson JL, Antman EM, Faxon DP, Fuster V, Halperin JL, Hiratzka LF, Hunt SA, Lytle BW, Nishimura R, Page RL and Riegel B. 2008 focussed update incorporated into the ACC/AHA 2006 guidelines for the management of patients with valvular heart disease: a report of the American College of Cardiology/American Heart Association Task Force on Practice Guidelines (writing committee to revise the 1998 Guidelines for the Management of Patients With Valvular Heart Disease): developed in collaboration with the Society of Cardiovascular Anesthesiologists: endorsed by the Society for Cardiovascular Angiography and Interventions and the Society of Thoracic Surgeons. *Circulation*. 2008;118:e523-e661.
10. Cardiac Surgery in the Adult.
11. Chan KMJ, Amirak E, Zakkar M, Flather M, Pepper JR, Punjabi PP. Ischemic mitral regurgitation: in search of the best treatment for a common condition. Prog Cardiovasc Dis. 2009;51:460–71.
12. Amirak E, Chan KMJ, Zakkar M, Punjabi PP. Current status of surgery for degenerative mitral valve disease. Prog Cardiovasc Dis. 2009;51:454–9.

2 Natural History and Pathophysiology of Functional Ischaemic Mitral Regurgitation

K.M. John Chan

Abstract

Functional ischaemic mitral regurgitation carries an adverse prognosis. Survival is worse compared to those without mitral regurgitation; increasing severity of mitral regurgitation is associated with progressively worse survival. It is primarily a disease of the left ventricle, occurring following myocardial infarction and ischaemia; remodelling and dilatation of the left ventricle pulls or restricts the mitral valve leaflets preventing them from coapting adequately and resulting in mitral regurgitation. Changes in mitral annular geometry and motion; mitral leaflet geometry and motion; papillary muscle geometry, function and viability; and left ventricular geometry, function and viability also occur in functional ischaemic mitral regurgitation.

Keywords

Functional ischaemic mitral regurgitation • Survival • Heart failure • Pathophysiology • Natural history

Natural History

Functional ischaemic mitral regurgitation has been reported in up to 40% of patients after myocardial infarction [1–3]. It is usually mild in severity and so is often undiagnosed [1, 3]. Its incidence may have decreased in recent years with increasingly earlier coronary artery revascularisation following myocardial infarction, either by primary percutaneous coronary intervention or in-patient coronary artery bypass graft surgery (CABG). It is a marker of adverse prognosis and patients with even mild functional ischaemic mitral regurgitation have a significantly increased risk of congestive heart failure and death compared to patients who do not have functional ischaemic mitral regurgitation after a myocardial infarction [1, 2, 4]. The SAVE study, for example, reported that 3 years after a myocardial infarction, the incidence of cardiovascular mortality

K.M.J. Chan, BM BS, MSc, PhD, FRCS CTh
Department of Cardiothoracic Surgery,
Gleneagles Hospital, Jalan Ampang,
Kuala Lumpur 50450, Malaysia
e-mail: kmjohnchan@yahoo.com

K.M.J. Chan (ed.), *Functional Mitral and Tricuspid Regurgitation*,
DOI 10.1007/978-3-319-43510-7_2

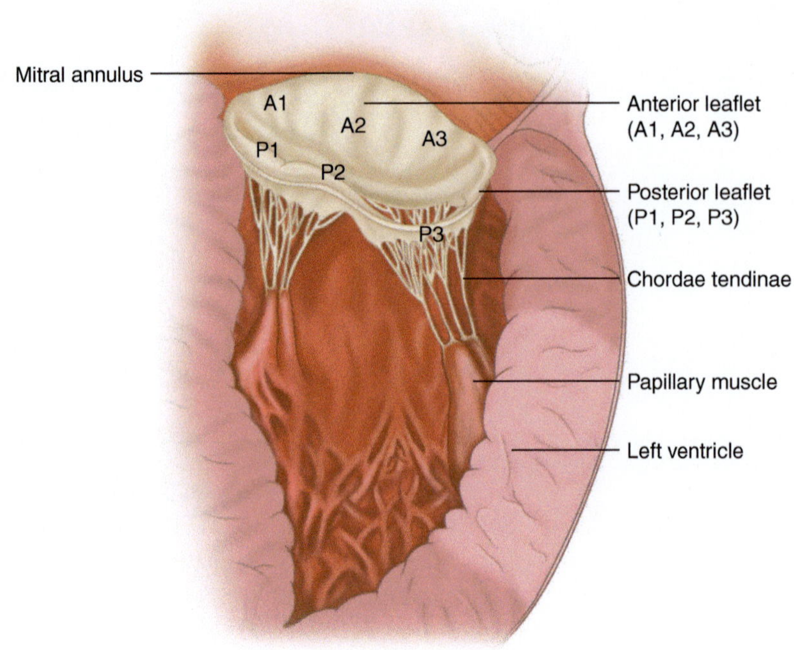

Fig. 2.1 The posterior mitral valve leaflet is tethered or restricted at P3 due to displacement of the posteromedial papillary muscle following an inferolateral myocardial infarction (Adapted from Chan et al. [5]. With permission from Elsevier)

in patients with mild functional ischaemic mitral regurgitation optimised on medical therapy was more than twice that of patients who did not have functional ischaemic mitral regurgitation (29 % vs 12 %, p<0.001) [2]. The presence of functional ischaemic mitral regurgitation was an independent predictor of cardiovascular mortality (OR 2.00, 95 % CI 1.23–3.04, p=0.002). The incidence of severe heart failure was 24 % in those with mild functional ischaemic mitral regurgitation compared to 16 % in those without functional ischaemic mitral regurgitation (p=0.015) [2]. More recently, Aronson et al. also reported a significantly increased incidence of severe heart failure in patients with mild functional ischaemic mitral regurgitation following myocardial infarction compared to those without functional ischaemic mitral regurgitation (HR 2.8, 95 % CI 1.8–4.2, p<0.001) [1]. The outcome is worse with increasing severity of functional ischaemic mitral regurgitation [3, 4]. Grigioni et al. reported a 5 year survival of 47 % in patients with mild functional ischaemic mitral regurgitation and only 29 % in those with moderate or severe functional ischaemic mitral regurgitation [4].

Pathophysiology

Functional ischaemic mitral regurgitation occurs as a result of impaired left ventricular contraction and dilatation following myocardial infarction which tethers the mitral valve leaflets preventing adequate leaflet coaptation. The mechanism of functional ischaemic mitral regurgitation has been studied extensively both in animals and humans. It is reported to be more common after inferior myocardial infarction where tethering of the posteromedial papillary muscle is thought to lead to tethering of the posterior mitral valve leaflet, mainly at the P3 scallop (Fig. 2.1) [6–9]. However, chordae tendinae from the posteromedial papillary muscle support both the anterior and posterior mitral valve leaflets (all of A3 and P3 and the medial halves of A2 and P2) [10]. Tethering of both mitral valve leaflets (A2, A3, P2 and P3) can therefore be expected following an inferior myocardial infarction. This may be important in the design of annuloplasty rings and in the surgical technique of repairing functional ischaemic mitral regurgitation.

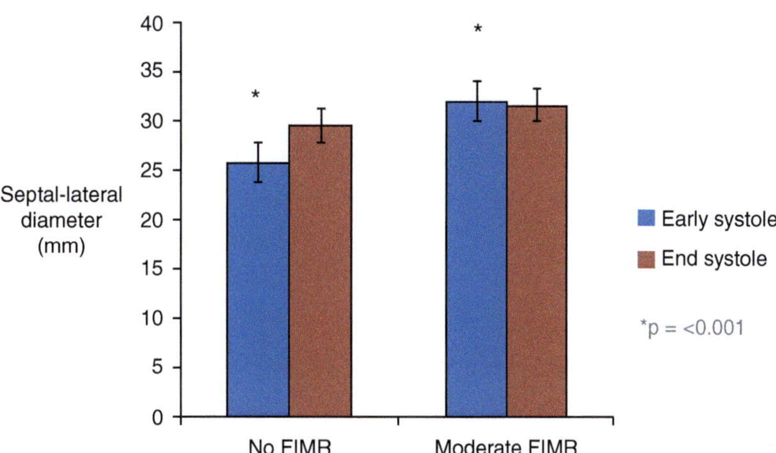

Fig. 2.2 Annular contractile function is absent in functional ischaemic mitral regurgitation (FIMR) in contrast to normal, where a 15 % reduction in the septal-lateral annular diameter occurs in early systole [23, 24]

Dilatation of the mitral annulus, both at the anterior fibrous trigone and the posterior muscular area, and flattening of its normal saddle shape, has been reported in functional ischaemic mitral regurgitation. These studies have largely been performed in animals and cadavers, and by echocardiography [6, 11–17]. Changes in the mitral annular geometry may be related to the degree of left ventricular remodelling and severity of mitral regurgitation in different patients, and may be related to the different stages of the cardiac cycle. Knowledge of this is important in the design of annuloplasty rings or bands, and in the practice of under-sizing the annuloplasty ring during surgery.

Functional ischaemic mitral regurgitation can also occur as a result of global left ventricular dilatation, usually following an anterior myocardial infarction, leading to displacement of both papillary muscles and tethering of both mitral valve leaflets [4, 9, 10, 18, 19]. However, it does not occur in all cases of ischaemic left ventricular dilatation, and further studies are needed to provide insights into this. It is possible that the development of functional ischaemic mitral regurgitation may be influenced by the degree and direction of papillary muscle displacement as a result of the dilated left ventricle, or an increased sphericity of the left ventricle, or decreased left ventricular contractility. Studies of the geometry, size, function and displacement of the papillary muscles and the left ventricle would provide valuable insights.

Animal studies have demonstrated that lateral displacement of papillary muscles occur in functional ischaemic mitral regurgitation [15]. Most echocardiographic studies have demonstrated lateral and posterior displacement of papillary muscles [7, 16, 19]. Some studies suggest that apical displacement of papillary muscles also occur [7, 19]. The role of papillary muscle dysfunction and infarction in the pathogenesis of functional ischaemic mitral regurgitation is also uncertain. It has been suggested that papillary muscle ischaemia or infarction may attenuate functional ischaemic mitral regurgitation as the loss of papillary muscle systolic contraction actually reduces leaflet tethering [8, 20–22]. The incidence of papillary muscle ischaemia or infarction is unknown.

Mitral Annular Geometry and Motion

The motion and geometry of the mitral annulus in the normal cardiac cycle is discussed in the previous chapter. In contrast to healthy subjects without functional ischaemic mitral regurgitation, in whom the mitral annular septolateral diameter decreased in size by about 15 % just before the start of left ventricular systole (phase VI of the cardiac cycle), and then increased in size towards the end of left ventricular systole just before leaflet opening (phase I of the cardiac cycle), the mitral annulus in patients with functional ischaemic mitral regurgitation remains a relatively constant size throughout the cardiac cycle (Fig. 2.2) [23–25].

In functional ischaemic mitral regurgitation, mitral annular function is impaired so that it fails to contract and reduce in size just before left ventricular systole. In normal subjects, the mitral annulus contracts and reduces in size just before left ventricular systole to increase the coaptation between the anterior and posterior mitral leaflets. This contractile function of the mitral annulus appears to be impaired in functional ischaemic mitral regurgitation and may be one of the mechanisms causing mitral incompetency [23, 24]. The mitral annulus is not necessarily dilated in functional ischaemic mitral regurgitation, although it may be. Rather, mitral annular function is impaired with reduced pre-systolic mitral annular contraction in its septolateral dimension. As a result, the mitral annulus is enlarged in the septolateral dimension at the onset of left ventricular systole, reducing leaflet coaptation.

The excursion of the mitral annulus towards the left ventricular apex during left ventricular systole in patients with functional ischaemic mitral regurgitation (phase I of the cardiac cycle) is significantly less than the corresponding values in healthy subjects [23, 24]. This finding again confirms reduced mitral annular function in functional ischaemic mitral regurgitation, although in this case, impaired left ventricular function is the likely contributing factor. The reduced excursion of the mitral annulus towards the left ventricular apex during left ventricular systole increases the tension on the mitral subvalvular apparatus during systole resulting in increased tethering of the mitral leaflets. This may be another mechanism contributing to mitral incompetency in functional ischaemic mitral regurgitation.

The mitral annulus in functional ischaemic mitral regurgitation shows impaired function with reduced septolateral contraction and reduced excursion towards the left ventricular apex and consequently, reduced recoil back towards the left atrium [24]. The mitral annulus in functional ischaemic mitral regurgitation is not necessarily dilated, at least in patients with less than severe functional ischaemic mitral regurgitation. Rather, the loss of pre-systolic mitral annular contraction results in a larger mitral annulus in the septolateral dimension at the onset of left ventricular systole, which may be an important mechanism reducing the surface of coaptation of the mitral valve leaflets [24]. Decreased mitral annular contraction in functional ischaemic mitral regurgitation has previously been documented using echocardiography [7, 16]. Some studies report that the mitral annulus is dilated in the septolateral direction but these studies did not analyse the mitral annular size throughout the cardiac cycle and it is possible the images were acquired at early systole [6, 16, 26]. It is also possible that patients in those studies had more severe mitral regurgitation and therefore more advanced disease.

In patients with more advanced disease with greater left ventricular dilatation, in addition to a loss of pre-systolic contraction, the mitral annulus may also dilate. Cadaveric studies have reported dilatation of both the anterior and posterior mitral annulus in advanced ischaemic cardiomyopathy [12]. Animal studies have also reported an increase in the septolateral mitral annular diameter in functional ischaemic mitral regurgitation, although the left ventricular remodelling in these animal models are likely to be more significant and exaggerated, compared to functional ischaemic mitral regurgitation patients, as the models involved complete acute ligation of the circumflex coronary artery [13, 15].

These findings lend support to the use of an under-sized complete rigid or semi-rigid annuloplasty ring for functional ischaemic mitral regurgitation, which reduces the size of the mitral annulus at the septolateral dimension and fixes its position in systole.

The excursion of the mitral annulus towards the left ventricular apex during left ventricular systole is also significantly reduced in patients with functional ischaemic mitral regurgitation compared to controls [24]. This observation has also been reported in another study using echocardiography [27]. As discussed in Chap. 1, the mitral annulus in normal subjects moves towards the apex of the left ventricle during left ventricular systole, and the left ventricle along with the papillary muscles it supports, moves towards the mitral annulus. Papillary muscle contraction occurs during this time to maintain mitral leaflet competency and prevent leaflet prolapse. The reduced excursion of the mitral annulus towards

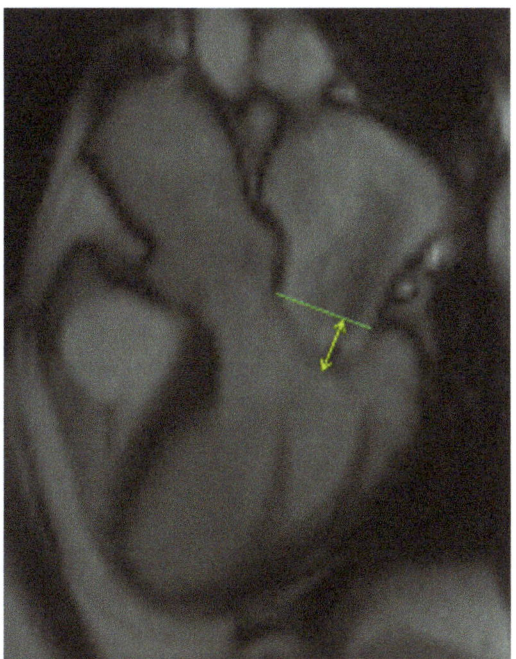

Fig. 2.3 The tethering distance is measured from the mitral annular plane to the coaptation point of the mitral leaflets

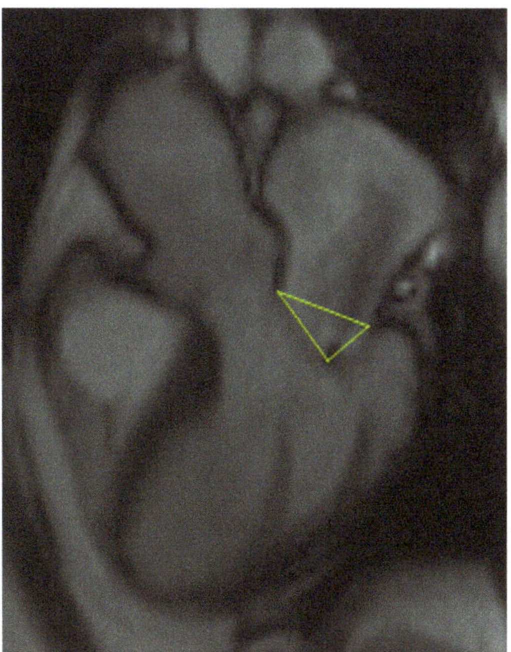

Fig. 2.4 The tethering area is measured as the area bounded by the mitral leaflets and the mitral annular plane

the left ventricular apex in functional ischaemic mitral regurgitation would have the effect of increasing tethering on the mitral valve leaflets. This is possibly an added mechanism contributing to functional ischaemic mitral regurgitation.

Mitral Leaflet Geometry and Motion

Leaflet restriction during systole, particularly of the posterior mitral leaflet at P3 is typical, although anterior leaflet restriction also occurs. In many cases, restriction of P2 is also present. Restriction of both the anterior and posterior mitral leaflets during left ventricular systole is present in most patients, with the most common scallops involved being A2-P2 and A3-P3. There is also restriction of leaflet mobility with the maximal separation of the mitral leaflets during diastole (in phase II of the cardiac cycle) being significantly less than that in healthy subjects [23, 24]. It was demonstrated in Chap. 1 that recoil of the mitral annulus towards the left atrium during atrial systole further increases leaflet separation. The reduced systolic excursion of the mitral annulus during left ventricular systole and resulting reduced atrial recoil of the annulus at the end of left ventricular systole may explain the reduced maximal separation of the mitral leaflets in functional ischaemic mitral regurgitation.

Restriction of the leaflets during systole results in an increase in the tethering distance and tethering area [26]. Most authors measure the tethering distance, which is the distance between the mitral annular plane and the point of coaptation of the mitral leaflets (Fig. 2.3). However, the difference between the tethering distance in functional ischaemic mitral regurgitation patients and healthy subjects may not always be large, and it may be better to measure the tethering area instead which gives a more reliable indicator of the degree of tethering throughout the mitral valve leaflets, rather than just at its coaptation point (Fig. 2.4) [24]. There is an increased tethering area and tethering distance between the plane of the mitral annulus and the mitral leaflets during systole. The size of the tethering area is correlated with left ventricular volumes; bigger left ventricles were associated with larger tethering areas [24].

The mitral leaflet in functional ischaemic mitral regurgitation shows restricted motion at systole with significant tethering away from the mitral annulus. Furthermore, the maximal separation of the mitral leaflets in diastole (Phase II of the cardiac cycle) is reduced, possibly due to decreased recoil of the mitral annulus in these patients [24]. As discussed in Chap. 1, recoil of the mitral annulus towards the left atrium may pull the mitral leaflets further apart. The maximal separation of the mitral valve leaflets during left ventricular diastole is decreased and may be related to impaired mitral annular function. Recent studies have also suggested that cellular changes occur in the mitral leaflet in mitral regurgitation with an increase in collagen synthesis and leaflet thickness, and it is possible that this may also contribute to its reduced motion and separation [28, 29].

Papillary Muscle Geometry, Function and Viability

Lateral and Posterior Displacement

During both left ventricular systole and diastole, the inter-papillary muscle distance (i.e., the distance between the anterolateral and posteromedial papillary muscles, Fig. 2.5), the posterior displacement of the posteromedial papillary muscle from the septum, and the lateral displacement of the posteromedial papillary muscle from the long axis midline of the left ventricular chamber are significantly greater in functional ischaemic mitral regurgitation compared to healthy subjects [23, 24].

These findings strongly demonstrate that in functional ischaemic mitral regurgitation, the geometry of the papillary muscles is altered with lateral displacement of the papillary muscles away from each other and from the midline of the left ventricular chamber, and posteriorly away from the LV-RV septum. This altered geometry of the papillary muscles is most marked at the end of left ventricular systole. The effect of such alterations in papillary muscle geometry would be to increase the tension on the chordae and the

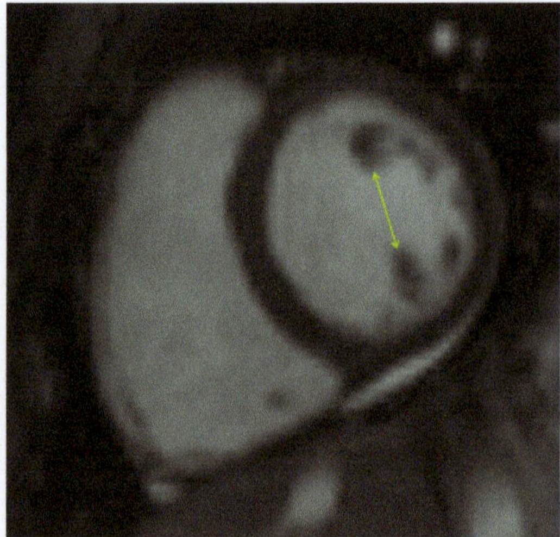

Fig. 2.5 Inter-papillary muscle distance

mitral leaflets during leaflet closure at the onset of left ventricular systole (phase VI of the cardiac cycle) resulting in increased mitral leaflet tethering. The cause of such alteration in the papillary muscle geometry may be related to increased left ventricular size and impaired left ventricular function, and to local remodelling of the left ventricle at the region of papillary muscle insertion.

Apical Displacement

The distance of the papillary muscles from the mitral annulus in functional ischaemic mitral regurgitation patients did not differ significantly from that in healthy subjects i.e., significant apical displacement of the papillary muscles did not occur significantly [23, 24]. In functional ischaemic mitral regurgitation, displacement of the papillary muscles occurs mainly laterally away from each other and from the long axis midline of the left ventricular chamber, and posteriorly away from the left ventricular septum, but not so much apically. Such lateral and posterior displacement of the papillary muscles causes tethering of the mitral leaflets and resulting leaflet restriction with reduced leaflet coaptation [24].

The displacement of the papillary muscles in functional ischaemic mitral regurgitation occurs predominantly laterally away from each other and from the long axis midline of the left ventricular chamber, and posteriorly, away from the left ventricular septum, causing leaflet tethering.

Significant apical displacement of the papillary muscles away from the mitral annulus did not occur. Contrary to common perception, significant displacement of the papillary muscles does not occur apically. This finding has also been reported in animal models where a posterior and lateral displacement of papillary muscles was observed, but not apical displacement [13, 15]. Yu et al. also previously reported an increased lateral separation between the papillary muscles in functional ischaemic mitral regurgitation as measured using cardiovascular magnetic resonance [18]. This study also reported an increased distance between the root of the posteromedial papillary muscle and the anterior mitral annulus, but not between the posteromedial papillary muscle and the posterior annulus, nor between the anterolateral papillary muscle and either the anterior or posterior mitral annulus. These findings therefore indicate posterolateral displacement of the posteromedial papillary muscle, rather than apical displacement in which all four measurements should show increased distance. The findings in Yu's study is therefore consistent with that reported in previous animal studies. An important distinction in these studies is that measurements were taken from the root of the papillary muscles in Yu's study whereas in other studies, measurements were taken from the tip of the papillary muscles. Measuring from the tip of the papillary muscles provides a more reliable indicator of the influence of papillary muscle geometry on functional ischaemic mitral regurgitation as it corrects for differences in papillary muscle length and function in different individuals [23]. Studies using echocardiography have also previously reported an increased distance between the papillary muscles and increased lateral and posterior displacement of the papillary muscles in functional ischaemic mitral regurgitation [7, 16, 19]. Interestingly, some of these studies also report an increased distance between the posteromedial papillary muscle head and the anterior mitral annulus, and have suggested that this indicated apical displacement of the papillary muscles [7, 9, 19]. However, neither the distance between the posteromedial papillary muscle and the posterior mitral annulus nor the distance between the anterolateral papillary muscle and the anterior or posterior mitral annulus showed increased distance in these studies, raising the possibility that this increased distance may represent posterolateral displacement of the papillary muscles rather than apical displacement.

These findings may be of relevance when considering recently described adjuncts to mitral annuloplasty for functional ischaemic mitral regurgitation. A recently described technique of a papillary muscle sling encircling both papillary muscles and approximating them to each other may prove useful, at least physiologically, as it would correct the lateral and posterior displacement of the papillary muscles [30]. Another surgical adjunct of placing a sling to approximate the posterolateral papillary muscle to the posterior mitral annulus may also show promise as this would correct the posterior displacement of the papillary muscles [31].

Papillary Muscle Function

Significant papillary muscle dysfunction is often present in functional ischaemic mitral regurgitation. The mean shortening of the papillary muscles in functional ischaemic mitral regurgitation is about 15% compared to 30–40% in normals [23, 24]. However, such papillary muscle dysfunction, resulting in an increased papillary muscle length at systole, is not the cause of the mitral regurgitation, but may on the contrary, help relieve some of the tethering effects of the displaced papillary muscles on the mitral leaflets. Papillary muscle contraction was reduced with a longer papillary muscle length in systole, which may help relieve leaflet tethering.

Papillary Muscle Viability

Papillary muscle infarction and fibrosis may also be present in functional ischaemic mitral regurgitation, particularly of the posteromedial papillary muscle. When present, papillary muscle function is significantly decreased in these papillary muscles [23]. Papillary muscle infarction is a recognised entity but its diagnosis is difficult and its incidence is unknown [21]. Its diagnosis using cardiovascular magnetic resonance was previously described in a

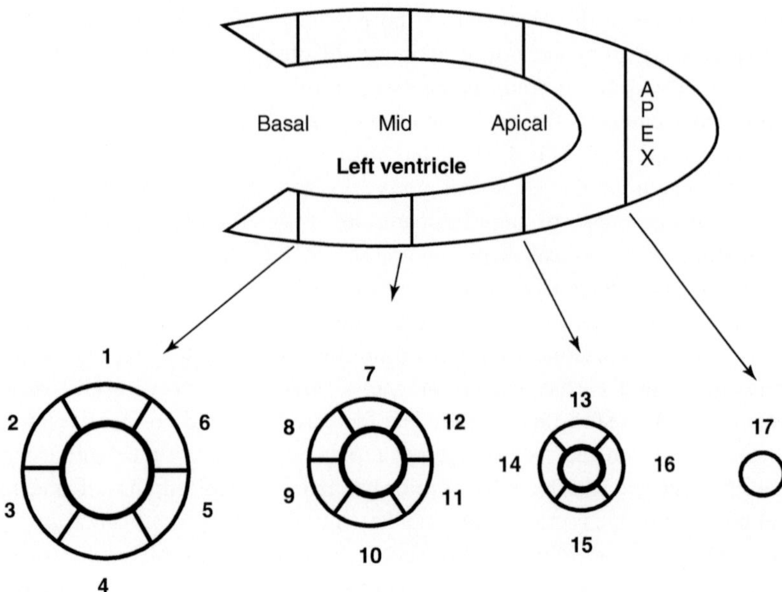

Fig. 2.6 The 17-segment left ventricular model used for regional wall motion and viability assessment

case report. [32] LGE in papillary muscles has previously been described in mitral valve prolapse where it appears to be confined to the tips of the papillary muscles, adjacent to the attachment of the chordae, and is likely to represent fibrosis. In functional ischaemic mitral regurgitation, LGE of the entire papillary muscles has been noted [23, 24].

Left Ventricular Function and Viability

Left ventricular volumes are typically larger in functional ischaemic mitral regurgitation and function impaired. Left ventricular volumes are typically correlated with the mitral leaflet tethering area. [23, 24] Regional wall motion abnormalities are typically present most marked in LV segments 4, 5, 10, 11, and 12, i.e., the basal inferior and basal inferolateral segments, the mid-inferior, mid-inferolateral and mid-superolateral segments i.e., the left ventricular segments which support the papillary muscles (Fig. 2.6) [24]. Evidence of previous myocardial infarction, as indicated by significant late gadolinium enhancement (LGE) is often present.

An association between LGE in the inferior left ventricular wall and functional ischaemic mitral regurgitation was previously reported in two studies and in one of them, an association was also found between LGE in the anterolateral wall and increasing severity of functional ischaemic mitral regurgitation, which may be attributable to additional increased left ventricular dilatation following an anterior myocardial infarct [26, 33]. Studies done on sheep have reported that functional mitral regurgitation occurs after an infarct in the inferior wall but not in the anterior or lateral walls [34].

Myocardial viability studies indicate that myocardial infarction of the inferior and lateral wall, and at the site of insertion of the papillary muscles to the left ventricle, are important contributing factors to the development of functional ischaemic mitral regurgitation. Myocardial infarction of these segments results in impaired regional myocardial contractility and local left ventricular remodelling. The normal geometry of papillary muscles which approximate towards each other and the midline of the left ventricular chamber during left ventricular systole is impaired, resulting in lateral and posterior displacement of the papillary muscles causing tethering of the mitral leaflets and impaired leaflet coaptation. Animal models suggest that these factors by themselves are not sufficient to cause significant mitral regurgitation, and dilatation of the left ventricle is necessary [35]. Remodelling of the infarcted left ventricular myocardium results in dilatation of the left ventricle and further displaces the papillary muscles laterally thereby increasing leaflet tethering. The severity of mitral regurgitation is increased further if an anterior myocardial infarction is also present due to more extensive left ventricular remodelling and dilatation. Furthermore, impaired pre-systolic mitral annular contraction ensues, further compromising mitral leaflet coaptation during left ventricular systole.

References

1. Aronson D, Goldsher N, Zukermann R, Kapeliovich M. Ischemic mitral regurgitation and risk of heart failure after myocardial infarction. Arch Intern Med. 2006;166:2362–8.
2. Lamas GA, Mitchell GF, Flaker GC, Smith SC, Gersh BJ. Clinical significance of mitral regurgitation after acute myocardial infarction. Circulation. 1997;96: 827–33.
3. Perez de Isla L. Prognostic significance of functional mitral regurgitation after a first non-ST-segment elevation acute coronary syndrome. Eur Heart J. 2006; 27:2655.
4. Grigoni F, Enriquez-Sarano M, Zehr KJ, Bailey KR. Ischemic mitral regurgitation. Long term outcome and prognostic implications with quantitative doppler assessment. Circulation. 2001;103:1759–64.
5. Chan KMJ, Amirak E, Zakkar M, Flather M, Pepper JR, Punjabi PP. Ischemic mitral regurgitation: in search of the best treatment for a common condition. Prog Cardiovasc Dis. 2009;51:460–71.
6. Kaji S, Nasu M, Yamamuro A, Tanabe K. Annular geometry in patients with chronic ischemic mitral regurgitation. Three dimensional magnetic resonance imaging study. Circulation. 2005;112:I-409–14.
7. Yiu SF, Enriquez-Sarano M, Tribouilloy C, Seward JB. Determinants of the degree of functional mitral regurgitation in patients with systolic left ventricular dysfunction. Circulation. 2000;102:1400–6.
8. Timek TA, Lai DT, Tibayan F, Liang D. Ischemia in three left ventricular regions: insights into the pathogenesis of acute ischemic mitral regurgitaiton. J Thorac Cardiovasc Surg. 2003;125:559–69.
9. Kumanohoso T, Otsuji Y, Yoshifuku S, Matsukida K. Mechanism of higher incidence of ischemic mitral regurgitation in patients with inferior myocardial infarction: quantitative analysis of left ventricular and mitral valve geometry in 103 patients with prior myocardial infarction. J Thorac Cardiovascu Surg. 2003;125:135–43.
10. Degandt AA, Weber PA, Saber HA, Duran CMG. Mitral valve basal chordae: comparative anatomy and terminology. Ann Thorac Surg. 2007;84:1250–5.
11. Ahmad RM, Gillinov M, McCarthy PM, Blackstone EH. Annular geometry and motion in human ischemic mitral regurgitation: novel assessment with three-dimensional echocardiography and computer reconstruction. Ann Thorac Surg. 2004;78:2063–8.
12. Hueb AC, Jatene FB, Moreira LFP, Pomerantzeff PM. Ventricular remodelling and mitral valve modifications in dilated cardiomyopathy: new insights from anatomic study. J Thorac Cardiovascu Surg. 2002;124.
13. Tibayan FA, Rodriguez F, Zasio MK, Bailey L. Geometric distortions of the mitral valvular-ventricular complex in chronic ischemic mitral regurgitation. Circulation. 2003;108:II-116–21.
14. Ryan LP, Jackson BM, Parish LM, Plappert TJ, St. John-Sutton MG, Gorman III JH, Gorman RC. Regional and global patterns of annular remodelling in ischemic mitral regurgitation. Ann Thorac Surg. 2007;84:553–9.
15. Jensen H, Jensen MO, Ringgaard S, Smerup MH, Sorensen TS, Kim WY, Sloth E, Wierup P, Hasenkam M, Nielsen SL. Geometric determinants of chronic functional ischemic mitral regurgitation: insights from three-dimensional cardiac magnetic resonance imaging. J Heart Valve Dis. 2008;17:16–23.
16. De Simone R, Wolf I, Mottl-Link S, Hoda R. A clinical study of annular geometry and dynamics in patients with ischemic mitral regurgitation: new insights into asymmetrical ring annuloplasty. Eur J Cardiothorac Surg. 2006;29:355–61.
17. Watanabe N, Ogasawara Y, Yamaura Y, Wada N, Kawamoto T. Mitral annulus flattens in ischemic mitral regurgitation: geometric differences between inferior and anterior myocardial infarction. A real-time 3-dimensional echocardiographic study. Circulation. 2005;112:I-458–62.
18. Yu H-Y, Su M-Y, Liao T-Y, Peng H-H. Functional mitral regurgitation in chronic ischemic coronary artery disease: analysis of geometric alterations of mitral apparatus with magnetic resonance imaging. J Thorac Cardiovascu Surg. 2004;128:543–51.
19. Agricola E, Oppizzi M, Maisano F, De Bonis M, Schinkel AFL. Echocardiographic classification of chronic ischemic mitral regurgitation caused by restricted motion according to tethering pattern. Eur J Echocardiogr. 2004;5:326–34.
20. Kaul S, Spotnitz WD, Glasheen WP, Touchstone DA. Mechanism of ischemic mitral regurgitation: an experimental evaluation. Circulation. 1991;84:2167–80.
21. Magnoni M. Reduction of mitral valve regurgitation caused by acute papillary muscle ischemia. Nat Clin Pract Cardiovasc Med. 2007;4:51.
22. Uemura T, Otsuji Y, Nakashiki K, Yoshifuku S. Papillary muscle dysfunction attenuates ischemic mitral regurgitation in patients with localized basal inferior left ventricular remodelling. J Am Coll Cardiol. 2005;46:113–9.

23. Chan KMJ, Wage RR, Symmonds K, Roussin I, Flather M, Pennell DJ, Prasad SK, Kilner PJ, Pepper JR. Mitral valve annular, leaflet and papillary muscle geometry and function in functional ischaemic mitral regurgitation: new insights from cardiovascular magnetic resonance. Circulation. 2011;124, A10987.
24. Chan KMJ. Ischaemic mitral regurgitation: randomised evaluation of surgical treatment and study of its pathophysiology and predictors of outcome. Cardiovascular Sciences, National Heart & Lung Institute, Imperial College London, PhD. 2012. p. 287.
25. Chan KMJ, Merrifield R, Wage RR, Symmonds K, Cannell T, Firmin DN, Pepper JR, Pennell DJ, Kilner PJ. Two-dimensional M-mode display of the mitral valve from CMR cine acquisitions: insights into normal leaflet and annular motion. J Cardiovasc Magn Reson. 2008;10 Suppl 1:A351.
26. Srichai MB, Grimm RA, Stillman AE, Gillinov AM, Rodriguez L, Lieber ML, Lara A, Weaver RT, McCarthy PM, White RD. Ischemic mitral regurgitation: impact of the left ventricle and mitral valve in patients with left ventricular systolic dysfunction. Ann Thorac Surg. 2005;80:170–8.
27. Daimon M, Saracino G, Gillinov AM, Koyama Y, Fukuda S, Kwan J, Song J-M, Kongsaerepong V, Agler DA, Thomas JD, Shiota T. Local dysfunction and asymmetrical deformation of mitral annular geometry in ischemic mitral regurgitation: a novel computerized 3D echocardiographic analysis. Echocardiography. 2008;25:414–23.
28. Dal-Bianco JP, Aikawa E, Bischoff J, Guerrero JL, Handschumacher MD, Sullivan S, Johnson B, Titus JS, Iwamoto Y, Wylie-Sears J, Levine RA, Carpentier A. Active adaptation of the tethered mitral valve: insights into a compensatory mechanism for functional mitral regurgitation. Circulation. 2009;120:334–42.
29. Stephens EH, Nguyen TC, Itoh A, Ingels NB, Miller DC, Grande-Allen KJ. The effects of mitral regurgitation alone are sufficient for leaflet remodelling. Circulation. 2008;118 Suppl 1:S243–9.
30. Hvass U, Tapia M, Baron F, Pouzet B. Papillary muscle sling: a new functional approach to mitral repair in patients with ischemic left ventricular dysfunction and functional mitral regurgitation. Ann Thorac Surg. 2003;75:809–11.
31. Kron IL, Green GR, Cope JT. Surgical relocation of the posterior papillary muscle in chronic ischemic mitral regurgitation. Ann Thorac Surg. 2002;74: 600–1.
32. Garcia-Fuster R, Estornell J, Rodriguez I, Estevez V. Papillary muscle infarction: the role of magnetic resonance imaging. Ann Thorac Surg. 2007;83: 1901–2.
33. Ancona GD, Biondo D, Mamone G, Marrone G, Pirone F, Santise G, Sciacca S, Pilato M. Ischemic mitral valve regurgitation in patients with depressed ventricular function: cardiac geometrical and myocardial perfusion evaluation with magnetic resonance imaging. Eur J Cardiothorac Surg. 2008;34:964–8.
34. Enomoto Y, Gorman III JH, Moainie S, Guy TS, Jackson BM, Parish LM, Plappert TJ, Zeeshan A, St. John-Sutton MG, Gorman RC. Surgical treatment of ischemic mitral regurgitation might not influence ventricular remodelling. J Thorac Cardiovasc Surg. 2005;129:504–11.
35. Otsuji Y, Handschumacher MD, Liel-Cohen N, Tanabe H, Jiang L, Schwammenthal E, Guerrero L, Nicholls LA, Vlahakes GJ, Levine RA. Mechanism of ischemic mitral regurgitation with segmental left ventricular dysfunction: three dimensional echocardiographic studies in models of acute and chronic progressive regurgitation. J Am Coll Cardiol. 2001;37: 641–8.

Echocardiographic Assessment of Functional Ischaemic Mitral Regurgitation

3

Shelley L. Rahman Haley

Abstract

The presence of functional ischaemic mitral regurgitation (FIMR) remains an important prognostic feature in the ischemic ventricle but the evaluation of the valve lesion and its associated hemodynamic effects can be complex and somewhat challenging. The cornerstone of diagnostic assessment is the echocardiogram, which provides anatomical and physiological detail, facilitating diagnosis, prognosis and planning of further management. During the past two decades, the roles of stress and strain imaging, transesophageal echocardiography and particularly of three-dimensional echocardiographic techniques have expanded the diagnostic armamentarium and provided considerable insights into the mechanisms of FIMR, hence improving not only diagnosis but also preoperative planning in the context of the multi-disciplinary heart team context.

Keywords

Functional mitral regurgitation • Ischemic mitral regurgitation • Transthoracic/transesophageal echocardiography • Three-dimensional echocardiography • Echocardiographic assessment of mitral regurgitation

Introduction

Echocardiography is the most important noninvasive imaging technique for evaluating the presence and severity of functional ischemic mitral regurgitation (FIMR). Its advantages over other techniques are manifold: its spatial resolution is sufficient to yield the necessary anatomical and morphological detail and hence accurately assess the mechanism of MR, and the temporal resolution combined with various Doppler techniques allows for in-depth physiological evaluation and ascertainment of the hemodynamic significance of the lesion [1, 2]. In addition, the widespread availability of echocardiography coupled with its safety mean that it is easily repeatable, which is

S.L.R. Haley, MA (Cantab), MD, FRCP, FESC
Harefield Echo Department, Royal Brompton & Harefield NHS Foundation Trust, Hill End Road, Harefield, Middlesex UB9 6JH, UK
e-mail: S.RahmanHaley@rbht.nhs.uk

K.M.J. Chan (ed.), *Functional Mitral and Tricuspid Regurgitation*,
DOI 10.1007/978-3-319-43510-7_3

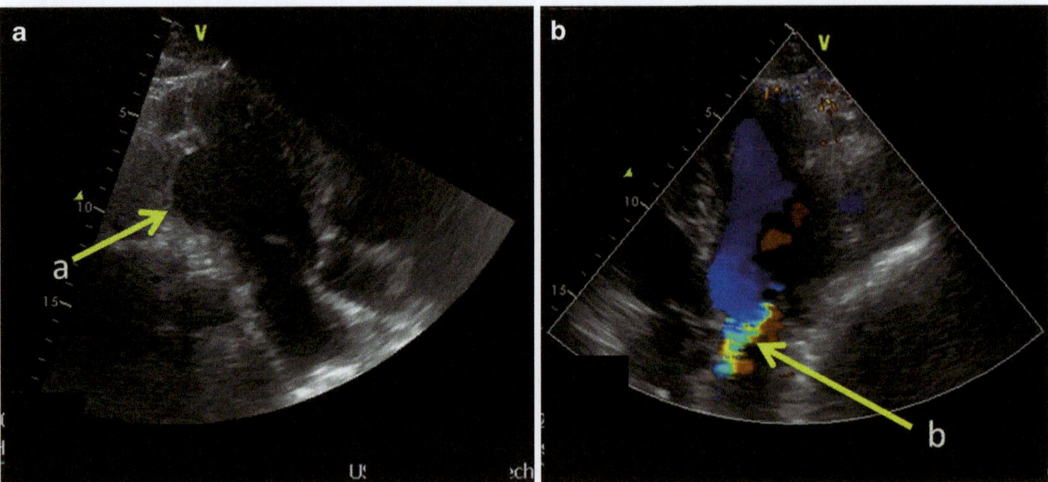

Fig. 3.1 (**a**) Dilatation of the basal inferior wall (*yellow arrow* **a**) as a result of myocardial infarction. (**b**) Jet of anteriorly-directed MR (*yellow arrow* **b**) resulting from restriction of the posterior leaflet secondary to inferior myocardial infarction

an important feature of any imaging investigation in patients with chronic conditions. Measurements are highly reproducible in laboratories with adequate quality-control systems in place – national and international systems of accreditation exist to ensure that departments which meet quality standards can be readily identified.

Ischemic heart disease may cause mitral regurgitation in both the acute and chronic situation. Acutely, in the first week after myocardial infarction (MI), there is the risk of papillary muscle rupture [3], and in addition segmental akinesis or dilatation of the myocardium may cause MR (Fig. 3.1a, b). MR after acute MI may be silent but is highly prognostically significant. One study used color Doppler echocardiography to show mild MR in 29 % and moderate-severe MR in 6 % of patients within 48 h of admission with acute MI. Any degree of MR was associated with increased 1 year mortality [4]. Perez de Isla et al. studied 300 consecutive patients by echocardiography after non-ST elevation MI and showed that MR was present in 42 % within the first week. Again, MR was a predictor of outcome over 14 months' follow up [5].

This chapter focuses on chronic FIMR, which is the result of remodeling of the ventricle over time after infarction.

The role of the echocardiocardiogram is threefold: first to confirm the diagnosis of FIMR, which encompasses a detailed assessment of the mechanism of regurgitation, the left ventricle and also exclusion or full description of other cardiac structural or functional abnormalities which may be contributing to the patient's presenting symptoms. Secondly, evaluation of severity by both qualitative and quantitative methods [6, 7] and finally (and increasingly important) the identification of prognostic features, such as those which predict the possibility of a less satisfactory outcome after surgical repair [8], and the presence of pulmonary hypertension (Fig. 3.2).

It must be noted that due to the complex, dynamic nature of FIMR, there is no one parameter which surmounts all others in terms of usefulness either diagnostically or prognostically: conventional 2-dimensional measurements and Doppler indices of regurgitation severity must be combined with the newer techniques of 3-dimensional and speckle-tracking echocardiography to provide an in-depth morphological assessment of valve anatomy and ventricular geometry, focusing on the effects of ischemic remodeling. The approach must be fully-comprehensive in every patient and the final conclusion is a synthesis of all the relevant information which can be used to inform clinical decision-making in a heart-team context [9].

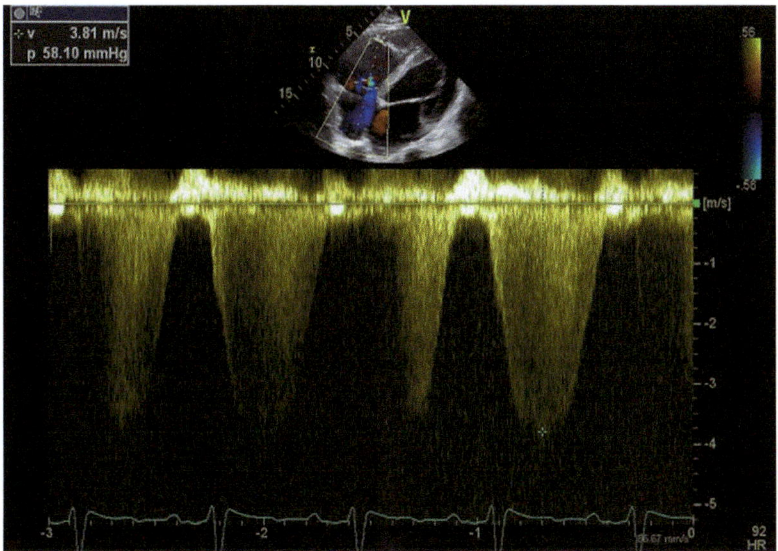

Fig. 3.2 Pulmonary hypertension in a patient with severe FIMR – the PASP is estimated as 4 V^2+RAPmmHg where V is the Vmax of the tricuspid regurgitant signal measured from the CW Doppler trace and RAP is right atrial pressure estimated from the size and inspiratory reactivity of the IVC

Diagnosis of FIMR and Quantification of Severity

Confirming a Diagnosis of Functional Ischemic MR by Echocardiography

Correctly identifying the mechanism of MR as functional and ischemic and correctly evaluating its severity can be surprisingly challenging. It is therefore fundamental to success that the echocardiologist has an in-depth understanding of the normal morphology and physiology of the mitral valve-LV complex [10]. The term "mitral valve-LV complex includes the leaflets, annulus, chordae, papillary muscles and supporting left ventricular myocardium, and the exact geometry required to produce perfect leaflet coaptation may be disrupted by abnormalities of any one of these components. Transthoracic echocardiography (TTE) may in many cases prove sufficient to confirm the diagnosis, but transesophageal echocardiography (TEE) is needed in cases where the ischemic mechanism is unclear and is also a useful adjunct for delineating the mechanism and quantifying morphological parameters in the pre- and perioperative patient thus allowing for advanced planning of individually-tailored intervention [11]. Guidelines state that all patients being considered for mitral intervention should undergo transesophageal echocardiography [19].

Many, but not all, patients will give a definite history of myocardial infarction and/or coronary artery disease. Before assessing the mitral valve itself, the echocardiographer must first make a thorough assessment of the left ventricle (LV), including wall thickness and diastolic and systolic chamber dimensions and volumes, either from 2-dimensional or 3-dimensional imaging (Fig. 3.3). The abnormality of the ventricle may be global dilatation or regional/segmental dysfunction (Fig. 3.4). Differentiation between the two is key to classification of the FIMR. Identification of a segmental wall motion abnormality suggesting previous infarction is often the key finding and the typically-affected segments are the basal and mid inferior and/or inferolateral segments [12]. These regional abnormalities can be very subtle, particularly if the infarct is subendocardial. In addition, in the presence of moderate or severe MR, the resulting hyperdynamic wall motion of other segments will tend to mask mild segmental abnormalities. The key is to have a high degree

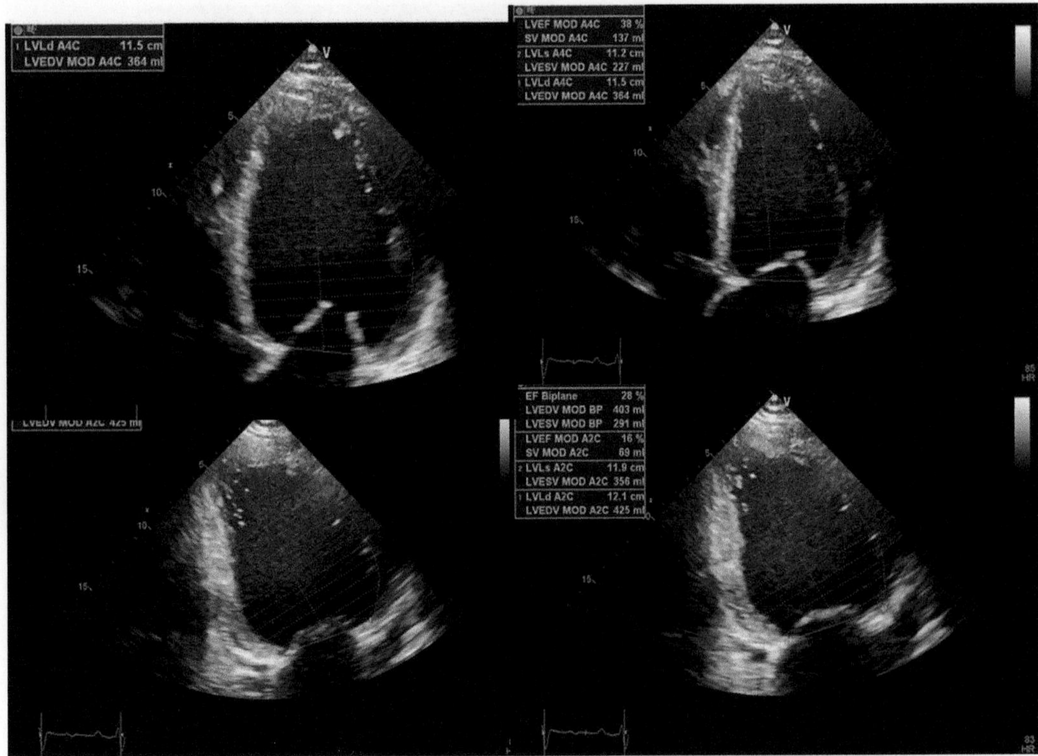

Fig. 3.3 Measuring volumes and LVEF by Simpson's Biplane Method of Discs in a patient with MR and very severely impaired LV function

of suspicion in any patient with a history of CAD or significant risk factors and to look for abnormalities of *thickening* rather than motion. Newer techniques such as analysis of basal rotational dynamics and segmental layered strain analysis by speckle-tracking echocardiography can be a useful adjunct if there is doubt about the presence of a segmental wall motion abnormality [13]. Cardiac magnetic resonance imaging has also proved to be helpful in these situations, in that late-enhancement with gadolinium contrast agents can identify areas of segmental partial thickness infarction, which may be revealed even in patients who do not have a confirmed history of myocardial infarction (Fig. 3.5) [14]. As infarction of the basal inferior and inferolateral segments is a predictor of recurrent MR after mitral ring annuloplasty this author recommends cardiac MRI in any patient with valve morphology consistent with FIMR but no history or obvious regional wall motion abnormality.

Leaflet Tethering

Leaflet tethering or restriction (the terms are used interchangeably) due to displacement of one or both papillary muscles (PM) is the key echocardiographic finding in FIMR. Tethering may be symmetrical, affecting both leaflets, when it is also referred to as "tenting" (Fig. 3.6) or asymmetrical, affecting only one leaflet (Fig. 3.7a) [15]. If only one leaflet is affected, it is more often the posterior leaflet, as the posteromedial papillary muscle tends to have a single-vessel blood supply and so inferior or inferolateral infarction is more likely to cause asymmetric tethering than anterior infarction – the P3 scallop can be restricted almost in isolation if an infarct is limited and well-circumscribed. The result is that the anterior leaflet coaptation zone or rough zone apposes the body of the posterior leaflet rather then its corresponding coaptation zone. This reduces the coaptation length and produces

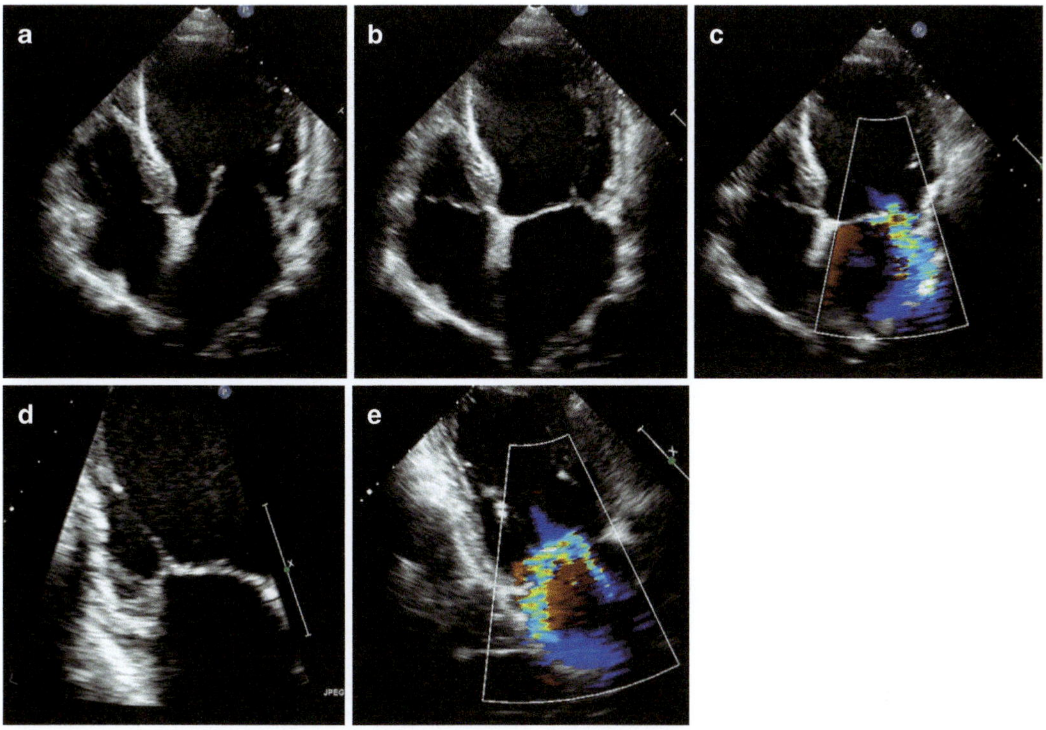

Fig. 3.4 Global and Regional Dysfunction causing FIMR. (Panel **a**) Globally-dilated ischaemic ventricle at end-diastole. (Panel **b**) Globally dilated ventricle at end-systole. (Panel **c**) Jet of functional ischaemic MR in association with globally-dilated ventricle. (Panel **d**) Zoomed PLAX image showing restricted posterior leaflet due to localised basal inferolateral infarction. (Panel **e**) posteriorly-directed jet of MR due to asymmetric tethering of the posterior leaflet

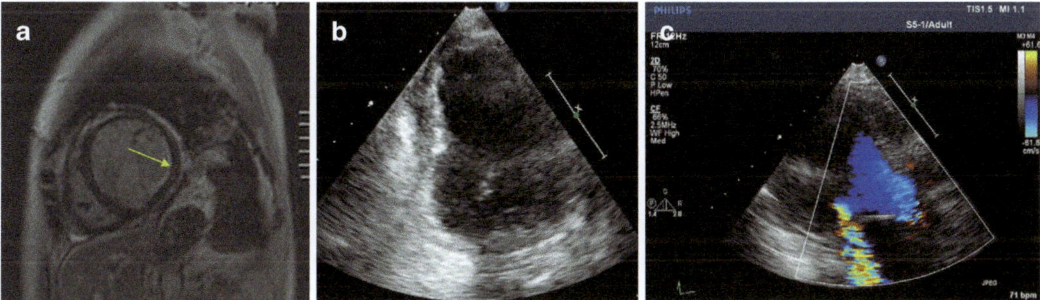

Fig. 3.5 (**a**) Cardiac magnetic resonance imaging with gadolinium contrast showing late-enhancement in the subendocardium of the basal posterolateral segment (*arrowed*) in a patient who presented with pulmonary oedema secondary to severe MR but with no history of previous myocardial infarction. (**b**) Apical 2-chamber view in the same patient showing infarcted basal inferior wall. (**c**) Colour jet of MR due to assymetric tethering of the posterior leaflet in this patient

an eccentric jet of mitral regurgitation – directed towards the restricted leaflet ie most commonly posteriorly-directed (Fig. 3.7b).

If the area of myocardial dysfunction is large and involves several segments, or if there is extensive ventricular remodeling, then LV dilatation may be global. The resulting apical displacement and increased separation of the papillary muscles causes both leaflets of the mitral valve to be tethered or tented into the LV. In these cases,

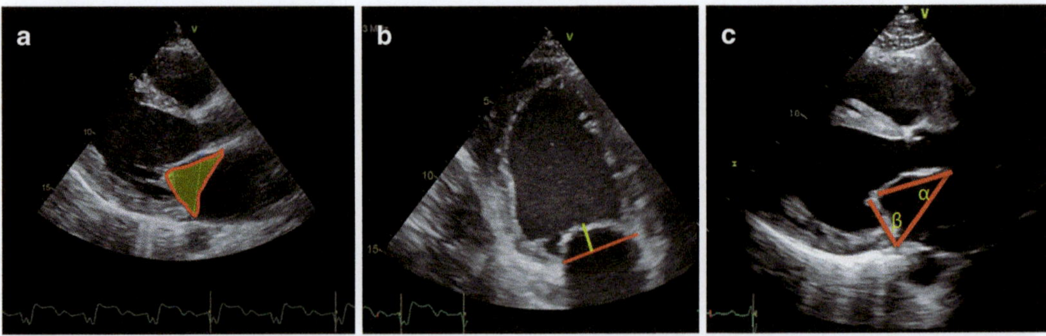

Fig. 3.6 Symmetrical tethering. (**a**) Deep symmetrical tethering of both anterior and posterior mitral leaflets shown in the parasternal long axis (PLAX) view by 2D Echo. The *yellow shaded area* is referred to as the tenting area. (**b**) Symmetrical tethering in a 2 chamber view. The *red line* is the annular plane and the *yellow line* indicates the tenting height/depth. (**c**) The anterior leaflet angle (α) is the angle subtended by the base of the anterior leaflet and the annular plane. The posterior leaflet angle (β) is that subtended by the base of the posterior leaflet and the annular plane. A posterior leaflet angle of >45° is associated with a higher rate of failure of mitral repair in FIMR

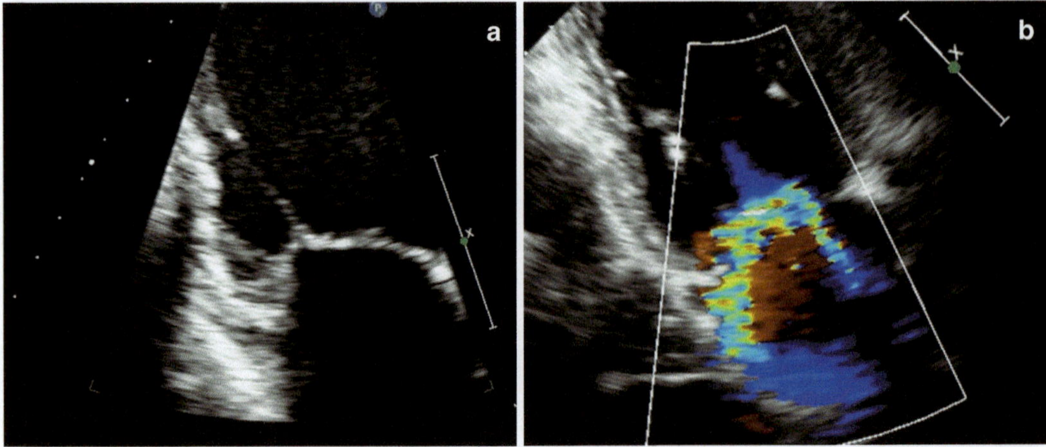

Fig. 3.7 Asymmetrical Tethering. Panel **a** shows tethering affecting the posterior leaflet in a zoomed parasternal long axis (PLAX) view; Panel **b** shows the corresponding jet of severe posteriorly-directed mitral regurgitation

the LV function is usually more severely impaired and the resultant mitral regurgitant jet is more central – though it is rarely absolutely central. There have been numerous studies investigating possible relationships between LV systolic dysfunction, dilatation and severity of FIMR. In an animal model it has been shown that systolic dysfunction in isolation does not cause MR, presumably because without the additional forces tethering the leaflets into the ventricle there is still sufficient force generated to produce sufficient leaflet coaptation. However, in the same model, when the LV was allowed to dilate, causing tethering of one or both leaflets, the result was MR. This confirms that the outward and apical displacement of the PMs is the key mechanism of FIMR. Other work in animal models suggests that ischemia or infarction of the PMs without displacement is not directly related to severity of FIMR. In a canine model there is poor correlation between reduced PM thickening and MR severity, and in another study FIMR was modeled by occlusion of the left circumflex artery in sheep. Ischemia and dysfunction of the PM in the ovine model correlated with reduced rather than increased MR, presumably due to reduction in tethering forces acting on the posterior leaflet. It is also recognized in humans that following inferior infarction, "waisting" or elongation of the posteromedial PM may prevent the occurrence or reduce the severity of FIMR. Gadolinium-enhanced cardiac MRI has also shown no firm correlation between PM infarction and FIMR.

The most important distinction to make is whether leaflet tethering is symmetrical or asymmetrical. In the context of limited inferior or inferolateral infarction, affecting one or two myocardial segments only, the outward displacement of the affected segments and distortion of the posterior annulus tethers only the posterior leaflet – often the P3 scallop is severely affected – and this produces a characteristic appearance which may be mistakenly interpreted by the less-experienced as "prolapse of the anterior mitral valve leaflet tip". In reality, the coaptation point does not come above the annulus, but failure of the tethered posterior leaflet to move upwards towards the annular plane results in the tip of the AMVL meeting the body of the PMVL. The resulting coaptation is highly inefficient and produces a highly-eccentric jet of IMR directed towards the tethered leaflet i.e., posteriorly around the posterior wall of the left atrium (LA). Tenting height, tenting area and tenting angles should also be measured in the parasternal long axis (PLAX) view or apical four chamber (A4Ch) view (Fig. 3.6). Tenting height (or depth – the terms are used interchangeably) is usually measured in the A4Ch view as the maximum mid-systolic distance from the coaptation point to the annular plane. This gives an assessment of the degree of apical shift of the coaptation point and reduction in coaptation length. The term "tenting angles" refers to the relationship between the base of the leaflets and the annular plane. The anterior leaflet angle is termed "α" and the posterior leaflet angle "β". Slices may be selected from 3D volumetric datasets to calculate tethering angles, but unfortunately these angles do vary depending on the exact slice selected and there is as yet no defined standard for how this should be done. In general terms, the greater the ratio of posterior leaflet angle to anterior leaflet angle, the greater the degree of asymmetric tethering, and increased asymmetry of tethering is associated with increased MR severity. A posterior leaflet angle of >45° is also important as a predictor of an unsatisfactory result after ring annuloplasty (see below). Tenting area is probably the most reproducible measurement as it is not dependent on delineation of one particular angle. It is defined as the area bounded by the anterior and posterior leaflets and the annular plane, usually in the PLAX view, and should be measured in mid-systole when the area is at a maximum. A tenting area of ≥ 4 cm^2 has been shown to be a predictor of moderate-severe FIMR over a 2-year period, and also of worsening of FIMR. In patients with systolic dysfunction, tenting area is a major determinant of FIMR severity, independent of global LV function or sphericity. This is probably because tenting area correlates with linear measures of PM displacement and thus acts as a surrogate marker for the severity of posterior and apical PM displacement. 3D volumetric datasets can be used to measure tenting volumes. However whether tenting areas or volumes are measured, it should be noted that for any given value of tenting area or volume, a greater degree of asymmetric tethering will be associated with more severe FIMR.

In addition to tethering of the leaflets due to PM displacement, the body of the anterior leaflet may also be tethered by its secondary chords, causing it to fold into a slight "V" shape in systole – sometimes called the "seagull sign", referring to the silhouette of a seagull's wings in flight. This form of asymmetric tethering is also associated with more severe FIMR.

Annular Dilatation

Dilatation of the annulus is often found in association with FIMR, as it can be caused by global LV dilatation or regional remodeling and exacerbated by increased LA size due to either chronically increased filling pressures or atrial fibrillation. Determining the size of the annulus is useful to the surgeon or interventionist and

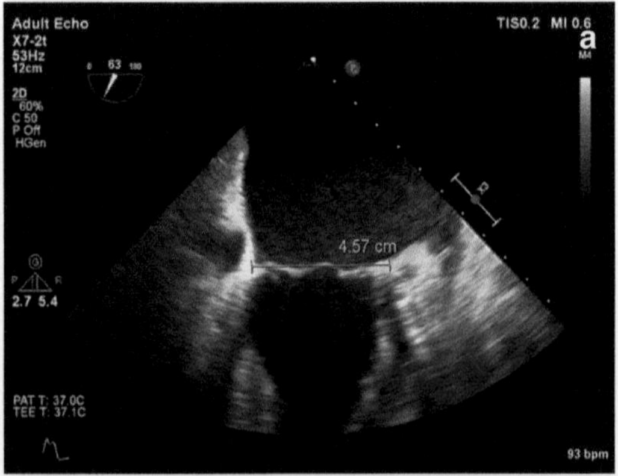

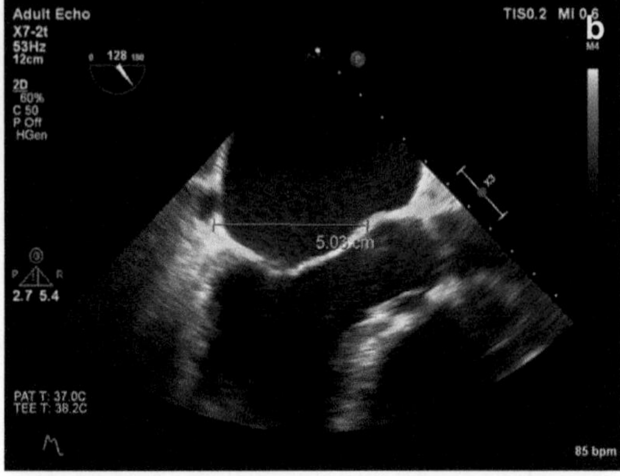

Fig. 3.8 Measuring the mitral annulus by TEE 60° (**a**) and 120° (**b**) views. Correct views for measuring dimensions of the mitral annulus during TEE. (**a**) The "bi-commissural" view, obtained at approximately 60° gives the dimension of the annulus across the commissures. (**b**) The 120° view gives the true AP annular dimension. If there is remodelling of the posterior wall and mitral annulus, then the AP dimension may almost equate to the dimension across the commissures, i.e., the mitral annulus becomes more circular

should be measured in at least two planes – across the commissures and in the antero-posterior direction. These are best appreciated from the 60° and 120° lower esophageal views by TEE (Fig. 3.8). Annular area can also be calculated assuming an elliptical shape by the formula $\boldsymbol{\pi(d/2)_A \times (d/2)_B}$ where A is the diameter of the long axis of the ellipse (ie across the commissures) and B is the short axis (anteroposterior diameter) or by using one of the widely available software analysis packages for quantification of the mitral valve. After infarction, reduced annular contraction correlates with increased MR severity.

The Mitral Leaflets

Although it is usually asserted that FIMR is a condition of the ventricle and not the valve itself, and that the leaflets are "normal", some work has suggested that over time, the leaflets do change in size and shape. In one study using 3D echocardiography to measure leaflet areas in humans, it was shown that total mitral leaflet area is greater in patients with FIMR than in patients without LV dilatation or previous infarction. However, the ratio of the total area to the "closing area" was decreased [16]. It has been postulated that the adaptation of the leaflets over time is due to reactivation of embryonic development pathways which allow the leaflets to enlarge and thicken, thus effectively remodeling the valve. Leaflet area can be appreciated well from 3-dimensional TOE datasets reconstructed using widely-available commercial analysis packages.

Assessment of Severity of Functional Ischemic Mitral Regurgitation

Echocardiographic assessment of the severity of functional ischemic mitral regurgitation is complicated by the dynamic nature of the condition, which is predominantly due to the changing function of the ventricle depending on pre and afterload. This load dependency means that there is no one parameter which alone indicates the severity of regurgitation. Clues to the severity can be gained both directly and indirectly and from all different modalities of echo. In this part of the chapter we will review each modality and what can be gained from it.

2-Dimensional Echocardiography

The dimensions and contractility of the LV can give the first clue to the severity. A reduced end-systolic dimension or volume is an indicator of hyperdynamic function due to a high degree of off-loading into the left atrium (LA) in severe MR. However, this can be confounded in the presence of severe ischemic impairment of LV function – infarcted myocardium is unable to contract so dimensions may not reflect the severity of MR. Annular size should always be measured and as this changes throughout the cardiac cycle, mid-systole is a reasonable point to do this. Dilatation of the annulus is a common finding in functional MR. The degree of tethering of the leaflet should be estimated and this is done by tracing the area bounded by the leaflets at end-systole and the annular plane. This "tenting area" is directly related to the chance of successful repair and so is vital information for the surgeon. The coaptation point and length should be measured. Only when the morphology of the valve has been fully delineated should other methods of echocardiography be used.

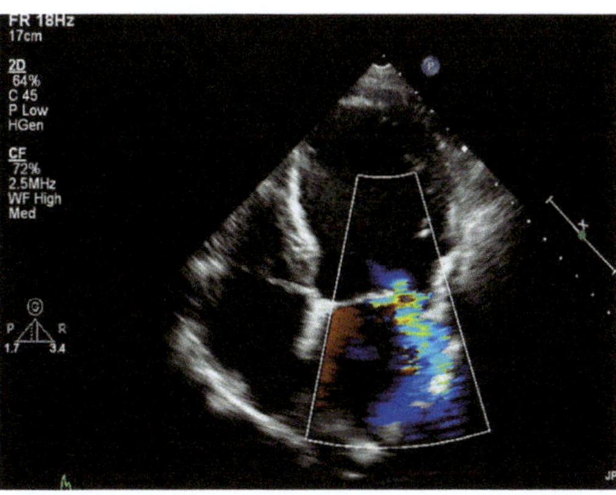

Fig. 3.9 Wall-hugging jets of MR often contain higher regurgitant volumes despite the relative slimness of the jet, which is due to the Coanda effect

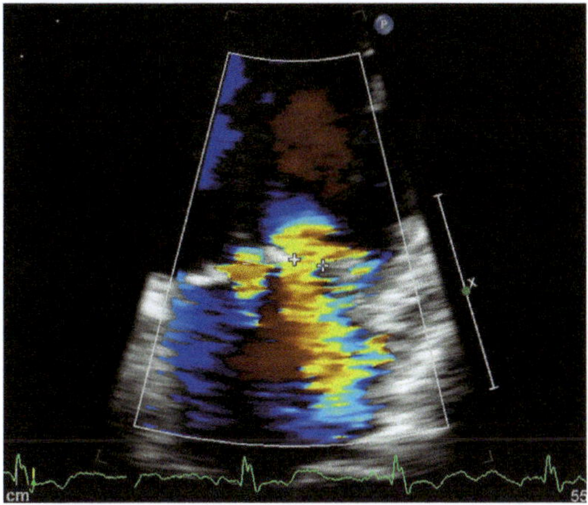

Fig. 3.10 2D vena contracta. The vena contracta (VC) is best measured in the PLAX view but in practical terms it tends to be measured in whichever view it is seen most clearly. This may lead to error as the VC width varies greatly depending on the plane chosen for measurement. 3D VC measurements have been shown to be more consistent

Color Doppler

Whilst the echocardiographic diagnosis of MR depends on the demonstration of a jet of mitral regurgitation on color flow Doppler imaging, this is not a good method of assessing severity. Nevertheless, there are some important clues which can be gained from an assessment of color flow.

Jet Direction and Area

The color jet alone is not a good indicator of severity. If imaged by 2-D echo it should be imaged in several planes to build up a 3-dimensional impression in the mind of the sonographer. An eccentric jet suggests asymmetric leaflet tethering and a more central jet is usually associated with global remodeling and annular dilatation. A jet which hugs the wall of the LA may appear to be very thin but as it is subject to the Coanda effect, whereby fluids are attracted to adjacent surfaces, the apparent slimness of the color jet is deceptive and these jets can be due to MR of significant volume [17] (Fig. 3.9). In broad terms, a jet with an area of $<4.0\ cm^2$ or which occupies $<20\,\%$ of the area of the left atrium is consistent with mild MR.

Vena Contracta

The vena contracta (VC) is the narrowest part of the jet, just as it emerges through the regurgitant orifice into the LA (Fig. 3.10). In theory it is a surrogate for the regurgitant orifice area. However, the regurgitant orifice is unlikely to be a regular shape in cross-section, so the VC width varies greatly depending on the plane chosen for its measurement. Parasternal views are recommended, but if this is not possible, it may be

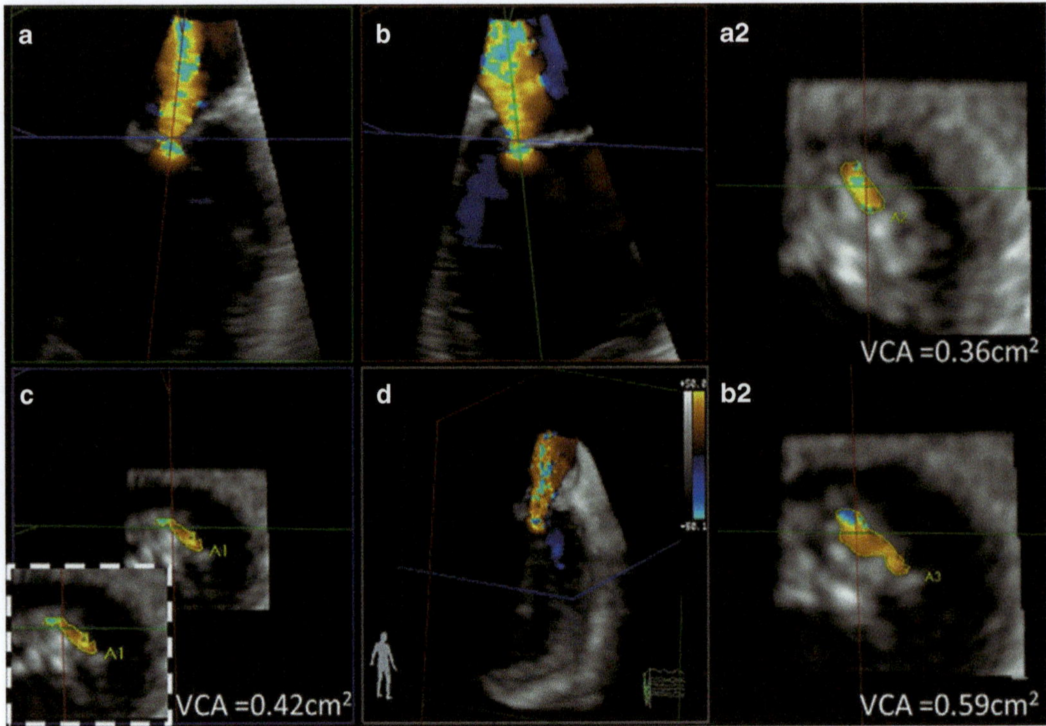

Fig. 3.11 3D Vena contracta. VCA Measurement Using 3D Color Full-Volume Acquisition by TEE. (**a**, **b**) Multiplanar reformatting to obtain the best view of the regurgitant jet and the vena contracta. (**c**) En face view of the vena contracta area (VCA) with planimetry. (**d**) Reformatted 3-dimensional (3D) volume illustrating the regurgitant jet. (**a2**) and (**b2**) illustrate the effect of a change in systolic phase and the location of the en face (*blue*) plane, respectively, on the VCA measurement. (From Thavendiranathan et al. [19]. With permission from Elsevier)

measured from the A4Ch or ALAX view (not the A2Ch view, as this typically tends to give a larger value). Values of ≤3 mm are consistent with mild MR and values ≥7 mm with severe MR but values in between fall into a grey area containing some mild, many moderate and some severe cases. Recently, the measurement of VC area (VCA) by 3D TEE has been shown to be consistent and reliable as a plane can be selected which gives a true cross-section through the jet at the point closest to the orifice [18]. A good description of how to do this practically can be found in the review by Thavendiranathan et al. [19] (Fig. 3.11).

Continuous Wave Doppler

The signal intensity of the Doppler trace through the regurgitant jet is directly related to the volume of blood it contains and hence the severity of MR. It may be best-appreciated in comparison with the antegrade flow signal intensity – if they are the same, or nearly so, then the regurgitation is likely to be severe. The CW Doppler mitral regurgitant trace can also be used to calculate the left ventricular dp/dt – the rate at which the LV is able to generate pressure, which is a good indicator of underlying mechanical contractility (Fig. 3.12b, c).

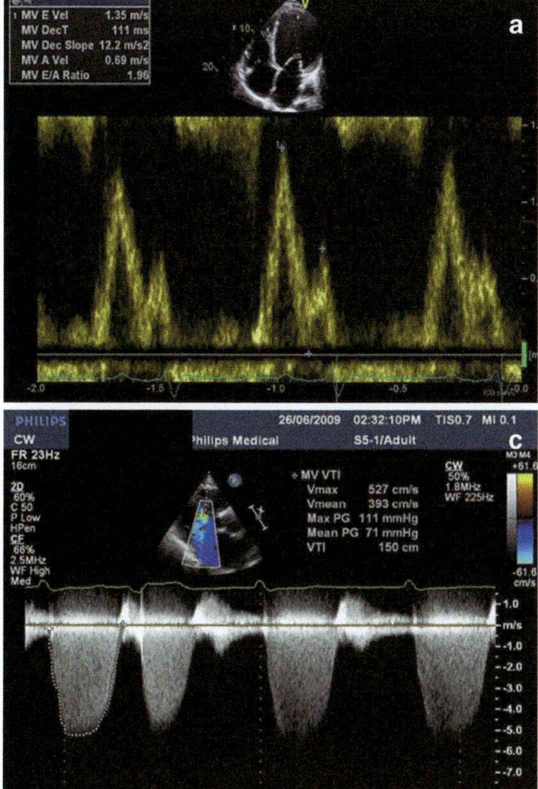

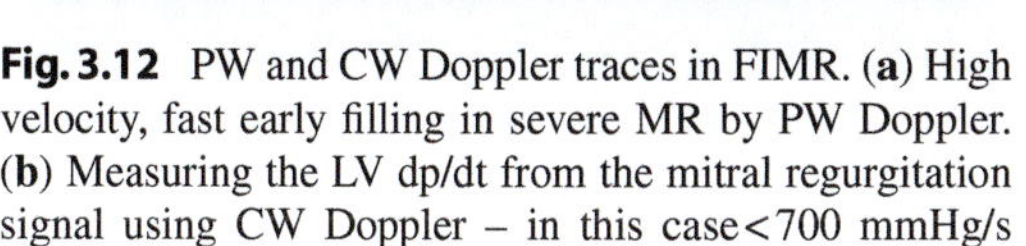

Fig. 3.12 PW and CW Doppler traces in FIMR. (**a**) High velocity, fast early filling in severe MR by PW Doppler. (**b**) Measuring the LV dp/dt from the mitral regurgitation signal using CW Doppler – in this case < 700 mmHg/s suggesting severe impairment of underlying myocardial contractility. (**c**) A dense, holodiastolic CW Doppler trace is consistent with severe MR

Pulsed Wave Doppler

Mitral regurgitation is associated with an increase in antegrade velocity due to increased flow volume across the valve in diastole. When severe MR is present, the E wave velocity in the awake patient will be ≥1.2 m/s in the absence of mitral stenosis or previous mitral repair/annuloplasty (Fig. 3.12a). Reduced forward (aortic) stroke volume is another finding in severe MR and can be calculated using PW Doppler in the LVOT with the sample volume placed 0.5 cm below (proximal to) the aortic valve (Fig. 3.13).

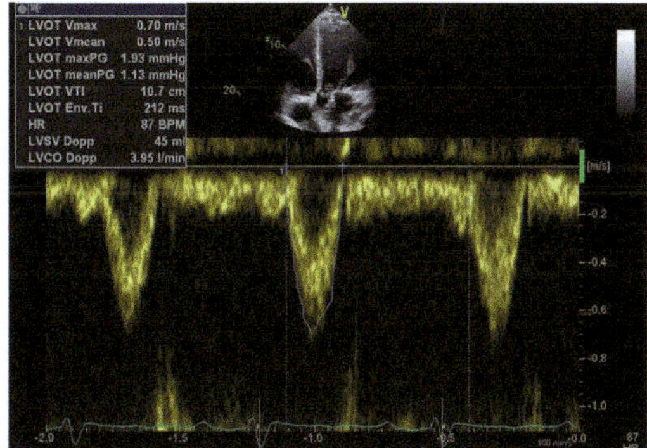

Fig. 3.13 Reduced forward flow in severe FIMR, evidenced by low LVOT VTI (normal range 15–25)

Pulmonary Vein Flow

A PW Doppler sample in a pulmonary vein at a distance from the jet will show blunting of the systolic wave in moderate MR and systolic reversal in severe MR. It can be tricky to obtain an accurate trace from TTE, especially as the MR jet may be directed towards the pulmonary vein most amenable to measurement, but it is almost always possible to assess pulmonary vein flow from TEE (Fig. 3.14).

Flow Convergence and Proximal Isovelocity Surface Area

When a fluid passes through a small circular orifice in a flat plate, flow accelerates just proximal to the orifice and the flow converges on the orifice in hemispheric shells of equal velocity. This region of accelerated flow can be seen on color Doppler imaging in the A4Ch view as an approximate hemisphere on the ventricular side of the regurgitant orifice. The image is optimized by adjusting the aliasing velocity until the radius of the hemisphere can be easily measured – this is termed the "PISA radius" (Fig. 3.15). The effective regurgitant orifice area (EROA) can be calculated from the following equation [$6.28 \times (PISA\ radius)^2 \times aliasing\ velocity$]/$MR\ V_{max}$ (*cm/s*). The EROA is not directly correlated with LVEF but is directly related to the extent of leaflet tethering [20]. To obtain regurgitant volume, multiply the EROA by the velocity-time integral of the signal (Box 3.1 PISA Calculation).

Mitral Regurgitant Volume Calculation from Stroke Volumes

Another method of calculating regurgitant volume is to subtract the aortic stroke volume

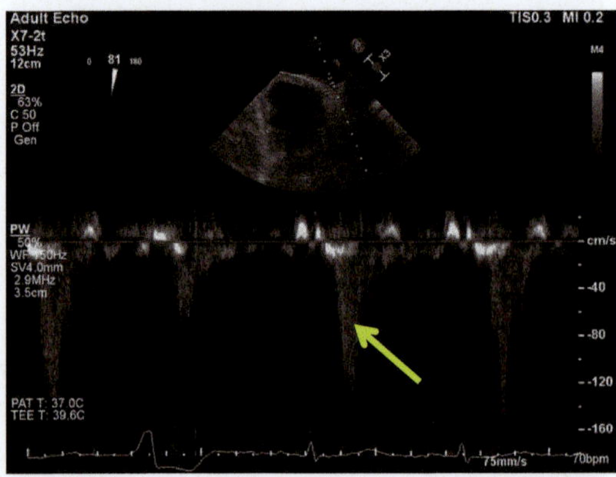

Fig. 3.14 Pulmonary vein systolic flow reversal in severe FIMR. Systolic flow reversal (*yellow arrow*) recorded in the left upper lobe pulmonary vein during transoesophageal echocardiography

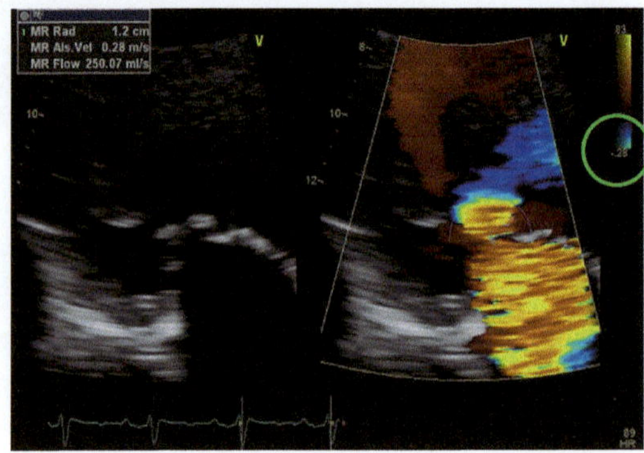

Fig. 3.15 Measuring the PISA radius in FIMR. The PISA radius (here 1.2 cm) is measured by turning down the colour baseline until a *yellow* hemisphere is seen on the ventricular side of the mitral valve. The Nyquist cutoff limit is shown at the top right of the screen (*green circle*)

Box 3.1. PISA Calculation

$$\text{EROA} = \frac{6.28 \times [\text{PISA Radius (cm)}]^2 \times \text{Nyquist cutoff}}{\text{MR } V_{\text{max}} \text{ (cm/s)}} \times 100\,(\text{mm}^2)$$

from CW Doppler trace

$$\text{Regurgitant volume} = \text{EROA} \times \text{VTI}_{\text{MR}}\ (\text{ml})$$

from the mitral inflow volume. First the mitral valve cross-sectional area must be calculated. This is done by measuring the mitral annulus diameter (d) at early or mid-diastole and using the formula $\pi(\mathbf{d/2})^2$ if a circular orifice is assumed or if an elliptical assumption is made then the annulus is measured in both the 2-chamber and 4-chamber views and the calculation becomes $\pi(\mathbf{d/2})_{(4Ch)} \times (\mathbf{d/2})_{(2Ch)}$. Inflow volume can be calculated by multiplying the cross-sectional area by the inflow VTI measured by PW Doppler at the annular plane. Similarly, LVOT stroke volume is calculated by measuring the LVOT diameter at mid-end systole and calculated using the formula above assuming a circular shape. Stroke volume is obtained by multiplying the cross-sectional area by the LVOT VTI measured by PW Doppler 5 mm below the aortic valve in the LVOT. These calculations make a number of geometric assumptions of varying validity, and also assume no disease of the aortic valve.

Synthesizing the information: Ischemic Versus Non-ischemic MR

The final report should contain all of the measurements along with a full description of all components of the mitral valve-LV complex. There should be a clear statement regarding the severity of the regurgitation. New guidelines for the management of patients with valvular heart disease were issued by the AHA/ACC in 2014, referring to this condition as "ischemic chronic secondary MR" [21]. In recognition of the fact that outcomes in patient with functional MR secondary to ischemic heart disease are worse than those in patients with the same degree of primary or degenerative MR, the current criteria for defining severity of FIMR are accordingly different (Box 3.2 – criteria from new ESC Statement).

Transesophageal Echocardiography

Transesophageal echocardiography of the native mitral valve should rarely, if ever, be required to

Box 3.2. Echo Criteria for the Definition of Severe MR

Qualitative	
Mitral valve morphology	Flail leaflet/ruptured papillary muscle
Color flow regurgitant jet	Very large central or eccentric jet adhering, swirling and reaching the posterior wall of the left atrium
Continuous wave signal of regurgitant jet	Dense/triangular
Flow convergence zone	Large[a]
Semi-quantitative	
Vena contracta width (mm)	>7 (>8 for biplane)/[a]
Pulmonary vein flow	Systolic flow reversal
Inflow	E-wave dominant >1.5 m/s[b]
TVI mitral/TVI aortic	>1.4
Quantitative	
EROA (mm^2)	> 40 (primary), > 20 (secondary)
Regurgitant volume (ml/beat)	> 60 (primary), > 30 (secondary)
Cardiac chamber enlargement	Left ventricle, left atrium

From De Bonis et al., Surgical and interventional management of mitral valve regurgitation: a position statement from the European Society of Cardiology Working Groups on Cardiovascular Surgery and Valvular Heart Disease. July 17, 2015. *European Heart Journal. By permission of Oxford University Press.* DOI: http://dx.doi.org/10.1093/eurheartj/ehv322

Nyquist limit 50–60 cm/s

TVI time-velocity integral, *EROA* effective regurgitant orifice area

[a]Average between apical four- and two-chamber views

[b]In the absence of mitral stenosis or other causes of elevated left atrial pressure

determine severity of FIMR. It should be used primarily as an adjunct to TTE in the detailed delineation of abnormal morphology and in order that intervention might be tailored to the individual patient. A comparison of TEE and TTE measurements relevant to the mechanism of functional ischaemic MR was made by analyzing images acquired in 196 patients enrolled in the Surgical Treatment For Ischemic Heart Failure (STICH) trial. Only a modest correlation was found between the two techniques for MR grade (r=0.52), for long axis tenting height (r=0.27), tenting area (r=0.35) and long axis mitral annular diameter (r=0.41). For this reason, TTE should be used primarily for determining the hemodynamic significance of FIMR, and TEE for mechanistic detail – the two tests are complementary [22]. For the surgeon, an expert opinion regarding the echo can be invaluable but it behoves the echocardiologist to become as familiar as possible with the relevant surgical techniques and appearances and to visit the operating theatre regularly in order to become familiar with the various techniques employed [23] and also because there is no better way of gaining feedback about the accuracy of the TEE findings than by seeing the valve being analysed in situ by the surgeon. TEE of the mitral valve should be done, whenever possible, in the awake or lightly sedated patient so that the physiology is not masked by the vasodilatory, hypotensive and myocardial depressant effects of heavy sedation or general anesthesia. With appropriate patient counselling and expectations management, "awake" TEE can be carried out with little or no sedation and the patient's full co-operation [24]. This is particularly valuable in the elderly, frail or co-morbid patient, in whom the major risk associated with TEE arises from the respiratory depressant effects of sedation. In the anesthetized patient, it can be assumed that all measurements of severity are at least one degree less than they would be in the awake situation [25]. Vasopressors may be used in the perioperative situation to increase the blood pressure to close-to-systolic levels in order to better appreciate the degree of MR [26].

TEE of the mitral valve should be carried out according to published protocols. 3-dimensional volumetric datasets should be acquired for offline analysis and reconstruction – commercial packages produce images which are highly-appreciable even by someone who is not expert at echo interpretation (Fig. 3.16).

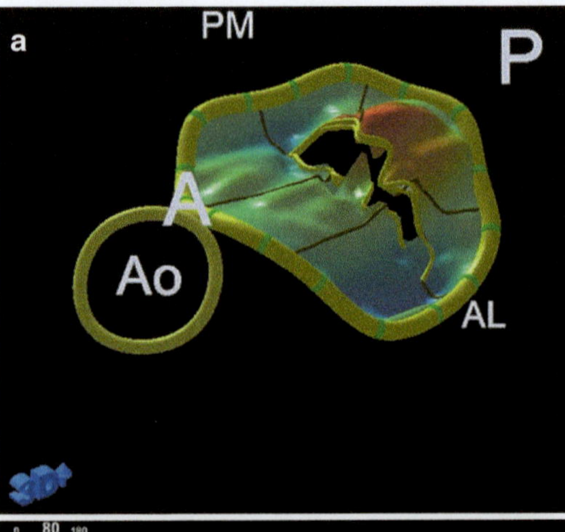

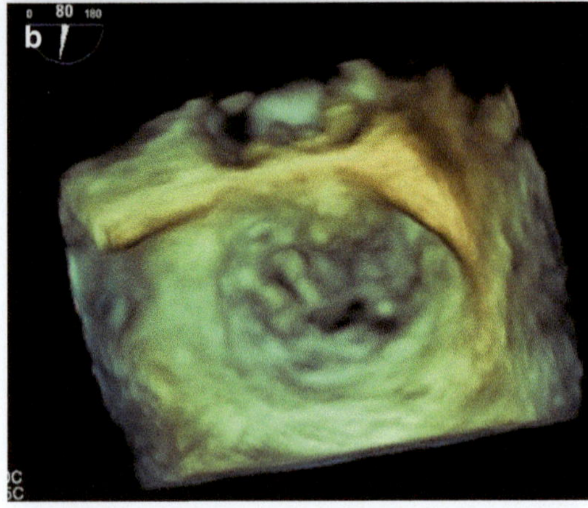

Fig. 3.16 (**a**) 3DTEE reconstruction of a mitral valve showing prolapse of the P2 scallop of the posterior leaflet. (**b**) En-face 3D "surgeon's" view of the mitral valve showing prolapsing anterior commissure

3-Dimensional Versus 2-Dimensional Techniques

Although most of the physiological information required to diagnose the severity of FIMR by echocardiography is available from conventional 2-dimensional imaging, and in particular, a thorough Doppler examination, 3-dimensional techniques have been shown to have certain advantages, especially in the measurement of irregular shapes such as vena contracta area, effective regurgitant orifice area and anatomical regurgitant orifice area as well as stroke volume [27]. Perhaps the greatest advantage is that the images are more intuitive and thus the anatomy is more easily and quickly appreciated by the less expert observer. 3DTEE allows the mitral valve to be displayed in an en-face view from the LA, oriented as the surgeon would see it (Fig. 3.16b). This facilitates heart team discussions and also communication in the operating theatre. 3DTEE has also been shown to have an advantage in facilitating analysis of the scallops of the mitral leaflets and correctly identifying the affected segments. Reconstructed 3D datasets allow better appreciation of changes in annular shape, particularly the degree of asymmetric annular distortion in FIMR and recent software permits direct measurements of length to be made from 3D images, so distances such as papillary muscle tethering lengths can be appreciated [28]. As a general rule, it makes sense to have as much information as possible to inform decision-making and 3DTEE should now be considered part of the routine assessment for all patients being considered for mitral valve intervention [29, 30].

Echocardiographic Predictors of Poor Outcome After Mitral Annuloplasty in FIMR

There remains controversy over whether there is benefit to mitral ring annuloplasty over mitral valve replacement in the patient with FIMR who is undergoing revascularization [31–34]. Medium-long term results are variable and ongoing LV remodeling with dilatation may lead to recurrence of FIMR. However, there are certain features which suggest the likelihood of an unsatisfactory result even in the short term. Parameters thought to predict recurrence of MR include indexed LV end-diastolic dimension of >6.5 cm or >3.5 cm/m^2, coaptation depth of >10 mm, posterior leaflet angle of >45° and scarring of the basal inferolateral segment shown by gadolinium-enhanced MRI [35] (Box 3.3). Some patients may be considered less suitable for surgery due to increased risk or other factors suggesting a less favorable outcome with surgical mitral repair and these patients may be considered for percutaneous mitral intervention. Echo criteria for suitability for percutaneous edge-edge (clip) intervention based on the results of the EVEREST II trial are shown in Box 3.4.

Box 3.3. Echo Predictors of Failure After Undersized Ring Annuloplasty for Secondary MR

Coaptation depth >1 cm
Systolic tenting area >2.5 cm^2
Posterior mitral leaflet angle >45°
Distal anterior mitral leaflet angle >25°
LV end-diastolic diameter >65 mm

Box 3.4. Suitability for Edge-Edge Percutaneous Repair Techniques

Favorable/eligible	Unfavorable/ineligible
Mod-severe MR Grade 3/4	Commissural lesions
Pathology in A2/P2 zone	Short posterior leaflet
Coaptation length ≥2 mm	Severe asymmetric tethering
Coaptation depth <11 mm	Calcification in grasping area
Flail gap <10 mm	Severe annular calcification
Flail width < 15 mm	Cleft
Mitral Valve orifice area >4 cm^2	Severe annular dilatation
Mobile leaflet length >1 cm	Severe LV remodeling
Large (>50 %) inter-commisanal extension of regurgitant jet	Severe myxomatous degeneration with multi-scallop prolapse

From De Bonis et al., Surgical and interventional management of mitral valve regurgitation: a position statement from the European Society of Cardiology Working Groups on Cardiovascular Surgery and Valvular Heart Disease. July 17, 2015. *European Heart Journal. By permission of Oxford University Press.* DOI: http://dx.doi.org/10.1093/eurheartj/ehv322

Stress Echocardiography in MR

Stress echocardiography can be very useful in the assessment of patients with mild or moderate FIMR who exhibit exertional symptoms [36, 37]. Bicycle exercise stress is recommended over pharmacological techniques for several reasons: firstly, physical exercise mimics the situations patients find themselves in when they experience symptoms, thus giving the cardiologist the opportunity to assess and objectively document exercise capacity and symptoms at first-hand. Secondly, the induction of ischemia may exacerbate leaflet tethering by causing increased LV dilatation or inducing a segmental wall motion abnormality, increasing the MR (Fig. 3.17). Finally, there is the opportunity to document exercise-induced pulmonary hypertension which has prognostic importance and may influence the timing of intervention [38]. There is some data suggesting that demonstration of contractile reserve by exercise stress testing can identify those more likely to have improved survival and functional capacity after mitral repair in patients with asymptomatic severe MR [39, 40].

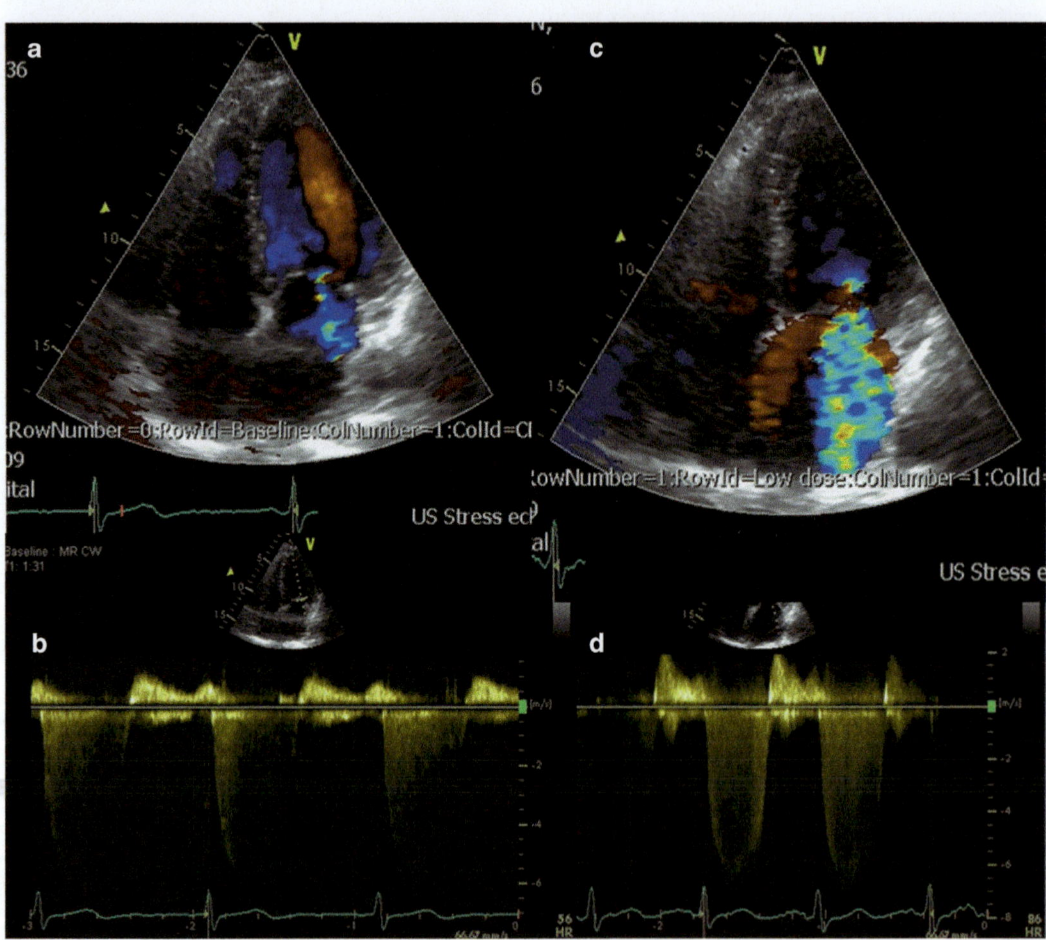

Fig. 3.17 (Panel **a**) colour flow Doppler at rest showing mild MR only *(arrow)*. (Panel **b**) CW Doppler trace corresponding to (**a**) shows mild MR. (Panel **c**) Colour flow Doppler during low dose dobutamine infusion plus submaximal exercise showing increased moderate+MR. (Panel **d**) CW Doppler trace corresponding to (**c**) shows moderate+MR

Limitations and Future Directions

Modern echocardiographic techniques and equipment are ideal for fully evaluating chronic ischemic mitral regurgitation. However, there are some limitations that remain. Without doubt, even with high levels of automation, image acquisition and quality are significantly operator-dependent and interpretation is also particularly dependent upon experience. The dynamic nature of FIMR means that any assessment of severity is only applicable to the loading conditions prevailing at that time. One area that remains challenging is the prediction of LV functional outcome after ring annuloplasty or mitral valve replacement [41]. Another is the identification of patients in whom there is a particularly high chance of early recurrence of MR – it is becoming apparent that this is more frequent after repair for FIMR than might have been realized over the past two decades and data is emerging that there may be no benefit in repair over replacement in FIMR. This area is likely to remain controversial for some time to come, due in part to the difficulties inherent in recruiting appropriate cohorts to randomized trials of surgical techniques (i.e., avoiding the limitation of study cohorts containing "low-risk" patients only – patients in whom neither treatment arm is likely to be hugely beneficial, resulting in "non-inferiority" or apparent equivalence of the two treatment arms). Newer techniques including strain imaging by speckle-tracking, multi-layered strain, atrial strain and analysis of rotational dynamics are likely to be increasingly important.

Summary

Echocardiographic assessment of functional ischemic mitral regurgitation is complex and challenging, due to the dynamic nature of the condition and the large number of parameters and features which must be considered. The final conclusions require a synthesis of qualitative and quantitative data from all modalities of transthoracic and transesophageal echocardiography, including M-mode, rest and stress 2- and 3-dimensional imaging, color flow Doppler and Doppler hemodynamic studies.

References

1. Otto CM. Textbook of clinical echocardiography. 3rd ed. Philadelphia, PA: Elsevier Saunders; 2013 ISBN-13: 978-0-7216-0789-4.
2. Zoghbi WA, Enriquez-Sarano M, Foster E, Grayburn PA, Kraft CD, Levine RA, et al. Recommendations for evaluation of the severity of native valvular regurgitation with two-dimensional and Doppler echocardiography. J Am Soc Echocardiogr. 2003;16(7):777–802.
3. Yamanishi H, Izumoto H, Kitahara H, Kamata J, Tasai K, Kawazoe K. Clinical experiences of surgical repair for mitral regurgitation secondary to papillary muscle rupture complicating acute myocardial infarction. Ann Thorac Cardiovasc Surg. 1998;4(2):83–6.
4. Feinberg MS, Schwammenthal E, Shlizerman L, et al. Prognostic significance of mild mitral regurgitation by color Doppler echocardiography in acute myocardial infarction. Am J Cardiol. 2000;86:903–7.
5. Perez de Isla L, Zamorano J, Quezada M, Almería C, Rodrigo JL, Serra V, et al. Prognostic significance of functional mitral regurgitation after a first non-ST-segment elevation acute coronary syndrome. Eur Heart J. 2006;27(22):2655–60.
6. Garbi M, Monaghan MJ. Quantitative mitral valve anatomy and pathology. Echo Res Pract. 2015;2: R63–72.
7. Zamorano JL, Fernández-Golfín C, González-Gómez A. Quantification of mitral regurgitation by echocardiography. Heart. 2015;101(2):146–54. doi:10.1136/heartjnl-2012-303498.
8. Konsaerepong V, Shiota M, Gillinov AM, Song J-M, Fukuda S, McCarthy PM, et al. Echocardiographic predictors of successful versus unsuccessful mitral repair in ischaemic mitral regurgitation. Am J Cardiol. 2006;98(4):504–8.
9. Dudzinski DM, Hung J. Echocardiographic assessment of ischemic mitral regurgitation. Cardiovasc Ultrasound. 2014;12:46.
10. Dal-Bianco JP, Levine RA. Anatomy of the mitral valve apparatus – role of 2D and 3D echocardiography. Cardiol Clin. 2013;31(2):151–64.
11. Hahn R. Recent advances in echocardiography for valvular heart disease. F1000Res. 2015;4(F1000 Faculty Rev):914.
12. Kumanohoso T, Otsuji Y, Yoshifuku S, Matsukida K, Koriyama C, Kisanuki A, et al. Mechanism of higher incidence of ischaemic mitral regurgitation in patients with inferior myocardial infarction: quantitative analysis of left ventricular and mitral valve geometry in 103 patients with prior myocardial infarction. J Thorac Cardiovasc Surg. 2003;125(1):135–43.

13. Zito C, Cusmà-Piccione M, Oreto L, Tripepi S, Mohammed M, Di Bella G, et al. In patients with post-infarction left ventricular dysfunction, how does impaired basal rotation affect chronic ischemic mitral regurgitation? J Am Soc Echocardiogr. 2013;26(10):1118–29.
14. Kwong RY, Sattar H, Wu H, Vorobiof G, Gandla V, Steel K, et al. Incidence and prognostic implication of unrecognized myocardial scar characterized by cardiac magnetic resonance in diabetic patients without clinical evidence of myocardial infarction. Circulation. 2008;118(10):1011–20.
15. Agricola E, Oppizzi M, Maisano F, De Bonis M, Schinkel AFL, Torracca L, et al. Echocardiographic classification of chronic ischemic mitral regurgitation caused by restricted motion according to tethering pattern. Eur J Echocardiogr. 2004;5:326–34.
16. Dal-Bianco P, Aikawa E, Bischoff J, Guerrero JL, Handschumacher MD, Sullivan S, et al. Active adaptation of the tethered mitral valve: insights into a compensatory mechanism for functional mitral regurgitation. Circulation. 2009;120:334–42.
17. Chen CG, Thomas JD, Anconina J, Harrigan P, Mueller L, Picard MH, Levine RA, Weyman AE. Impact of impinging wall jet on color Doppler quantification of mitral regurgitation. Circulation. 1991;84:712–20.
18. Zeng X, Levine RA, Hua L, Morris EL, Kang Y, Flaherty M, et al. Diagnostic value of vena contracta area in the quantification of mitral regurgitation severity by color Doppler 3D echocardiography. Circ Cardiovasc Imaging. 2011;4(5):506–13.
19. Thavendiranathan P, Phelan D, Collier P, Thomas JD, Flamm SD, Marwick TH. Quantitative assessment of mitral regurgitation: how best to do it. JACC Cardiovasc Imaging. 2012;5(11):1161–75.
20. Yiu SF, Enriquez-Sarano M, Tribouilloy C, Seward JB, Tajik AJ. Determinants of the degree of functional mitral regurgitation in patients with systolic left ventricular dysfunction: a quantitative clinical study. Circulation. 2000;102:1400–6.
21. Nishimura RA, Otto CM, Bonow RO, Carabello BA, Erwin 3rd JP, Guyton RA, O'Gara PT, Ruiz CE, Skubas NJ, Sorajja P, Sundt 3rd TM, Thomas JD. ACC/AHA Task Force Members 2014 AHA/ACC guideline for the management of patients with valvular heart disease: a report of the American College of Cardiology/American Heart Association Task Force on Practice Guidelines. Circulation. 2014;129(23):e521–643.
22. Grayburn PA, She L, Roberts BJ, Golba KS, Mokrzycki K, Drozdz J, Cherniavsky A, Przybylski R, Wrobel K, Asch FM, Holly TA, Haddad H, Yii M, Maurer G, Kron I, Schaff H, Velazquez EJ, Oh JK. Comparison of transesophageal and transthoracic echocardiographic measurements of mechanism and severity of mitral regurgitation in ischemic cardiomyopathy (from the surgical treatment of ischemic heart failure trial). Am J Cardiol. 2015;116(6):913–8.
23. Jensen H, Jensen MO, Nielsen SL. Surgical treatment of functional ischaemic MR. J Heart Valve Dis. 2015;24(1):30–42.
24. Report from the Education Committee of the British Society of Echocardiography: Richard Wheeler (Lead Author), Richard Steeds (Chair), Gill Wharton, Bushra Rana, Richard Wheeler, Nicola Smith, et al. http://www.bsecho.org/recommendations-for-safe-practice-in-sedation/.
25. Grewal KS, Malkowski MJ, Piracha AR, Astbur JC, Kramer C, Dianzumba S, Reichek N. Effect of general anesthesia on the severity of mitral regurgitation by transesophageal echocardiography. Am J Cardiol. 2000;85:199–203.
26. Mihalatos DG, Gopal AS, Kates R, Toole RS, Bercow NR, Lamendola C, Berkay SH, Damus P, Robinson N, Grimson R, Shen K, Reichek N. Intraoperative assessment of mitral regurgitation: role of phenylephrine challenge. J Am Soc Echocardiogr. 2006;19(9):1158–64.
27. Jain S, Malouf JF. Incremental value of 3-D transesophageal echocardiographic imaging of the mitral valve. Curr Cardiol Rep. 2014;16(1):439.
28. Fattouch K, Murana G, Castrovinci S, Mossuto C, Sampognaro R, Borruso MG, et al. Mitral valve annuloplasty and papillary muscle relocation oriented by 3-dimensional transesophageal echocardiography for severe functional mitral regurgitation. J Thorac Cardiovasc Surg. 2012;143(4 Suppl):S38–42.
29. Ben Zekry S, Nagueh SF, Little SH, Quinones MA, McCulloch ML, Karanbir S, Herrera EL, Lawrie GM, Zoghbi WA. Comparative accuracy of two- and three-dimensional transthoracic and transesophageal echocardiography in identifying mitral valve pathology in patients undergoing mitral valve repair: initial observations. J Am Soc Echocardiogr. 2011;24(10):1079–85.
30. Golba K, Mokrzycki K, Drozdz J, Cherniavsky A, Drobel K, Roberts BJ, et al. STICH TEE Substudy Investigators. Mechanisms of functional mitral regurgitation in ischemic cardiomyopathy determined by transesophageal echocardiography (from the Surgical Treatment for Ischemic Heart Failure Trial). Am J Cardiol. 2013;112(11):1812–1818.
31. Smith PK, Puskas JD, Ascheim DD, Voisine P, Gelijns AC, Moskowitz AJ, et al. Cardiothoracic Surgical Trials Network Investigators. Surgical treatment of moderate ischemic mitral regurgitation. N Engl J Med. 2014;371(23):2178–88.
32. Acker MA, Daganais F, Goldstein D, Kron IL, Perrault LP. Severe ischaemic MR: repair or replace. J Thorac Cardiovasc Surg. 2015;150(6):1425–7.
33. Tolis Jr G, Sundt 3rd TM. Surgical strategies for management of mitral regurgitation: recent evidence from randomized controlled trials. Curr Atheroscler Rep. 2015;17(12):67.
34. LaPar DJ, Acker MA, Gelijns AC, Kron IL. Repair or replace for severe ischemic mitral regurgitation: prospective randomized multicenter data. Ann Cardiothorac Surg. 2015;4(5):411–6.
35. Flynn M, Curtin R, Nowicki ER, Rajeswaran J, Flamm SD, Blackstone EH, Mihaljevic T. Regional wall motion abnormalities and scarring in severe

functional ischemic mitral regurgitation: a pilot cardiovascular magnetic resonance imaging study. J Thorac Cardiovasc Surg. 2009;137(5):1063–70.
36. Lancellotti P, Magne J. Stress testing for the evaluation of patients with mitral regurgitation. Curr Opin Cardiol. 2012;27(5):492–8.
37. Garbi M, Chambers J, Vannan MA, Lancellotti P. Valve stress echocardiography: a practical guide for referral, procedure, reporting, and clinical implementation of results from the HAVEC group. JACC Cardiovasc Imaging. 2015;8(6):724–36.
38. Lancellotti P, Magne J, Dulgheru R, Ancion A, Martinez C, Piérard LA. Clinical significance of exercise pulmonary hypertension in secondary mitral regurgitation. Am J Cardiol. 2015;115(10):1454–61.
39. Lee R, Haluska B, Leung DY, Case C, Mundy J, Marwick TH. Functional and prognostic implications of left ventricular contractile reserve in patients with asymptomatic severe mitral regurgitation. Heart. 2005;91(11):1407–12.
40. le Polain de Waroux JB, Pouleur AC, Vancraeynest D, Pasquet A, Gerber BL, El Khoury G, Noirhomme P, Robert A, Vanoverschelde JL. Early hazards of mitral ring annuloplasty in patients with moderate to severe ischemic mitral regurgitation undergoing coronary revascularization: the importance of preoperative myocardial viability. J Heart Valve Dis. 2009;18(1):35–43.
41. Song JM, Kang SH, Lee EJ, Shin MJ, Lee JW, Chung CH, et al. Echocardiographic predictors of left ventricular function and clinical outcomes after successful mitral valve repair: conventional two-dimensional versus speckle-tracking parameters. Ann Thorac Surg. 2011;91(6):1816–23.

Assessment of Functional Mitral Regurgitation by Cardiovascular Magnetic Resonance

4

Philip Kilner and Afshin Khalatbari

Abstract

In functional mitral regurgitation the leaflets of the mitral valve appear morphologically normal but do not close adequately due to left ventricular disease, either ischaemic or cardiomyopathic. While echocardiography generally remains the first line modality for investigation of mitral regurgitation, cardiovascular magnetic resonance (CMR) has complementary and additional roles. It enables assessment of the regurgitant fraction, mitral annular dimensions, left and right ventricular volumes and function, the effects of MR on the left atrium and pulmonary arteries, any pathology in other heart valves and the extent and distribution of any scarring and hence the viability of the left ventricle. CMR also contributes to assessment of the reparability of the mitral valve. This chapter covers the CMR acquisition methods used, some relevant approaches to image analysis and, finally, the limitations and strengths of CMR relative to echocardiography.

Keywords

Functional mitral regurgitation • Dilated cardiomyopathy • Chronic ischaemic mitral regurgitation • Viability • Cardiac MRI • Tricuspid regurgitation

Introduction

Mitral regurgitation (MR) is generally classified as organic (or primary) and functional (or secondary).

In organic MR, the main pathology is intrinsic disease in the mitral valve apparatus and the leaflets often look abnormal. The most common causes of organic mitral regurgitation are degenerative disease (e.g. Barlow's disease, fibroelastic deficiency, Marfan's syndrome,

P. Kilner, MD, PhD
CMR Unit, Royal Brompton Hospital, Sydney Street, London SW3 6NP, UK
e-mail: p.kilner@rbht.nhs.uk

A. Khalatbari, MD, PhD, MRCP (UK) (✉)
Department of Cardiac Diagnostics, Liverpool Heart and Chest Hospital, Liverpool L14 3PE, UK
e-mail: Afshin.khalatbari@lhch.nhs.uk; AfshinKhalatbari@doctors.org.uk

K.M.J. Chan (ed.), *Functional Mitral and Tricuspid Regurgitation*,
DOI 10.1007/978-3-319-43510-7_4

Ehlers- Danlos syndrome), rheumatic disease, endocarditis, ruptured papillary muscle, and congenital abnormalities such as cleft mitral valve.

In functional mitral regurgitation, the leaflets appear morphologically normal and open well in diastole, but cannot close (coapt) adequately in systole. This is caused by disease in the left ventricle which affects the function of the papillary muscles and also dilates the mitral annulus. The most common causes of functional mitral regurgitation are ischaemia and cardiomyopathies particularly dilated cardiomyopathy (DCM). It is therefore important to remember that in functional mitral regurgitation the underlying problem is in the left ventricle not the mitral valve.

While echocardiography remains the gold standard for the diagnosis and quantification of mitral regurgitation, CMR is considered to be the gold standard for the assessment of left ventricular size and systolic function. CMR has the additional ability to detect scar or fibrosis in the myocardium, which helps to assess myocardial viability in the case of ischaemic MR and to identify the underlying aetiology of disease in the left ventricle in the case of cardiomyopathies. The presence of myocardial fibrosis on preoperative CMR (in both ischaemic and non-ischaemic patterns; see below) is associated with increased postoperative risk of significant arrhythmia, cardiac pacing, and readmission to intensive care unit [1].

A thorough assessment of functional mitral regurgitation is feasible with CMR. The aims of the investigation are to:

1. Confirm the presence and mechanism of MR.
2. Quantify the severity of MR.
3. Assess mitral annulus.
4. Assess the left ventricular (LV) structure and function.
5. Assess the right ventricular (RV) structure and function and the tricuspid valve.
6. Look for consequences of MR on the left atrium and pulmonary arteries.
7. Look for significant pathology in other valves.
8. Comment on the reparability of the mitral valve. Assess the risk of repair failure if mitral valve repair is to be considered.
9. Assess left ventricular myocardial viability

In this chapter we will first discuss the CMR protocol for the assessment of mitral regurgitation and then explain how to analyse the images to provide answers to the above questions. The same protocol can be used for the assessment of organic mitral regurgitation by CMR.

Imaging Protocol

Scout Imaging

Transaxial, coronal, sagittal.

Thoracic Structures

Acquire transaxial set of steady state free precession (SSFP) or fast spin echo images through the chest. Use the still images to plan the cine images.

Standard Cine Images of the Heart

Acquire end expiratory breath hold steady state free precession (bSSFP) cine images of 2-chamber, 3-chamber (also known as left ventricular outflow tract view), 4-chamber, and short axis stack. Slice thickness 6–8 mm, with 2–4 mm interslice gaps to equal 10 mm.

Mitral Valve Stack

The mitral valve stack allows assessment of the scallops of both mitral leaflets for tethering, prolapse or regurgitation.

(a) Choose a basal short axis slice where mitral valve can be seen well (Fig. 4.1a).
(b) Acquire contiguous stack of oblique slices, 5 mm thickness, aligned orthogonal to the central part of the line of coaptation (Fig. 4.1b). Start from the superior (i.e., anterolateral) commissure adjacent to A1-P1 and progress towards the inferior (i.e., posteromedial) commissure adjacent

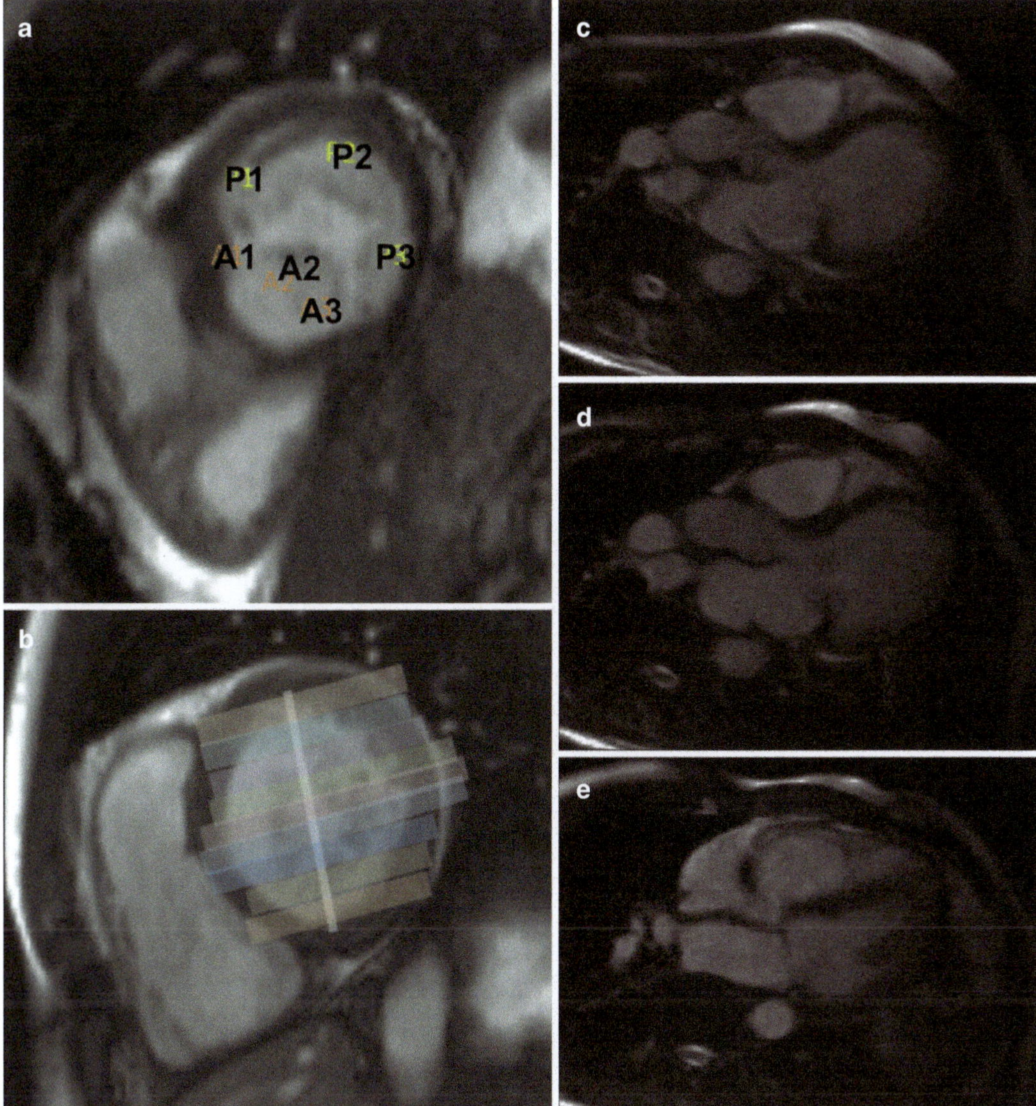

Fig. 4.1 (**a**) A basal short axis slice showing the half open leaflets of the mitral valve, with the P1, P2 and P3 scallops of the posterior leaflet. (**b**) A contiguous stack of oblique slices of 5 mm thickness is aligned orthogonal to the central part of the line of coaptation, covering the extent of the valve. (**c–e**) Three of the slices are shown which show the A1-P1, A2-P2 and A3-P3 regions of the valve, respectively

to A3-P3. Slices should be 5 mm in thickness with no gap. Typically 8–10 slices cover the length of the valve. Three are illustrated (Fig. 4.1c–e).

(c) Acquire further pair of oblique slices orthogonal to the oblique line of leaflet coaptation at each end of the valve adjacent to the commissures (across A1-P1 and A3-P3)

Aortic and Pulmonary Flow Study

Phase contrast through-plane velocity mapping of aortic and main pulmonary artery flow is performed. The velocity encoding (VENC) should be adapted to actual velocity using the lowest velocity without aliasing. The flow velocity and volume should be measured perpendicular to the vessel distal to valve leaflet tips. A useful anatomical landmark for the aortic flow is to measure the flow just above the sinotubular junction at end systole. The recorded net forward volumes are used to calculate regurgitant volume and regurgitant fraction (see below). Because coronary flow does not pass though this slice, the aortic flow measured is typically about 5 % less than main pulmonary artery flow in the absence of a shunt.

In-plane/Through-Plane Fast Low Angle Shot (FLASH) of Mitral Valve (Optional)

FLASH cine acquisitions can have higher sensitivity than bSSFP for the visualisation of the regurgitant jets, depending on their echo time and other aspects of sequence design. A specific FLASH sequence may therefore be found useful for identification of the number, origin, and direction of the regurgitation jet (s), with possible qualitative assessment of the severity of regurgitation.

Phase Velocity Mapping of MR (Optional)

Through-plane phase velocity mapping of the mitral inflow gives a measurement of the anterograde velocity of the mitral inflow which is equal to mitral E and A velocities on pulsed wave Doppler echocardiography. Similar to echo, the measurement should be performed just distal to the tips of the mitral leaflets in diastole. The velocity encoding (VENC) should be adapted to actual velocity using the lowest velocity without aliasing. In addition, as an alternative to the FLASH approach, through-plane breath hold velocity mapping can be used, placed immediately on the atrial side of the closed MV, orthogonal to the jet(s), to map the locations and number of regurgitant lesions. Although MR jet velocity is expected to be higher, a VENC of 250 cm/s is usually adequate because of partial volume averaging, and can result in more effective visualisation than too high a VENC.

Viability

Assessment of myocardial viability and any scar or fibrosis is based on the late enhancement of the myocardium following gadolinium contrast injection. Gadolinium contrast is injected intravenously at a dose of 0.1–0.2 mmol/kg. After 8–10 min wait, the late gadolinium enhanced (LGE) images are acquired. Same views as for cine imaging (except for the mitral valve stack images) should be acquired. Slice thickness is the same as for cine imaging. In-plane resolution is about 1.4–1.8 mm. The acquisition duration per R-R interval should be below 200 ms but should be less in the setting of tachycardia to avoid image blurring. Inversion time is set to null myocardium. We recommend routine use of phase sensitive inversion recovery (PSIR) sequence in addition to magnitude images. The PSIR sequence requires less frequent adjustment of the inversion time (TI) and is particularly useful when the TI used to acquire the magnitude images was not optimal. Read out is usually every other heartbeat. It should be modified to every heartbeat in bradycardic patients and to every third heartbeat in tachycardic patients.

Analysis of the Images

Assess Mitral Valve Structure

Mitral leaflets and the mitral apparatus should be assessed on the 2-chamber, 3-chamber (i.e., LVOT view), 4-chamber, basal short axis, and MV stack cine images for any evidence of thickening, calcification, prolapse, restriction or tethering of the leaflets. The mitral valve stack images help to localise the pathology to mitral leaflet scallops (A1-A3, P1-P3) according to Carpentier's nomenclature. In functional mitral regurgitation, the leaflets appear structurally normal but the mitral annulus is often dilated. Annular dilatation is present when the anteroposterior (AP) diameter is more than 35 mm or the AP diameter/anterior leaflet length ratio is more than 1.3.

The following measurements can be readily performed on CMR (similar to echocardiography) and help to quantify the extent of LV remodelling and the severity of altered geometry of the mitral valve, as well as the risk of postoperative failure of mitral valve repair.

- **In LVOT view**:
  (a) The length of the anterior and posterior leaflets and the anterior-posterior (AP) diameter of the mitral annulus (Fig. 4.2a). Severe annular dilatation (annular diameter >50 mm) is a predictor of operation failure.
  (b) Basal anterior septum in diastole (Fig. 4.2b). A septal bulge of more than 15 mm in thickness is a predictor of SAM and LVOT obstruction after repair.
  (c) C-Sept: C-Sept is the shortest distance between the basal septal bulge and the coaptation point in systole (Fig. 4.2c). Coaptation point is the point where the mitral leaflets coapt in systole. C-sept <2.5 cm is a predictor of SAM and LVOT obstruction after mitral valve repair. This is because the mitral valve repair procedure usually includes ring annuloplasty. The implantation of the ring moves the whole mitral valve anteriorly towards the LVOT and increases the risk of SAM and LVOT obstruction.
  (d) Aorto-mitral angle in systole and diastole. The aorto-mitral angle is the angle between the mitral annular plane and the aortic annular plane. When the aorto-mitral angle is more than 120°, the risk of SAM and LVOT obstruction following repair would be low. The sharper the aorto-mitral angle, the higher the risk of SAM and LVOT obstruction following repair.
- **In 4 chamber view**:
  (a) Tenting area: This is the area between the mitral annular plane and the mitral leaflets in mid systole in the 4 chamber view (Fig. 4.3a). A tenting area of more than 2.5 cm^2 is a predictor of unsuccessful repair. This is because a large tenting area implies that the leaflets are pulled down severely by the papillary muscles which itself means the LV is severely dilated and remodelled, and if the remodelling continues after the operation the patient will develop severe MR again.

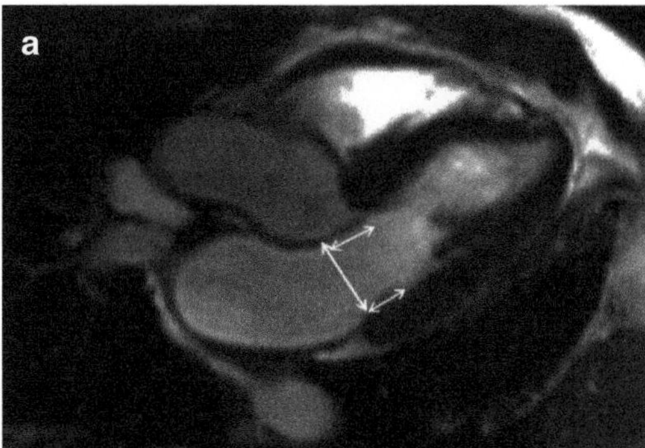

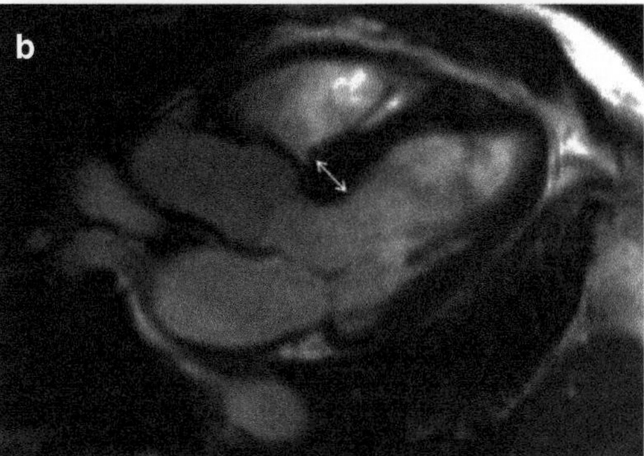

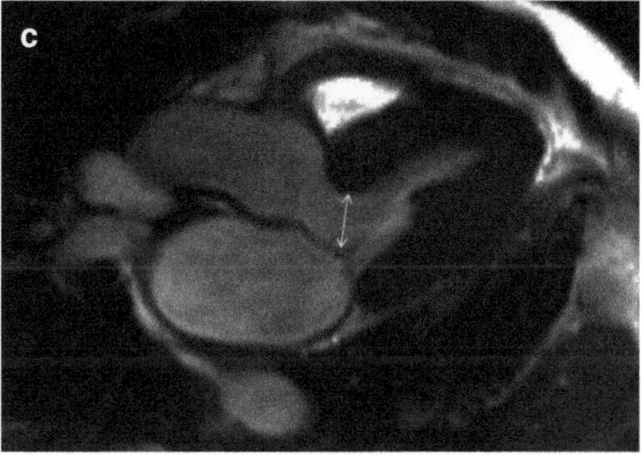

Fig. 4.2 The panels each show a frame of 3-chamber cines in which functionally relevant measurements can be made. (**a**) The lengths of the anterior and posterior leaflets of the mitral annulus and its anterior-posterior diameter. (**b**) The thickness of the basal septum at end diastole. (**c**) The shortest distance between the basal septal bulge and the coaptation point. The aorto-mitral angle, being the angle between the mitral annular plane and the aortic annular plane, can also be measured in systole and diastole. When the aorto-mitral angle is more than 120°, the risk of SAM and LVOT obstruction following repair would be low. The more acute the aorto-mitral angle, the higher the risk of SAM and LVOT obstruction following repair

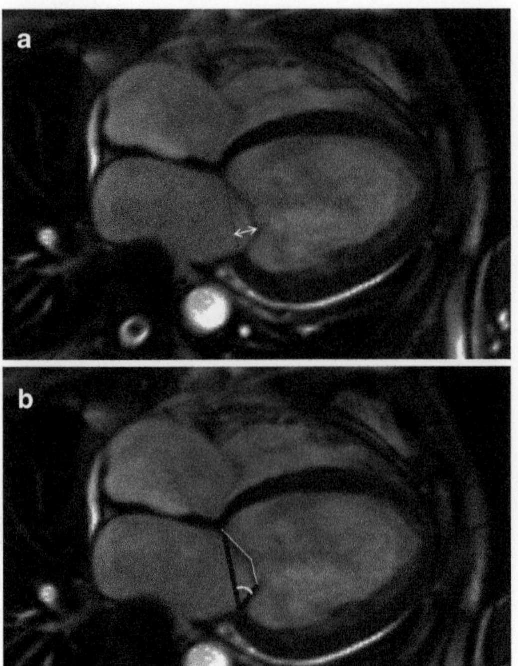

Fig. 4.3 In a four chamber view (**a**), the tenting area is the area between the mitral annular plane and the mitral leaflets in mid systole. The coaptation distance is the longest distance between the coaptation point and the mitral annular plane in systole. The posterior leaflet angle (**b**) is the angle which is the largest angle between the mitral annular plane and the posterior leaflet in mid-systole

(b) Coaptation distance: This is the longest distance between the coaptation point and the mitral annular plane in systole. A coaptation distance more than 1 cm predicts unsuccessful surgery and post-operative MR (Fig. 4.3b)

(c) Posterior leaflet angle: The posterior leaflet angle which is the largest angle between the mitral annular plane and the posterior leaflet in mid-systole is another indicator of LV remodelling and displacement of the papillary muscles. A posterior leaflet angle of more than 45° predicts unsuccessful operation (Fig. 4.3b).

– **In short axis view**:

The intercommissural diameter of the mitral annulus can be measured from the basal LV short axis view of the mitral valve (Fig. 4.4).

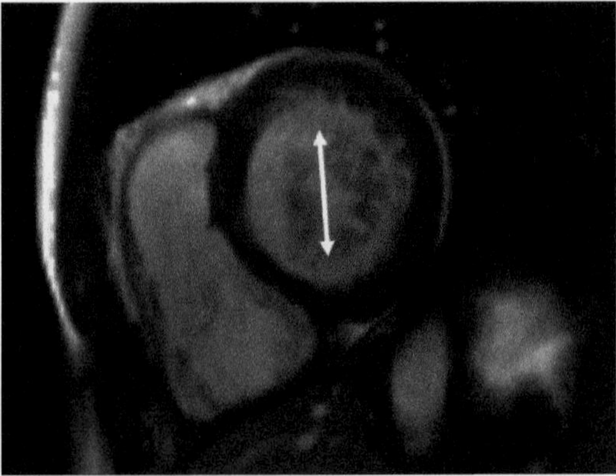

Fig. 4.4 The intercommissural diameter of the mitral annulus as measured from the basal LV short axis view of the mitral valve

There are two papillary muscles in the left ventricle: the anterolateral papillary muscle and the posteromedial papillary muscle. Both papillary muscles should be assessed for rupture, infarction, fibrotic elongation, and displacement. Due to the limited spatial resolution of MRI, chordae tendineae are usually not seen unless they are thickened.

Confirm the Presence and Mechanism of MR

The MR jet can be seen readily on the bSSFP and FLASH cine sequences.

Functional MR in DCM In functional MR secondary to DCM, both leaflets are symmetrically tethered which leads to a symmetrical tenting pattern of the mitral valve in systole (Fig. 4.3c). The same pattern can be seen in patients with ischaemic cardiomyopathy due to both anterior and inferoposterior infarction (see below). In dilated cardiomyopathy, functional MR is a consequence of:

(a) Apical displacement of the papillary muscles. This leads to tethering of both mitral leaflets towards the apex (Carpentier type IIIb).

(b) Dilatation of the mitral annulus so that the leaflets cannot reach each other to coapt in systole (Carpentier type I).

(c) Reduced contraction of the mitral annulus in systole. The normal contraction of the mitral annulus in systole (decrease in annular area in systole) is 25 % [2].
(d) Dysfunction of the LV and papillary muscles as part of the cardiomyopathic process.
(e) Dyssynchronous contraction of the papillary muscles and the left ventricle especially in the presence of left bundle branch block.

Functional MR in chronic ischaemic MR Chronic ischaemic MR is a consequence of previous myocardial infarction (MI) which has led to focal adverse remodelling of the left ventricle and the papillary muscle(s). Chronic ischaemic MR is commonly seen in one of the following patterns:

1. Following inferolateral MI: The inferoposterolateral left ventricular wall and the posteromedial papillary muscle (Carpentier type IIIb) are affected. In these patients the posterior leaflet appears tethered to the infarcted wall and the tenting pattern is asymmetrical. The MR jet is eccentric and posteriorly directed.
2. Following MI in more than one coronary territory: Chronic ischaemic MR can also be seen in ischaemic cardiomyopathy due to previous myocardial infarction in more than one coronary territory. In these patients there is global LV adverse remodelling and both papillary muscles are displaced and dysfunctional. This leads to tethering of both mitral leaflets and therefore the regurgitation jet is centrally directed.
3. It is also possible to see fibrotic elongation of an infarcted papillary muscle which will lead to prolapse of the affected mitral leaflet (Carpentier type 2).

Acute myocardial infarction can be complicated by rupture of a papillary muscle and lead to flail mitral leaflet and acute severe mitral regurgitation. This form of "acute ischaemic MR" which is a cardiac emergency is best classified under "organic MR". The affected patient is usually unwell and in pulmonary oedema and unlikely to be able to lie flat for 30–40 min for a CMR study. These patients are best assessed with echocardiography.

Quantify the Severity of MR

Similar to echocardiography, the severity of mitral regurgitation is initially assessed visually. The presence of an eccentric wall-hugging jet or the presence of a jet core indicates severe mitral regurgitation. To quantify the severity of mitral regurgitation with CMR, regurgitant volume and regurgitant fraction are calculated. The best and the most reproducible way of calculating mitral regurgitant volume (MRV) with CMR is to subtract the aortic forward stroke volume (AoSV) from LV stroke volume (LVSV), (Eq. 4.1). Care must be taken to perform these measurements meticulously. This formula can be used even in the presence of aortic regurgitation:

$$MRV(ml) = LVSV - AoSV \tag{4.1}$$

The regurgitant fraction (RF) is the ratio of the MRV divided by the LVSV multiplied by 100 (Eq. 4.2):

$$RF(\%) = \frac{MRV}{LVSV} \times 100 \tag{4.2}$$

Another way of calculating the mitral regurgitant volume is by subtracting the RV stroke volume (RVSV) from the LV stroke volume (Eq. 4.3). This is a less reliable method because RVSV is less reproducible compared to LVSV. Moreover, associated tricuspid regurgitation which often accompanies severe MR, or the presence of aortic or pulmonary regurgitation, invalidates the use of RVSV to determine MRV. Therefore, this formula can only be used in the absence of significant regurgitation in the other valves.

$$MRV(ml) = LVSV - RVSV \tag{4.3}$$

There are not yet established criteria for grading by CMR. However, regurgitant fractions (RF) calculated from CMR acquisitions have been correlated with echocardiographic grading in 83 patients with mitral regurgitation [3], although relatively few of these had more than moderate regurgitation. In the absence of established criteria for CMR, the findings of this study, derived from LV volume and ascending aortic flow measurements, can be noted: mild=RF≤15 %, moderate=RF 16–24 %, moderate-severe=RF 25–42 %, severe=RF >42 %. If the regurgitant volume is more than 60 ml, the mitral regurgitation is severe.

Assess the Left Ventricular Structure and Function

From the bSSFP cine images, the left ventricle should be assessed for its shape, size, and systolic function. Spherical remodelling of left ventricular shape, dilatation of the left ventricle with displacement of the papillary muscles, and impaired left ventricular systolic function are all important contributors to the development of functional mitral regurgitation.

(a) Left ventricular shape: The normal left ventricle has a bullet-shaped geometry. In advanced stages of dilated and ischaemic cardiomyopathies, adverse myocardial remodelling leads to spherical remodelling of the left ventricular shape and the left ventricle looks more like a balloon than a bullet. Spherical remodelling is associated with adverse outcomes and worse prognosis because a spherically remodelled left ventricle is less likely to improve in response to medical or surgical treatment. The degree of left ventricular sphericity can be assessed visually. It can also be quantified with the measurement of "sphericity index" which is the ratio of maximum cavity diameter and cavity length in systole and diastole (Eq. 4.4):

$$Sphericity\,index = LV\ diameter\ /\ LV\ length \tag{4.4}$$

The normal ranges for sphericity index are given in Table 4.1 [4]. As it can be seen from the figures, women have more spherical ventricles than men.

Table 4.1 Normal left ventricular sphericity index range in the adult

	Men	Women
Sphericity index, diastole	0.35±0.06 (0.22, 0.48)	0.4±0.07 (0.27, 0.53)
Sphericity index, systole	0.20±0.05 (0.10, 0.29)	0.23±0.068 (0.09, 0.36)

(b) Left ventricular size: left ventricular end-diastolic and end-systolic volumes are calculated from the stack of short axis cine images using a computer-aided analysis package and are indexed for body surface area.

Left ventricular internal diameters in end systole and end diastole should also be measured and reported. This is because the current guidelines for the timing of mitral valve surgery in mitral regurgitation refer to the left ventricular internal diameters rather than volumes. Also most cardiologists and cardiac surgeons are more familiar with left ventricular diameter values than left ventricular volumes. Left ventricular internal diameters should be measured from the basal short axis slice immediately basal to the tips of the papillary muscles. Alternatively, the measurements can be performed from the 3-chamber (LVOT) view similar to parasternal long axis view in echocardiography.

(c) Left ventricular function: Assessment of the left ventricular systolic function begins with visual analysis of left ventricular global and segmental function. Wall motion is described as hyperkinetic, normal, hypokinetic, akinetic, and dyskinetic.

Unlike organic severe mitral regurgitation where the left ventricle is initially hyperdynamic, in functional mitral regurgitation the left ventricular function is either regionally or globally impaired. Regional wall motion abnormalities and abnormal myocardial wall thinning in a coronary territory suggest previous myocardial infarction. Inferoposterior myocardial infarctions in the RCA or LCx territories commonly affect the posterolateral papillary muscle and lead to chronic ischaemic mitral regurgitation. In these patients, the posterior mitral leaflet appears tethered to the infarcted segment and the regurgitation jet is posteriorly directed.

Quantitative analysis of the LV systolic function is based on the measurement of the LV end-diastolic and end-systolic volumes by the computer-aided analysis package as described above. LV ejection fraction, stroke volume, and cardiac output are calculated and reported. It is of utmost importance that these measurements are performed meticulously because the calculated LV stroke volume is used to quantify mitral regurgitant volume and fraction.

Assess the Right Ventricular Structure and Function and the Tricuspid Valve

Assessment of the RV begins with visual analysis of RV structure and function.

In normal subjects, RV looks smaller than LV in the 4-chamber view. When the RV looks larger than LV, it is dilated. When the RV looks larger than LV and forms the apex of the heart, it is severely dilated.

It is important to take note of any RV hypertrophy as it can be a sign of pulmonary hypertension. RV hypertrophy is defined as RV free wall thickness >5 mm.

It is also important t to look for systolic and/or diastolic flattening of the ventricular septum. Flattening of the septum makes the LV cavity look like the letter "D". Systolic flattening of the ventricular septum is a sign of RV pressure overload e.g., due to pulmonary hypertension and in the absence of primary disease in the lungs or pulmonary vasculature, indicates significant left heart disease e.g., severe mitral regurgitation. Diastolic flattening of the ventricular septum is a sign of RV volume overload and is commonly seen in severe tricuspid regurgitation, severe pulmonary regurgitation, and severe left to right intracardiac shunt e.g., large atrial septal defect. Depending on the chronicity of the underlying pathology, the RV systolic function may be hyperdynamic, normal, or globally impaired.

Pathological regional wall motion abnormalities are not common in RV and if present are usually due to either previous myocardial infarction (right coronary artery territory) or arrhythmogenic right ventricular cardiomyopathy. Regional wall motion abnormality in the RV free wall is common around the insertion point of the moderator band and is considered to be a normal variant.

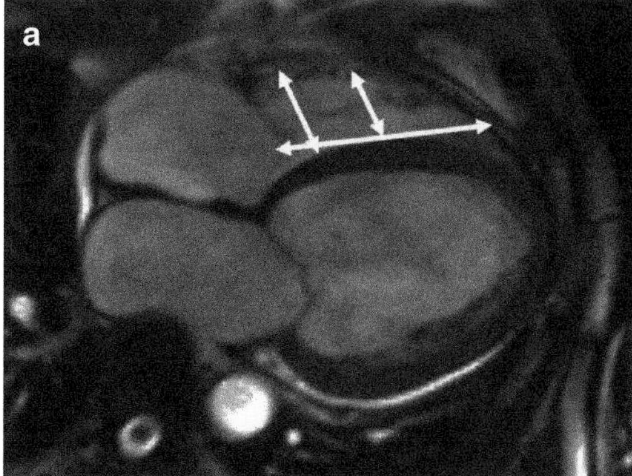

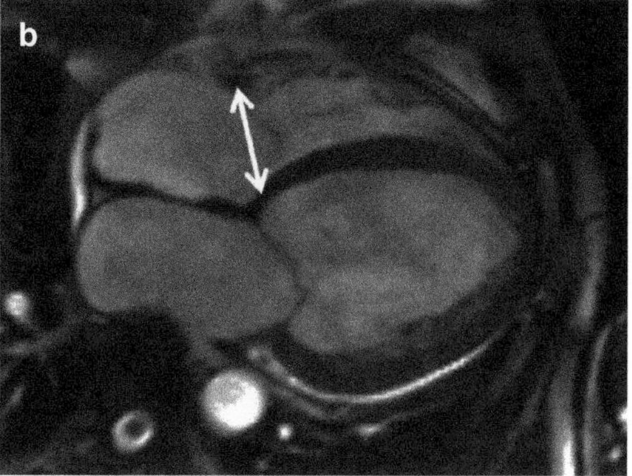

Fig. 4.5 (**a**) in a four chamber view, internal diameters of the RV (base, mid, length) can be measured, as in echocardiography. (**b**) The antero-posterior diameter of the annulus can also be measured

For the quantitative analysis of the RV size and systolic function, RV end-diastolic and end-systolic volumes, stroke volume, and ejection fraction are calculated from the stack of short axis cine images using a computer-aided analysis package. All measurements except for the ejection fraction are indexed for body surface area. RV volumes can also be measured from a transaxial stack of the heart. RV internal diameters (base, mid, length) can be measured from the 4-chamber view in a similar fashion to echocardiography (Fig. 4.5a).

Severe tricuspid regurgitation is most commonly functional and due to annular dilatation secondary to RV and/or right atrial dilatation. Severe tricuspid regurgitation can gradually make itself worse by causing RV volume overload which leads to further dilatation of RV and tricuspid annulus. It is important to report tricuspid regurgitation and assess its severity. The severity of tricuspid regurgitation can be assessed visually. It can also be quantified by subtracting the pulmonary stroke volume from RV stroke volume (Eqs. 4.5 and 4.6):

$$\text{Tricuspid regurgitant volume} = \text{RV stroke volume} - \text{pulmonary stroke volume} \quad (4.5)$$

$$\text{Tricuspid regurgitant fraction} = \frac{\text{Tricuspid regurgitant volume}}{\text{RV stroke volume}} \quad (4.6)$$

Tricuspid annulus diameter can be measured in 4-chamber view and should be mentioned in the report (Fig. 4.5b). In patients who are candidates for mitral valve surgery, most surgeons consider concomitant restrictive ring annuloplasty of the tricuspid valve if there is more than mild tricuspid regurgitation and the tricuspid annular diameter is more than 4 cm.

Look for Consequences of MR on the Left Atrium and Pulmonary Arteries

Severe MR is usually associated with dilatation of the left atrium. Severe MR can also be associated with pulmonary hypertension which manifests itself with dilatation of the pulmonary arteries on transaxial images.

Look for Significant Pathology in Aortic and Pulmonary Valves

It is important to exclude significant aortic stenosis, aortic regurgitation, and significant disease of the pulmonary valve because it may change the management plan. Both aortic and pulmonary valves should be assessed visually on the cine images of the LVOT and RVOT. If the cine images indicate pathology, the valve should be thoroughly assessed with short axis cine image of the valve to assess opening valve area (in the case of valvular stenosis) and/or coaptation failure (in the case of valvular regurgitation). Appropriate flow studies should be performed with phase contrast velocity mapping to quantify the severity of valve disease.

Assess Left Ventricular Myocardial Viability and Contractile Reserve

Myocardial fibrosis and viability is assessed using LGE studies. Assessment of myocardial viability is particularly important in patients with ischaemic MR and can affect the clinician's decision regarding revascularisation or conservative treatment. The aim of viability testing is to make a distinction between reversible and irreversible myocardial injury. If the damage to the myocardium is reversible, revascularisation can improve LV and papillary muscle function and lead to improvement in the severity of MR. Remember that in the context of LGE studies, the term "non-viable" is used to predict low likelihood of improvement in contractility following revascularisation and the so-called "non-viable" myocardial segments often have an epicardial rim of non-infarcted myocardium.

Further assessment of myocardial viability and LV contractile reserve is possible with low dose dobutamine infusion (see below). In patients with impaired left ventricular systolic function, this information helps to predict the likelihood of reverse LV remodelling after mitral valve repair.

In non-ischaemic cardiomyopathies, assessment of the pattern of myocardial fibrosis can be helpful in determining the underlying aetiology.

(a) LGE studies: The pattern and extent of LGE should be assessed. For most clinical indications, visual assessment is sufficient. The LGE pattern may be ischaemic or non-ischaemic:
  (a) Ischaemic pattern: is characterised by subendocardial hyperenhancement in a coronary artery perfusion territory. The location and extent of subendocardial scar is reported using the American Heart Association 17-segment model. Comparison of the LGE images with the corresponding cine images is recommended for correct interpretation of viability. The average transmural extent of the LGE is estimated within each myocardial segment and represents the transmural extent of the non-viable myocardium. LGE transmurality is reported as 0 %, 1–25 %, 26–50 %, 51–75 %, 76–100 %. There is an inverse relation between the transmural extent of LGE and the likelihood of improvement in contractility after revascularisation. The smaller the % thickness of LGE, the higher the likelihood of increased contractility after revascularisation (Table 4.2).
  (b) Non-ischaemic pattern: usually spares the subendocardium and is limited to the mid- wall or epicardium. If the subendocardial hyperenhancement is global, then a non-ischaemic pathology such as amyloidosis or endomyocardial fibrosis is more likely. In dilated cardiomyopathy, mid-wall fibrosis is seen in 40–50 % of patients and is more common in the ventricular septum.

(b) Contractile reserve:

The left ventricular contractile reserve can be assessed using low dose dobutamine stress at 5 and 10 mcg/kg/min.

Table 4.2 Relationships between the % LGE transmurality and the likelihood of functional recovery after revascularisation

% LGE transmurality	Likelihood of functional recovery post-revascularisation (%)
0	80
1–25	60
26–50	40
51–75	10
>75	~0

The Relative Strengths and Limitations of CMR

Among its several strengths, magnetic resonance is arguably the most versatile of the imaging modalities. This is by virtue of the control afforded at tissue level, by magnetic field gradient applications, over the interactions of radio signals with the spins of protons in relation to their surroundings. The unpaired protons of hydrogen occur mainly in the water of blood and tissues, and in fat. The radio signals that convey energy and information to and from them through the body are non-destructive and non-ionising. As long as precautions are taken to avoid the possible dangers that might be associated with metal objects or wires in the magnet, CMR is safe and non-invasive. However, the versatility, complex physics and elaborate technology of CMR mean that it is best performed in specialised units, with significant costs associated.

The large, unrestricted fields of view of CMR give relatively comprehensive access to the several structures and flow features relevant to functional MR. Of note, the mitral annulus, leaflets, chordae, papillary muscles, their insertions in the LV wall, and the tissue characteristics and mobility of the myocardial wall itself are all relevant to adequate assessment, as well as visualisation of the regurgitant jets. All these, except typically for more linear chordae, can be visualised and interrogated by CMR. However, the spatial resolution of typical acquisitions may be suboptimal. Although the pixel size (typically about

1.2×1.5 mm) can give clear images with good blood-tissue contrast, the thickness of the image slice (typically 5–8 mm for cine imaging) needs to be borne in mind, particularly when imaging thin structures such as valve leaflets or narrow jets. These can nevertheless be seen well if the imaging plane lies perpendicular to the plane or line of the structure, which then minimises the effects of partial volume averaging.

CMR allows arguably the most accurate and reproducible measurements of LV cavity volumes and stroke volume, LV mass and aortic flow, which together enable quantification of mitral regurgitation. However, such quantification is indirect and dependent on more than one type of measurement, so it is important to recognise possible sources of error.

Unfortunately, CMR image quality tends to be compromised by irregularity of heart rhythm, notably atrial fibrillation. This is because the cine images are typically acquired, with ECG triggering, over the 10–25 heartbeats of a single breath-hold. Beat-to-beat variations of structural position and flow degrade image quality, particularly of the finer structures and features. This includes any vegetations of endocarditis, which are rarely seen adequately by CMR.

The heavy equipment and magnetic field of CMR mean that it is not available for bedside or intra-operative investigation.

In conclusion, while echocardiography generally remains the favoured modality for imaging and assessing mitral valve disease, CMR has complementary strengths. Not only does it offer an alternative in patients with limited ultrasonic access, but it can also add information, particularly on ventricular volumetric assessment and myocardial tissue characterisation.

References

1. Chaikriangkrai K, Lopez-Mattei JC, Lawrie G, Ibrahim H, Quinones MA, Zoghbi W, Little SH, Shah DJ. Prognostic value of delayed enhancement cardiac magnetic resonance imaging in mitral valve repair. Ann Thorac Surg. 2014;98:1557–63.
2. Lancellotti P, Lebrun F, Piérard LA. Determinants of exercise-induced changes in mitral regurgitation in patients with coronary artery disease and left ventricular dysfunction. J Am Coll Cardiol. 2003;42:1921–8.
3. Gelfand EV, Hughes S, Hauser TH, Yeon SB, Goepfert L, Kissinger KV, Rofsky NM, Manning WJ. Severity of mitral and aortic regurgitation as assessed by cardiovascular magnetic resonance: optimizing correlation with Doppler echocardiography. J Cardiovasc Magn Reson. 2006;8:503–7.
4. Nadine Kawel-Boehm, Alicia Maceira, Emanuela R Valsangiacomo-Buechel, Jens Vogel-Claussen, Evrim B Turkbey, Rupert Williams, Sven Plein, Michael Tee, John Eng and David A Bluemke. Normal values for cardiovascular magnetic resonance in adults and children. J Cardiovasc Magn Reson. 2015;17:29.

5 Cardiac Resynchronization Therapy for Functional Ischaemic Mitral Regurgitation

Marta Sitges and Bàrbara Vidal

Abstract

Functional mitral regurgitation (MR) is a common finding in patients with heart failure (HF). It results from an imbalance between closing and tethering forces that ensure valve competence as a consequence of systolic dysfunction and altered geometry of the left ventricle (LV). In some patients, mechanical asynchrony in chamber contraction might be present and also contributes to the development of MR, either leading to diastolic MR, systolic MR or both.

Cardiac resynchronization therapy (CRT) has the potential to reverse the vicious cycle resulting in MR worsening, specifically in those patients with abnormal electrical conduction leading to disturbances in mechanical contraction. CRT leads to LV reverse remodeling and reduces morbidity and mortality, in addition to symptoms and exercise capacity improvement. CRT can effectively reduce functional MR by improving mechanical dyssynchrony in cardiac contraction, which leads to improve LV systolic and diastolic function, and also by inducing reverse LV remodeling which in turn restores the abnormal geometry of the mitral valve apparatus. There is growing evidence that CRT can be considered as a first line treatment in patients with HF and severe secondary MR who have mechanical dyssynchrony amenable to be electrically corrected with CRT.

Keywords

Functional mitral regurgitation • Cardiac resynchronization therapy • Left ventricle remodeling • Dyssynchrony • Heart failure • Pacing • Cardiomyopathy • Systolic dysfunction • Predictors • Mortality

M. Sitges, MD, PhD (✉) • B. Vidal, MD, PhD
Cardiology Department, Cardiovascular Institute,
Hospital Clinic, Institut d'Investigacions
Biomèdiques August Pi i Sunyer (IDIBAPS),
University of Barcelona, Barcelona, Spain
e-mail: msitges@clinic.ub.es

K.M.J. Chan (ed.), *Functional Mitral and Tricuspid Regurgitation*,
DOI 10.1007/978-3-319-43510-7_5

Abbreviations

CRT	Cardiac resynchronization therapy
ECG	Electrocardiogram
HF	Heart failure
LBBB	Left bundle branch block
LV	Left ventricle
LVEF	Left ventricular ejection fraction
MR	Mitral regurgitation

Principles of Treatment

Pathogenesis of functional mitral regurgitation (MR) involves multiple factors, including increased mitral leaflet tethering due to the outward displacement of the papillary muscles caused by global and regional left ventricular (LV) remodeling, decreased LV closing forces and deformation of the whole mitral apparatus including the annulus [1, 2]. In some patients with heart failure, differences in the timing of cardiac chamber or even between myocardial segments contraction, namely mechanical dyssynchrony, can contribute to the development of more insufficiency of the mitral valve. Dyssynchrony may cause the increase in functional MR in several pathways: the presence of global LV dyssynchrony may decrease the efficiency of LV contraction and thus, decrease the LV closing force acting on the mitral leaflets. Also, dyssynchronous contraction of the papillary muscle insertion sites at the LV free wall may induce geometric distortion of the mitral valve apparatus. Finally, dyssynchronous contraction of the LV basal segments may render a non-simultaneous contraction of the papillary muscles and adjacent LV walls, resulting in uneven timing of leaflet coaptation [3]. Also, the presence of atrioventricular dyssynchrony with abnormal atrioventricular coupling may lead to diastolic MR (Fig. 5.1), as well as the presence of interventricular dyssynchrony, which induces an abnormal motion of the interventricular septum, may provoke the inadequate closure of the mitral leaflets.

Improvement in papillary muscles dyssynchrony [4] together with an increase in the rate of LV pressure increase [5], which counteracts tethering forces and leads to more effective mitral valve closure with the consequent reduction of the MR orifice area, explains the immediate decrease of MR with CRT-activation [6, 7]. It has

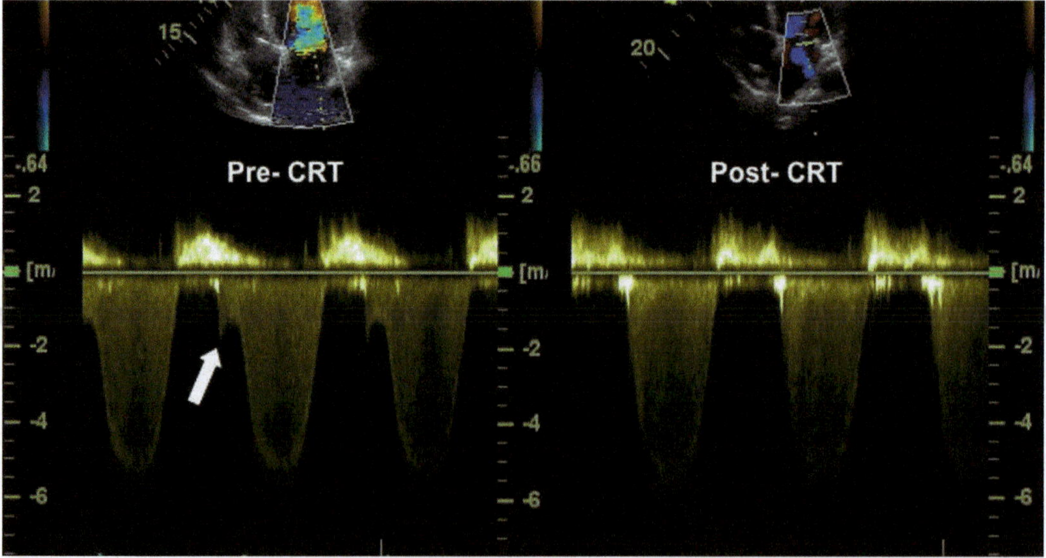

Fig. 5.1 *On the left panel*, a continuous wave Doppler signal of a mitral regurgitation with a presystolic component can be observed that disappears with the pacemaker activation as shown *on the right panel*. On the other hand, the signal intensity is reduced after CRT activation, suggesting an improvement of the regurgitation severity

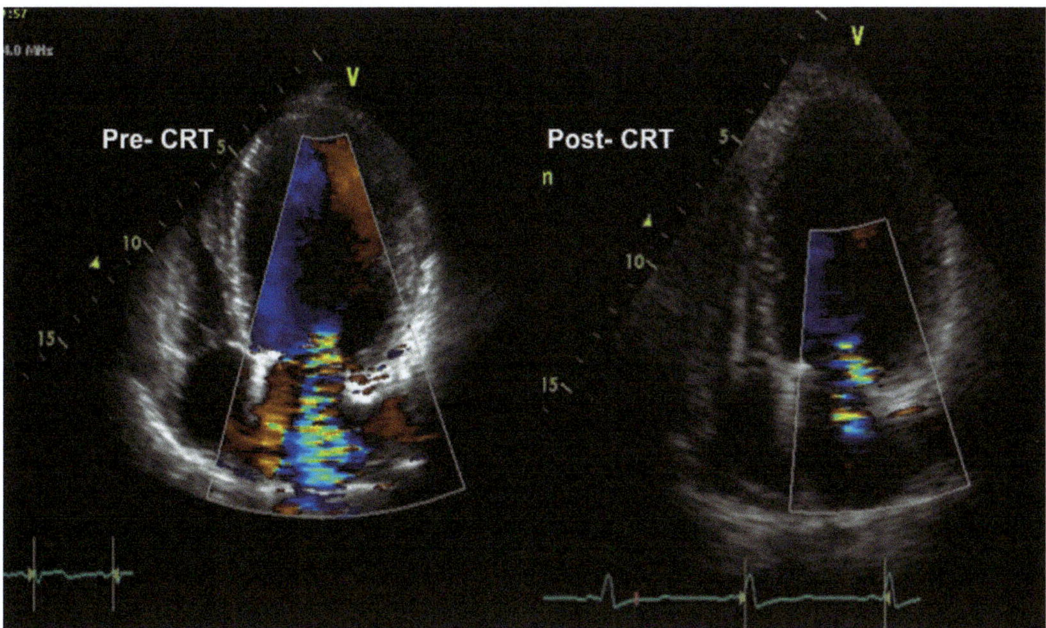

Fig. 5.2 Mitral regurgitation improvement after 6-month CRT. Reduction in the left ventricle volume can also be observed

also been observed an acute beneficial change in MV geometry after CRT in patients who would be responders in the follow-up (defined by echocardiographic criteria as a reduction in end-systolic LV volume >15 %) [5]. This acute effect on the mitral valve is pacing dependent as the interruption of CRT causes an immediate recurrence of MR [4]. Another described acute effect of CRT is the correction of the atrioventricular delay in CRT that eliminates diastolic or pre-systolic MR, when present.

In the mid-long run, the reduction of MR induced by CRT can also extend in relation to a global (LV volumes) and local (mitral valve geometry) resynchronization-related reverse remodeling [7] (Fig. 5.2).

Another factor that has to be considered in the response to CRT, including MR improvement, is the presence of myocardial viability. Traditionally, it has been accepted that patients with ischemic cardiomyopathy, large scar tissue and particularly with severe MR at baseline, present lesser LV reverse remodeling and clinical response at follow-up when treated with CRT [8]. Other studies show that ischemic patients do also respond to CRT but to a lesser extent [9]. This discrepancy between studies suggests that response to CRT is a multifactorial process and that the presence and location of myocardial viability is an important factor together with the presence of a mechanical abnormality that is amenable to be electrically corrected [10]. A direct relationship between the extent of myocardial contractile recruitment during a stress echo and the extent of LV remodeling has been shown. Also, the precise status of the myocardium at the site of the lead placement is important; in this sense some studies have shown that the coincidence of the site of the lead implantation on scar tissue is related to a poorer response to CRT [11].

Indications

According to current Guidelines [12], CRT is indicated in symptomatic HF patients in functional class II-IV despite receiving optimal medical treatment, severe left ventricle systolic dysfunction with a left ventricular ejection fraction (LVEF) ≤35 % and presenting with a wide QRS on the ECG (QRS width ≥ 120 ms) preferably with a LBBB pattern.

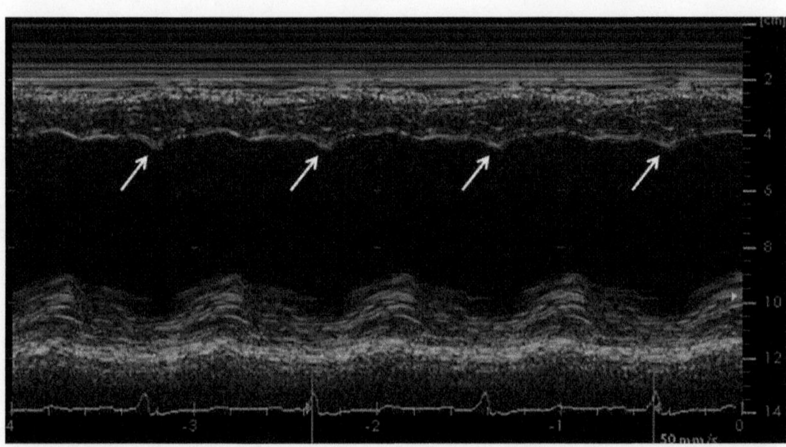

Fig. 5.3 M-mode scan across the left ventricle depicting the typical motion of the septum in patients with intraventricular dyssynchrony that correspond to the septal flash. The septal flash (*arrows*) can be detected in M-mode imaging as an early rapid contraction and relaxation of the interventricular septum. The lateral wall contraction is delayed

Use of CRT to treat functional MR without fulfilling the previous conditions is still not contemplated in the guidelines, although growing evidence exists about the benefits of CRT in reducing the severity of mitral regurgitation by at least one degree, and for this reason, the possibility to postpone surgical treatment in the CRT-responder patients. The pooled data from 5 major studies including more than 350 patients treated with biventricular pacing, followed up for more than 6 months, showed a decrease in the amount of MR by 30–40 % [13].

Identification of patients who will benefit with CRT treatment is still a matter of controversy, despite recent approaches based on understanding the mechanisms leading to cardiac dyssynchrony amenable to be electrically corrected have been proposed. Some studies [10, 14] have demonstrated that the presence of a correctable mechanical abnormality is almost mandatory to obtain a positive response with CRT. The presence of a septal flash (Fig. 5.3) is the mechanical abnormality that can be most easily corrected with CRT and most related to a clear response. Moreover, patients without any mechanical abnormality are largely non-responders. It is important to use an integral approach when assessing cardiac dyssynchrony, taking into account all kinds of possible subtypes of dyssynchrony, since all of them are potentially correctable with CRT and can lead to a substantial improvement in patient outcome. The presence of these mechanical abnormalities is an independent predictor of echocardiographic response and midterm cardiovascular mortality, along with creatinine level and LV diameters, which reflect severity and evolutive status of the disease. A correctable mechanical abnormality not only detects patients with a higher probability of reverse remodeling, but also has a real impact on survival. However, the extent of response will be variable depending on other baseline parameters such as myocardial substrate (viability), underlying disease (renal insufficiency), and clinical status [10].

Some authors have also tried to identify baseline characteristics that may point to the best candidates for CRT regarding MR reduction after CRT. In this sense a very severe MR with a baseline tenting area of >3.8 cm^2 would identify patients in whom CRT would not be effective to reduce MR, suggesting that the more advanced LV remodeling and the more distorted LV geometry, the lower the probability of effective treatment for functional MR [7] (Fig. 5.4). The fact is that response to CRT is modulated by several factors and acute and long-term benefits depend not only on the presence of LV dyssynchrony but also on the extent of residual myocardial viability in ischemic patients and severity of MR.

A less invasive percutaneous approach to treat MR in non-responder patients to CRT using the Mitraclip device has been recently proposed in order to avoid a high-risk surgery in this population of very fragile patients [15].

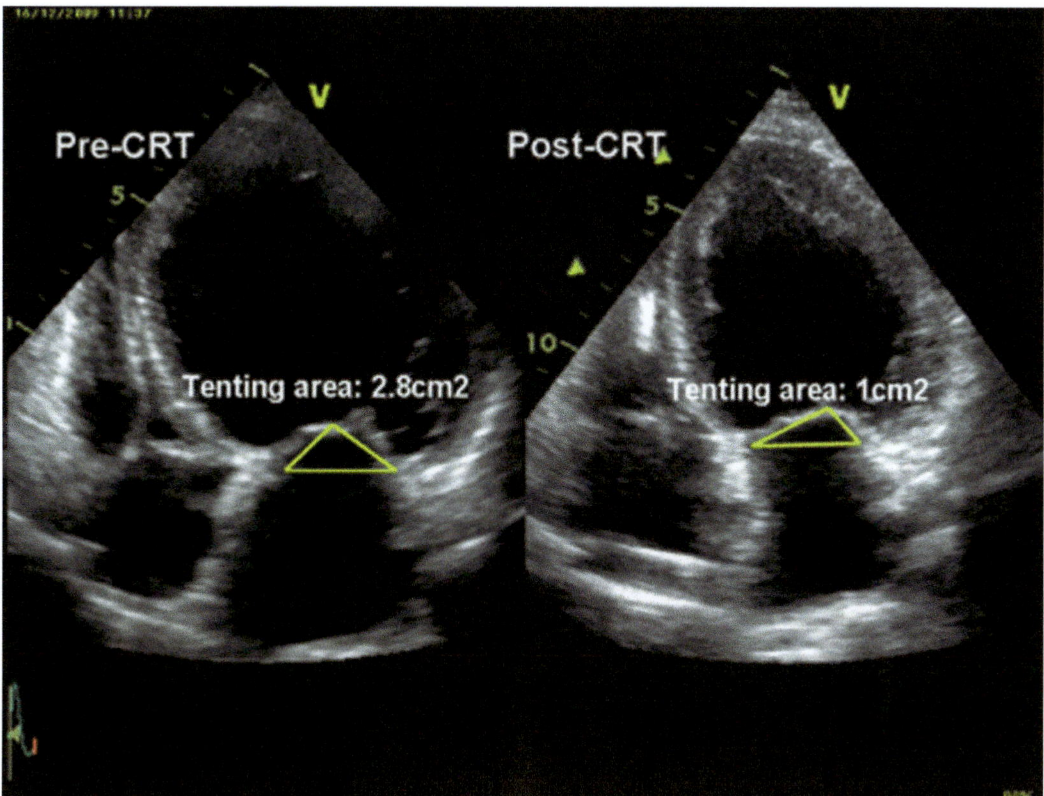

Fig. 5.4 The changes of mitral geometry together with left ventricle remodeling explain the reduction of mitral regurgitation with CRT. A baseline tenting area of >3.8 cm^2 would identify patients in whom CRT would not be effective to reduce MR

Results of Treatment

Large prospective studies have demonstrated the additional clinical benefit of CRT in HF patients medically treated with suboptimum response. CRT results in improvement in symptoms, quality of life and survival in patients with advanced heart failure and wide QRS [16, 17], especially if associated to a cardioverter - defibrillator [18, 19]. Echocardiographically, a progressive LV reverse remodelling (with even normalization of LV dimensions) is found with a reduction in LV volumes and dyssynchrony. Moreover, a significant reduction of MR severity of at least one degree is expected in around 30–40 % of the patients [4] independently of the etiology of the underlying cardiomyopathy [7]. These benefits, which are very congruent in all published studies, have helped to expand the indications of CRT, and nowadays, the tendency is to start CRT in less advanced stages of heart failure patients.

The influence of MR severity on CRT response is also conflicting. Some investigators have shown that patients with severe MR have less chance of a positive response to CRT [13, 20, 21]. Others, like from those participating in the CARE-HF study, which was a randomized trial including a large number of patients, conversely showed that patients who did not respond to CRT were likely to have less MR as compared to responders [22]. Nonetheless, the presence of severe MR at baseline is usually associated with lower response to CRT as it usually indicates a more advance stage of the disease (50 % clinical and 40 % echocardiographic response instead of 70 and 50 %) [7].

The reduction in MR severity with CRT typically occurs within the first days after starting

CRT [6] and can be expected even until the first 3-months follow-up; however, it is very unlikely to happen after that period [4]. This MR reduction behavior has two important implications: firstly, patients who present MR improvement of at least one degree at 3-months with CRT will probably continue to be CRT responders at mid-long term and no further intervention will be required. Secondly, patients who persist with severe MR at 3-months follow-up, and are candidates for surgery, do not benefit from waiting longer because no positive response is expected anymore at mid-long term and another treatment approach should be proposed, if possible.

Which Patient Should Have This Procedure

According to current Guidelines [12], CRT is indicated for patients with symptomatic heart failure in NYHA class II-IV despite receiving optimum medical treatment, with an LVEF <35 % and a wide QRS in the ECG. All these patients could benefit from CRT therapy, specially if they have not achieved the point of no return in the evolution of the heart failure syndrome: what it seems clear, is that patients presenting with too dilated ventricles, specially of an ischemic origin, too severe MR and a very severe reduction of LVEF [9] have a very low chance of improving with the therapy.

Although some discrepancies exist, the presence of a severe MR reduces the probability of clinical response to CRT, which decreases from 70 % back to 50 %. On the other hand, it is also known that around 30–40 % patients with severe MR respond to the therapy. Complementary information about the presence of dyssynchrony, viability of the LV myocardium, magnitude and transmurality of the scar and the functional etiology of MR can help us to better select the candidate patient for CRT.

Once the device is implanted, an acute benefit on MR reduction is expected. Most patients experience acute improvement confirmed echocardiographically at 3–6 months follow-up. At this point, typically no more improvement is to be expected, and if the patient persists with severe MR, surgery has to be planned. In high risk patients a less invasive approach with Mitraclip can be also proposed (Fig. 5.5).

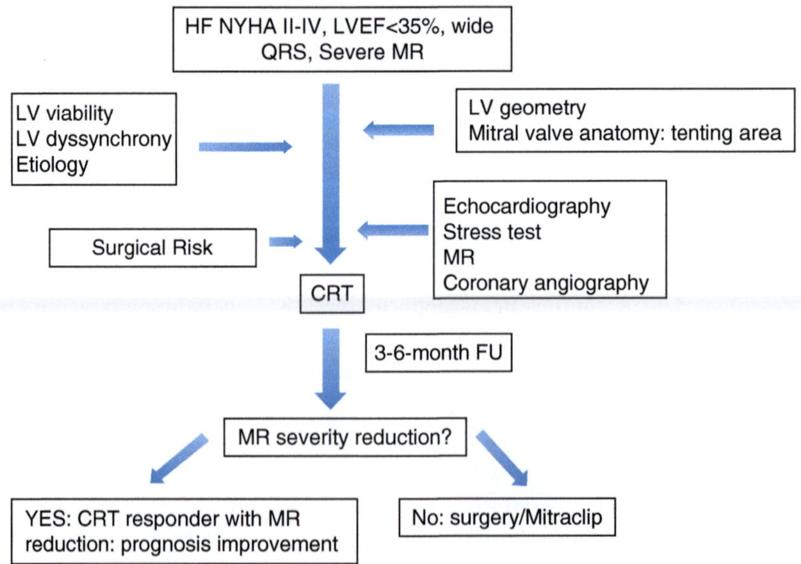

Fig. 5.5 Proposed management algorithm to select which patient should have this procedure

References

1. Levine RA, Schwammenthal E. Ischemic mitral regurgitation on the threshold of a solution: from paradoxes to unifying concepts. Circulation. 2005;112(5):745–58.
2. Otsuji Y, Handschumacher MD, Schwammenthal E, Jiang L, Song JK, Guerrero JL, Vlahakes GJ, Levine RA. Insights from three-dimensional echocardiography into the mechanism of functional mitral regurgitation: direct in vivo demonstration of altered leaflet tethering geometry. Circulation. 1997;96(6):1999–2008.
3. Liang YJ, Zhang Q, Fang F, Lee AP, Liu M, Yan BP, Lam YY, Chan GC, Yu CM. Incremental value of global systolic dyssynchrony in determining the occurrence of functional mitral regurgitation in patients with left ventricular systolic dysfunction. Eur Heart J. 2013;34(10):767–74.
4. Di Biase L, Auricchio A, Mohanty P, Bai R, Kautzner J, Pieragnoli P, Regoli F, Sorgente A, Spinucci G, Ricciardi G, Michelucci A, Perrotta L, Faletra F, Mlcochová H, Sedlacek K, Canby R, Sanchez JE, Horton R, Burkhardt JD, Moccetti T, Padeletti L, Natale A. Impact of cardiac resynchronization therapy on the severity of mitral regurgitation. Europace. 2011;13(6):829–38.
5. Solis J, McCarty D, Levine RA, Handschumacher MD, Fernandez-Friera L, Chen-Tournoux A, Mont L, Vidal B, Singh JP, Brugada J, Picard MH, Sitges M, Hung J. Mechanism of decrease in mitral regurgitation after cardiac resynchronization therapy: optimization of the force-balance relationship. Circ Cardiovasc Imaging. 2009;2(6):444–50.
6. Verhaert D, Popovic ZB, De S, Puntawangkoon C, Wolski K, Wilkoff BL, Starling RC, Tang WH, Thomas JD, Griffin BP, Grimm RA. Impact of mitral regurgitation on reverse remodeling and outcome in patients undergoing cardiac resynchronization therapy. Circ Cardiovasc Imaging. 2012;5(1):21–6.
7. Sitges M, Vidal B, Delgado V, Mont L, Garcia-Alvarez A, Tolosana JM, Castel A, Berruezo A, Azqueta M, Pare C, Brugada J. Long-term effect of cardiac resynchronization therapy on functional mitral valve regurgitation. Am J Cardiol. 2009;104(3):383–8.
8. Sutton MG, Plappert T, Hilpisch KE, Abraham WT, Hayes DL, Chinchoy E. Sustained reverse left ventricular structural remodeling with cardiac resynchronization at one year is a function of etiology: quantitative Doppler echocardiographic evidence from the Multicenter InSync Randomized Clinical Evaluation (MIRACLE). Circulation. 2006;113(2):266–72.
9. Vidal B, Sitges M, Delgado V, Mont L, Díaz-Infante E, Azqueta M, Paré C, Tolosana JM, Berruezo A, Tamborero D, Roig E, Brugada J. Influence of cardiopathy etiology on responses to cardiac resynchronization therapy. Rev Esp Cardiol. 2007;60(12):1264–71.
10. Doltra A, Bijnens B, Tolosana JM, Borràs R, Khatib M, Penela D, De Caralt TM, Castel MA, Berruezo A, Brugada J, Mont L, Sitges M. Mechanical abnormalities detected with conventional echocardiography are associated with response and midterm survival in CRT. J Am Coll Cardiol Img. 2014;7:969–79.
11. Sénéchal M, Lancellotti P, Magne J, Garceau P, Champagne J, Philippon F, O'Hara G, Moonen M, Dubois M. Impact of mitral regurgitation and myocardial viability on left ventricular reverse remodeling after cardiac resynchronization therapy in patients with ischemic cardiomyopathy. Am J Cardiol. 2010;106(1):31–7.
12. Russo AM, Stainback RF, Bailey SR, et al. ACCF/HRS/AHA/ASE/HFSA/SCAI/SCCT/SCMR 2013 appropriate use criteria for implantable cardioverter-defibrillators and cardiac resynchronization therapy: a report of the American College of Cardiology Foundation appropriate use criteria task force, Heart Rhythm Society, American Heart Association, American Society of Echocardiography, Heart Failure Society of America, Society for Cardiovascular Angiography and Interventions, Society of Cardiovascular Computed Tomography, and Society for Cardiovascular Magnetic Resonance. J Am Coll Cardiol. 2013;61:1318–68.
13. Vinereanu D. Mitral regurgitation and cardiac resynchronization therapy. Echocardiography. 2008;25(10):1155–66.
14. Parsai C, Bijnens B, Sutherland GR, Baltabaeva A, Claus P, Marciniak M, Paul V, Scheffer M, Donal E, Derumeaux G, Anderson L. Toward understanding response to cardiac resynchronization therapy: left ventricular dyssynchrony is only one of multiple mechanisms. Eur Heart J. 2009;30(8):940–9.
15. Auricchio A, Schillinger W, Meyer S, Maisano F, Hoffmann R, Ussia GP, Pedrazzini GB, van der Heyden J, Fratini S, Klersy C, Komtebedde J, Franzen O, PERMIT-CARE Investigators. Correction of mitral regurgitation in nonresponders to cardiac resynchronization therapy by MitraClip improves symptoms and promotes reverse remodeling. J Am Coll Cardiol. 2011;58(21):2183–9.
16. Abraham WT, Fisher WG, Smith AL, Delurgio DB, Leon AR, Loh E, Kocovic DZ, Packer M, Clavell AL, Hayes DL, Ellestad M, Trupp RJ, Underwood J, Pickering F, Truex C, McAtee P, Messenger J, MIRACLE Study Group, Multicenter InSync Randomized Clinical Evaluation. Cardiac resynchronization in chronic heart failure. N Engl J Med. 2002;346(24):1845–53.
17. Cleland JG, Daubert JC, Erdmann E, Freemantle N, Gras D, Kappenberger L, Tavazzi L, Cardiac Resynchronization-Heart Failure (CARE-HF) Study Investigators. The effect of cardiac resynchronization on morbidity and mortality in heart failure. N Engl J Med. 2005;352(15):1539–49.
18. Gold MR, Daubert JC, Abraham WT, Hassager C, Dinerman JL, Hudnall JH, Cerkvenik J, Linde C.

Implantable defibrillators improve survival in patients with mildly symptomatic heart failure receiving cardiac resynchronization therapy: analysis of the long-term follow-up of remodeling in systolic left ventricular dysfunction (REVERSE). Circ Arrhythm Electrophysiol. 2013;6(6):1163–8.

19. Linde C, Gold MR, Abraham WT, St John Sutton M, Ghio S, Cerkvenik J, Daubert C, REsynchronization reVErses Remodeling in Systolic left vEntricular dysfunction Study Group. Long-term impact of cardiac resynchronization therapy in mild heart failure: 5-year results from the REsynchronization reVErses Remodeling in Systolic left vEntricular dysfunction (REVERSE) study. Eur Heart J. 2013;34(33):2592–9.
20. Díaz-Infante E, Mont L, Leal J, García-Bolao I, Fernández-Lozano I, Hernández-Madrid A, Pérez-Castellano N, Sitges M, Pavón-Jiménez R, Barba J, Cavero MA, Moya JL, Pérez-Isla L, Brugada J, SCARS Investigators. Predictors of lack of response to resynchronization therapy. Am J Cardiol. 2005;95(12):1436–40.
21. Cabrera-Bueno F, García-Pinilla JM, Peña-Hernández J, Jiménez-Navarro M, Gómez-Doblas JJ, Barrera-Cordero A, Alzueta-Rodríguez J, de Teresa-Galván E. Repercussion of functional mitral regurgitation on reverse remodelling in cardiac resynchronization therapy. Europace. 2007;9(9):757–61.
22. Cleland J, Freemantle N, Ghio S, Fruhwald F, Shankar A, Marijanowski M, Verboven Y, Tavazzi L. Predicting the long-term effects of cardiac resynchronization therapy on mortality from baseline variables and the early response a report from the CARE-HF (Cardiac Resynchronization in Heart Failure) Trial. J Am Coll Cardiol. 2008;52(6):438–45.

Treatment of Functional Ischemic Mitral Regurgitation by Coronary Artery Bypass Grafting

6

Michael Sean Mulvihill and Peter K. Smith

Abstract

This chapter reviews recent developments in the treatment of ischemic mitral regurgitation. Recent and ongoing studies have added to our understanding of this dynamic disease process. We discuss current investigations on outcomes of new and established approaches, including adjunctive surgical techniques.

Keywords

Ischemic Mitral Regurgitation (IMR) • Revascularization • Mitral Valve Repair (MVR) • Coronary Artery Bypass Grafting (CABG) • Left Ventricular Reverse Remodeling

Introduction

Mitral regurgitation (MR) represents the most frequent valvular heart disease in the United States. Ischemic mitral regurgitation (IMR) is common after myocardial infarction and results in significantly increased risk for congestive heart failure and death. It is usually mild in severity and consequently may go undiagnosed [1]. While outcomes are worse with increasing IMR severity, even mild IMR portends a significantly increased risk of cardiovascular mortality. The Survival and Ventricular Enlargement (SAVE) study reported a cardiovascular mortality incidence of 29 % at 3.5 years after MI in those developing IMR, compared to 12 % in those without IMR ($P<0.001$) [2]. The dynamic nature of IMR makes assessment and treatment selection challenging.

Pathophysiology of IMR

Pathologic condition in any one or more of the components of the mitral valve apparatus may lead to mitral regurgitation; however, the mitral valve is

M.S. Mulvihill, MD
Department of General and Thoracic Surgery, Duke University School of Medicine, DUMC 3443 Duke South Room 3581, White Zone, Durham, NC 27710, USA
e-mail: mike.mulvihill@dm.duke.edu

P.K. Smith, MD (✉)
Division of Cardiovascular and Thoracic Surgery, Duke University School of Medicine, DUMC 3442, Durham, NC 27710, USA
e-mail: peter.smith@dm.duke.edu

K.M.J. Chan (ed.), *Functional Mitral and Tricuspid Regurgitation*,
DOI 10.1007/978-3-319-43510-7_6

normal in structure in most cases of IMR. The definition of ischemic (functional) mitral regurgitation by the classic Carpentier triad requires the following: (1) patient with known coronary artery disease and a global or regional wall motion abnormality; (2) echocardiographic evidence for restricted leaflet motion in systole and/or annular dilatation, and (3) valve leaflet tethering but otherwise macroscopically normal leaflets [3]. Mitral regurgitation in the ischemic and dysfunctional LV further increases atrial pressure, which may lead to both pulmonary hypertension [4] and heart failure [5].

IMR is largely due to left ventricular dysfunction and dilatation. Because chordae are non-extensible, papillary-muscle displacement exerts traction on leaflets [6]. Subsequent dilatation of the mitral annulus contributes to IMR by distracting the mitral leaflets and preventing appropriate leaflet coaptation. IMR occurs due to papillary muscle rupture in a small minority of cases. More commonly, local LV remodeling in the region of papillary muscles attachment results in displacement and thus alteration of mitral valve coaptation. Commonly, myocardial infarction involving the right or circumflex coronary arteries will result in greater displacement of the posterior compared to the anterior papillary muscle [7]. This results in greater posterior leaflet tethering. After anterior MI, apical displacement of papillary muscles may result in apical tethering of both mitral valve leaflets and central mitral regurgitation [8].

Multiple lines of evidence suggest that MR in the setting of ischemic disease is associated with poor outcome [1, 5, 9, 10]. Still disputed is whether IMR intrinsically causes poor outcome or whether IMR is a surrogate for left ventricular alterations which themselves are responsible for poor outcomes. However, the association of severe ischemic mitral regurgitation with poor outcomes independent of ejection fraction, age, and presentation all suggest that regurgitation itself is a major contributor to poor outcomes.

Treatment Options

While modest improvements have been made in recent years, rates of morbidity and mortality with intervention in IMR remain high [11, 12]. Overall suboptimal outcomes reflect uncertainty with respect to surgical indications. With transcatheter interventional treatments for mitral regurgitation primarily in the experimental phase, surgery is the treatment recommended by management guidelines [13]. The most recently published ACC/AHA guidelines for CABG and Valve Disease avoid a formal decision algorithm for the treatment of IMR and at present lag behind the best available clinical evidence. 2014 guidelines advise that a concomitant mitral valve repair procedure be considered in patients with chronic moderate secondary MR undergoing other cardiac surgery (*Level of Evidence*: *C*) [14]. In this chapter, the use of coronary artery revascularization by way of CABG alone in the treatment of ischemic mitral regurgitation will be reviewed. The decision to add a concomitant mitral valve procedure will be fully discussed in the next chapter. Most broadly, the best clinical evidence available at this time support the use of revascularization with CABG alone for the treatment of moderate ischemic mitral regurgitation. We do not recommend the routine inclusion of a concomitant mitral valve procedure to CABG for the treatment of moderate ischemic mitral regurgitation.

Coronary Artery Revascularization

Reported hospital mortality in patients with IMR undergoing CABG varies widely from 1.0 to 12.5 %, due to differences in baseline comorbidities, LV size and LV function [15–18]. While percutaneous coronary intervention (PCI) continues to be offered to some patients at high risk for conventional open CABG, this modality often fails to address the persistently occluded coronary arteries common in IMR patients. Ellis and colleagues reported a 28 % rate of complete revascularization with PCI in this population [19]. Ellis and colleagues suggest that maximally complete revascularization by CABG may offer better outcomes since most IMR patients suffer from severe multivessel coronary artery disease.

The response of IMR to coronary revascularization alone is known to be variable. Among patients with moderate IMR undergoing CABG alone, Lam and colleagues report a 22 % progression to severe IMR at 6 weeks [17]. By contrast, Tolis and colleagues report a similar population of patients undergoing CABG alone for mild-moderate IMR and show improvement at 3 year follow-up of MR grade from 1.7 to 0.5 [18]. This variation in outcome is hypothesized to relate to the completeness of revascularization, a standpoint supported by recent observational studies [20]. LV contractile reserve may also play a role, in that successful CABG will restore viable LV segments in the region of papillary muscle attachment that may relieve tethering of the mitral valve. Recent work examining cardiac remodeling has revealed no change in MR grade among patients without improvement in LV function or LV size following isolated CABG for IMR, supporting the thesis that maximal restoration of perfusion to viable myocardium is prerequisite for successful remodeling [16, 21, 22].

Five year survival in patients with moderate IMR undergoing CABG alone varies from 50 % [18] to 87 % [16] in recent observational studies. Survival after CABG in the IMR population is generally decreased compared to those patients undergoing isolated CABG without MR [17, 23, 24]. In their most recent work, Grossi and colleagues report that even mild IMR is an independent risk factor for worsening survival after CABG [24]. Examination of over 3000 patients treated at Duke University revealed a graded effect with increasing MR associated with increasing mortality after CABG [23]. These data again highlight that patients with increasing degrees of MR often present as more comorbid than patients without MR. Patients with MR had worse NYHA functional class and lower ejection fraction. These patients were more likely to suffer from renal insufficiency, and were more likely to have had an intra-aortic balloon pump (IABP) in place preoperatively. These factors have made appropriate risk stratification and propensity analysis challenging in determining the best course of therapy. Fortunately, recent prospective work has sought to clarify treatment strategies for this patient population.

Revascularization with CABG Alone for Ischemic MR

In patients with moderate IMR, there has been considerable controversy with respect to the appropriate course of therapy. In particular, the decision to perform a valve procedure in addition to revascularization with CABG has been the subject of much debate. The benefit of concomitant mitral valve intervention has hinged on an assessment of the extent to which revascularization alone can adequately improve valvular function. Proponents of CABG alone note that revascularization can promote left ventricular remodeling, leading to a decreased LV chamber size, restored functional integrity of the subchordal mitral valve apparatus, and thereby decreasing mitral regurgitation. Importantly, the kinetics and rate of remodeling remain to be fully elucidated. This is of particular importance in the evaluation of short-term outcomes following CABG, as near-term evaluation may not fully capture the benefit of coronary artery bypass surgery. Those who favor combined CABG and mitral intervention note that isolated CABG in the presence of scar and non-viable myocardium may not result in remodeling after revascularization, therefore necessitating mitral intervention as regurgitation will not improve despite revascularization. Recently, both updated observational studies and prospective clinical trial data have clarified the risks and benefits of each strategy in this patient population.

Castleberry et al. retrospectively reviewed patients at a single institution carrying a diagnosis of coronary artery disease and moderate or severe mitral regurgitation from 1990 to 2009 [25]. A total of 4989 patients were stratified by medical therapy alone, PCI, CABG, or CABG with concomitant mitral valve repair or replacement. After a median follow up period of 5.37 years, lower mortality was observed in patients treated with revascularization (by PCI, CABG, or CABG plus mitral valve repair or replacement) in comparison to medical therapy. Patients treated with CABG alone demonstrated the lowest risk of death.

Three prospective clinical trials now corroborate many of the findings first identified in

Table 6.1 Prospective studies comparing isolated CABG and CABG+MVR for the treatment of moderate ischemic mitral regurgitation

Study	Fattouch et al.		Chan et al. (RIME)		Smith et al. (CTSN)	
Years	2003–2007		2007–2011		2009–2013	
Treatment arm	Isolated CABG	CABG+MVR	Isolated CABG	CABG+MVR	Isolated CABG	CABG+MVR
Subjects	54	48	39	34	151	150
Primary endpoints	NYHA class II or greater		Change in peak oxygen consumption at 1 year		LVESI (mL/m^2) at 1 year	
	43.70 %	15.5 %*	0.8±2.9	3.3±2.3**	46.1±22.4	49.6±31.5
<u>One year outcomes</u>						
Mortality (%)	1.9 %	4.2 %	5.0 %	9.0 %	7.3 %	6.7 %
Stroke (%)					1.3 %	4.0 %
Heart failure readmission			8.0 %	3.0 %	13.2 %	14.7 %
NYHA class III or IV			15.0 %	4.0 %	10.3 %	7.9 %

CABG coronary artery bypass graft, *MVR* mitral valve repair, *MR* mitral regurgitation, *LVESVI* left ventricular end-systolic volume index, *NYHA* New York Heart Association Class of Heart Failure
*P<0.01; **P<0.001

the retrospective databases (Table 6.1). The first to publish (in 2009), Fattouch et al. reported a single center Italian study of 102 patients of which 48 underwent CABG with concomitant MVR, while 54 underwent CABG alone [26]. Primary endpoints were NYHA functional class to assess clinical status, and assessment of extent of reversal of left ventricular remodeling by way of echocardiographic assessment (TTE) of left ventricular end-systolic diameter (LVESD), left ventricular end-diastolic diameter (LVEDD) and ejection fraction. At 1 year, addition of MVR to CABG resulted in lower NYHA functional class (15.5 % of patients undergoing CABG with MVR vs. 43.7 % of patients undergoing CABG alone experiencing NYHA class II or greater symptoms). CABG-alone patients experienced higher rates of post-operative MR and had no significant change in LVESD or LVEDD at the conclusion of the study, while CABG with MVR patients exhibited reversal of left-ventricular remodeling as evidenced by a decrease in both LVESD and LVEDD. Subjects had no difference in ejection fraction nor survival, though the study was underpowered for the detection of survival differences.

The 2012 Randomized Ischemic Mitral Evaluation (RIME) trial randomized a total of 73 patients in the United Kingdom and Poland with moderate MR by echocardiography to isolated CABG vs CABG with concomitant MVR [27]. The study was concluded after 73 patients of a planned 100 after the primary endpoint – peak oxygen consumption – was reached after 1 year. Peak oxygen consumption has previously been recognized as a clinically-relevant measure of functional capacity. Patients undergoing CABG+MVR had a 22 % increase in peak oxygen consumption at 1-year compared to a 5 % increase in patients undergoing isolated CABG. Patients undergoing CABG+MVR had a median NYHA functional class of I, compared to median class of II in the isolated CABG group at the conclusion of the follow up period. The RIME study did not identify any difference in overall survival between the treatment arms, though again a small sample size and short duration of follow up limit the scope of long-term conclusions. Overall, the RIME study supported the addition of a mitral intervention in addition to revascularization with CABG.

Most recently, Smith et al. have reported the results of the largest trial to date designed to ascertain if the potential benefits of a combined CABG and mitral procedure outweigh the increased risks of the added intervention [28]. The Cardiothoracic Surgical Trials Network randomly assigned 301 patients across multiple centers with moderate ischemic mitral regurgitation as determined by transthoracic echocardiography to CABG alone or CABG plus mitral-valve repair (combined procedure). The primary end point was the left ventricular end-systolic volume index (LVESVI). At 1 year, significant reductions in the LVESVI were observed in both arms of the trial, but the addition of a mitral-valve repair to CABG did not result in a higher degree of left ventricular reverse remodeling. 69 % of patients in the CABG-alone group had no mitral regurgitation or mild regurgitation at 1 year, as compared with 89 % of patients in the combined procedure group. These findings suggest that revascularization alleviates reversible ischemia in both groups. Clinical outcomes at 1 year, including functional status, quality of life, mortality, need for mitral-valve reoperation, and major adverse cardiac or cerebrovascular events did not differ significantly between groups. The combined-procedure group did experience a higher rate of serious neurologic events and had a higher rate of supraventricular arrhythmias, likely related to the atriotomy mandated by the mitral valve procedure. Given that the addition of a mitral-valve repair to CABG did not result in a higher degree of left ventricular remodeling, but did lead to an increased number of untoward events, the trial did not show a clinically meaningful advantage of adding mitral repair to CABG.

The results of these three studies are in conflict. Taken together in recent meta-analysis, the addition of MVR to CABG in patients with moderate ischemic mitral regurgitation does reduce residual MR grade in short-term outcomes, but does so with a simultaneous increase in morbidity and does not offer improvement in mortality or other clinically-meaningful metrics. The opposing outcomes reached by these trials may reflect differences in the end points assessed, the methods of classifying mitral regurgitation, and baseline characteristics such as rates of prior myocardial infarction and duration of mitral regurgitation from initial diagnosis to trial enrollment. While there may well exist a patient population with moderate ischemic mitral regurgitation that will optimally benefit from CABG with concomitant mitral valve procedure in terms of survival, functional status, or symptoms, this patient population has not yet been conclusively identified in the literature. At present, a concomitant mitral valve procedure should not be routinely added to CABG for the treatment of moderate ischemic mitral regurgitation. Longer-term analyses of these trials will be of great value and will yield further insight into the long-term impact of revascularization in IMR. In particular, further assessment of the degree to which CABG can yield both long-term reversal of ventricular remodeling and improvement in clinical outcomes will be of extreme importance. Taken together, the best available evidence to date supports isolated CABG in the short term for the treatment of moderate ischemic mitral regurgitation. These data should be considered in the context of the individual patient who is evaluated for the treatment of ischemic mitral regurgitation in order to best identify an appropriately risk-stratified and individualized treatment plan.

References

1. Lamas GA, Mitchell G, Flaker GC, et al. Clinical significance of mitral regurgitation after acute myocardial infarction. Circulation. 1997;96:827–33.
2. Aronson D, Goldsher N, Zukermann R, et al. Ischemic mitral regurgitation and risk of heart failure after myocardial infarction. Arch Intern Med. 2006;166:2362–8.
3. Carpentier A. Cardiac valve surgery—the "French correction". J Thorac Cardiovasc Surg. 1983;86:323–37.
4. LA Pierard LP. The role of ischemic mitral regurgitation in the pathogenesis of acute pulmonary edema. N Engl J Med. 2004;351:1627–34.
5. Grigioni F, Detaint D, Avierinos J, Scott C, Tajik J, Enriquez-Sarano M. Contribution of ischemic mitral regurgitation to congestive heart failure after myocardial infarction. J Am Coll Cardiol. 2005;45(2):260–7.
6. Hung J, Guerrero J, Handschumacher MD, Supple G, et al. Reverse ventricular remodeling reduces ischemic mitral regurgitation: echo-guided device application in the beating heart. Circulation. 2002;106:2594–600.
7. Kaji S, Nasu M, Yamamuro A, et al. Annular geometry in patients with chronic ischemic mitral regurgitation. Three-dimensional magnetic resonance imaging study. Circulation. 2005;112(Suppl I):I-409–14.

8. Yu H-Y, Su M-Y, Liao T-Y, et al. Functional mitral regurgitation in chronic ischemic coronary artery disease: analysis of geometric alterations of mitral apparatus with magnetic resonance imaging. J Thorac Cardiovasc Surg. 2004;128:543–51.
9. Bursi F, Enriquez-Sarano M, Nkomo VT, Jacobsen SJ, Weston SA, Meverden RA, Roger VL. Heart failure and death after myocardial infarction in the community: the emerging role of mitral regurgitation. Circulation. 2005;111:295–301.
10. Lancellotti P, Troisfontaines P, Toussaint AC, Pierard LA. Prognostic importance of exercise-induced changes in mitral regurgitation in patients with chronic ischemic left ventricular dysfunction. Circulation. 2003;108:1713–17.
11. Grossi EA, Bizekis C, LaPietra A, et al. Late results of isolated mitral annuloplasty for "functional" ischemic mitral insufficiency. J Card Surg. 2001;16:328–32.
12. Johnston DR, Gillinov A, Blackstone EH, Griffin B, Stewart W, Sabik 3rd JF, Mihaljevic T, Svensson LG, Houghtaling PL, Lytle BW. Surgical repair of posterior mitral valve prolapse: implications for guidelines and percutaneous repair. Ann Thorac Surg. 2010; 89(5):1385–94.
13. Bonow RO, Carabello B, Chatterjee K, et al. ACC/AHA 2006 guidelines for the management of patients with valvular heart disease: a report of the American College of Cardiology/American Heart Association Task Force on Practice Guidelines (Writing Committee to Revise the 1998 Guidelines for the Management of Patients With Valvular Heart Disease) developed in collaboration with the Society of Cardiovascular Anesthesiologists endorsed by the Society for Cardiovascular Angiography and Interventions and the Society of Thoracic Surgeons. J Am Coll Cardiol. 2006;48:1–148.
14. Nishimura RA, Otto CM, Bonow RO, Carabello BA, Erwin 3rd JP, Guyton RA, O'Gara PT, Ruiz CE, Skubas NJ, Sorajja P, Sundt 3rd TM, Thomas JD. 2014 AHA/ACC guideline for the management of patients with valvular heart disease: a report of the American College of Cardiology/American Heart Association Task Force on Practice Guidelines. J Thorac Cardiovasc Surg. 2014;148(1):e1–e132.
15. Aklog L, Filsoufi F, Flores KQ, Chen RH, Cohn LH, Nathan NS, Byrne JG, Adams DH. Does coronary artery bypass grafting alone correct moderate ischemic mitral regurgitation? Circulation. 2001;104(90001):I-68–75. doi:10.1161/hc37t1.094706.
16. Kang DH, et al. Mitral valve repair versus revascularization alone in the treatment of ischemic mitral regurgitation. Circulation. 2006;114(1 Suppl):I499–503.
17. Lam B-K, Gillinov A, Blackstone EH, et al. Importance of moderate ischemic mitral regurgitation. Ann Thorac Surg. 2005;79:462–70.
18. Tolis GA, Korkolis D, Kopf GS, et al. Revascularization alone (without mitral valve repair) suffices in patients with advanced ischemic cardiomyopathy and mild-moderate mitral regurgitation. Ann Thorac Surg. 2002;74:1476–81.
19. Ellis SG, Whitlow P, Raymond RE, Schneider JP. Impact of mitral regurgitation on long-term survival after percutaneous coronary intervention. Am J Cardiol. 2002;89:315–18.
20. Campwala SZ, Bansal R, Wang N, et al. Mitral regurgitation progression following isolated coronary artery bypass surgery: frequency, risk factors, and potential prevention strategies. Eur J Cardiothorac Surg. 2006;29:348.
21. Buja P, Tarantini G, Bianco FD, et al. Moderate-to severe ischemic mitral regurgitation and multivessel coronary artery disease: impact of different treatment on survival and rehospitalization. Int J Cardiol. 2006;111:26–33.
22. Jones RH, Velazquez E, Michler RE, et al. Coronary bypass surgery with or without surgical ventricular reconstruction. N Engl J Med. 2009;360(17):1705–17.
23. Schroder JN, Williams M, Hata JA, et al. Impact of mitral valve regurgitation evaluated by intraoperative transesophageal echocardiography on long-term outcomes after coronary artery bypass grafting. Circulation. 2005;112(9_suppl):I-293–8. doi:10.1161/circulationaha.104.523472.
24. Grossi EA, Crooke G, Di Giorgi PL, et al. Impact of moderate functional mitral insufficiency in patients undergoing surgical revascularization. Circulation. 2006;114:I573.
25. Castleberry AW, Williams JB, Daneshmand MA, Honeycutt E, Shaw LK, Samad Z, Lopes RD, Alexander JH, Mathew JP, Velazquez EJ, Milano CA, Smith PK. Surgical revascularization is associated with maximal survival in patients with ischemic mitral regurgitation: a 20-year experience. Circulation. 2014;129(24):2547–56. doi:10.1161/CIRCULATIONAHA.113.005223.
26. Fattouch K, Guccione F, Sampognaro R, Panzarella G, Corrado E, Navarra E, Calvaruso D, Ruvolo G. POINT: efficacy of adding mitral valve restrictive annuloplasty to coronary artery bypass grafting in patients with moderate ischemic mitral valve regurgitation: a randomized trial. J Thorac Cardiovasc Surg. 2009;138(2):278–85.
27. Chan KM, Punjabi PP, Flather M, Wage R, Symmonds K, Roussin I, Rahman-Haley S, Pennell DJ, Kilner PJ, Dreyfus GD, Pepper JR. Coronary artery bypass surgery with or without mitral valve annuloplasty in moderate functional ischemic mitral regurgitation: final results of the Randomized Ischemic Mitral Evaluation (RIME) trial. Circulation. 2012;126(21): 2502–10.
28. Smith PK, Puskas JD, Ascheim DD, Voisine P, Gelijns AC, Moskowitz AJ, Hung JW, Parides MK, Ailawadi G, Perrault LP, Acker MA, Argenziano M, Thourani V, Gammie JS, Miller MA, Pagé P, Overbey JR, Bagiella E, Dagenais F, Blackstone EH, Kron IL, Goldstein DJ, Rose EA, Moquete EG, Jeffries N, Gardner TJ, O'Gara PT, Alexander JH, Michler RE. Surgical treatment of moderate ischemic mitral regurgitation. N Engl J Med. 2014;371(23):2178–88. doi:10.1056/NEJMoa1410490.

Treatment of Functional Ischemic Mitral Regurgitation by Mitral Valve Repair and Coronary Artery Bypass Grafting

7

K.M. John Chan and John R. Pepper

Abstract

Functional ischemic mitral regurgitation is most commonly repaired by mitral annuloplasty. Important surgical principles must be followed when repairing ischaemic mitral valves by annuloplasty to ensure a durable long term repair. When these principles are followed, a durable, long term repair is achievable. Recent randomized controlled trials have given insights into the groups of patients who would benefit most from concomitant mitral annuloplasty and coronary artery bypass graft surgery. Risk factors for recurrent mitral regurgitation following mitral annuloplasty have been identified; these patients may require additional adjunctive repair procedures or a mitral valve replacement.

Keywords

Functional ischemic mitral regurgitation • Mitral annuloplasty • Mitral valve repair • Coronary artery bypass graft surgery • Functional capacity

Principles of Treatment

The aim of mitral valve repair for mitral regurgitation is to restore the surface of coaptation of the two mitral valve leaflets, thereby, making the valve competent. In functional ischaemic mitral regurgitation, the mitral valve leaflets are normal in structure. The normal mitral valve leaflets are pulled apart, either as a result of a dilated mitral annulus or left ventricle, or due to tethering consequent upon poor contraction of the left ventricle in the region where the papillary muscles attach [1–3]. The surface of coaptation can be restored by reducing the size of the mitral

K.M.J. Chan, BM BS, MSc, PhD, FRCS CTh (✉)
Department of Cardiothoracic Surgery,
Gleneagles Hospital, Jalan Ampang,
Kuala Lumpur 50450, Malaysia
e-mail: kmjohnchan@yahoo.com

J.R. Pepper, MChir, FRCS
Department of Cardiothoracic Surgery,
Royal Brompton Hospital, Sydney Street,
London SW3 6NP, UK
e-mail: J.Pepper@rbht.nhs.uk

K.M.J. Chan (ed.), *Functional Mitral and Tricuspid Regurgitation*,
DOI 10.1007/978-3-319-43510-7_7

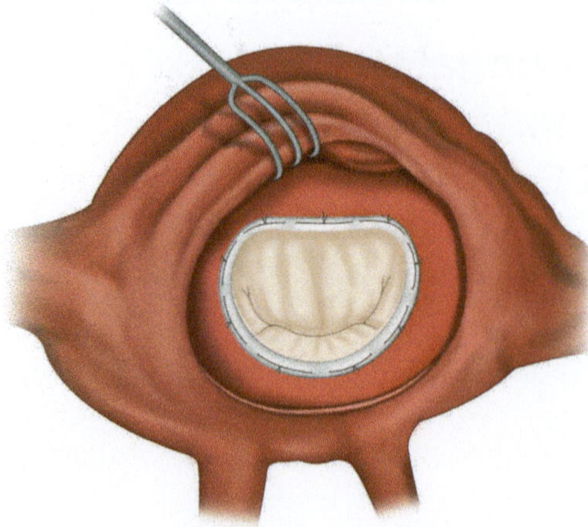

Fig. 7.1 Mitral annuloplasty. The size and shape of the annuloplasty ring restores normal mitral annular size and geometry resulting in improved mitral leaflet coaptation and competence (Adapted from Chan et al. [4]. With permission from Elsevier)

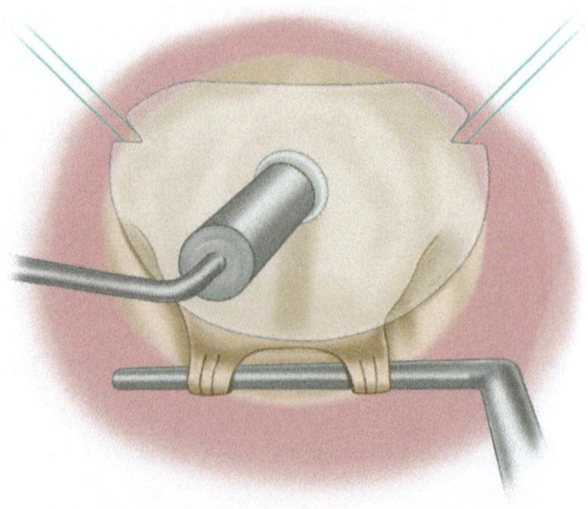

Fig. 7.2 Sizing the annuloplasty ring. The annuloplasty ring is sized by measurement of the distance between the fibrous trigones and the size of the anterior mitral valve leaflet (Adapted from Chan et al. [4]. With permission from Elsevier)

annulus, especially in the septolateral dimension. This can be achieved by implanting a ring onto the mitral annulus (mitral annuloplasty) (Fig. 7.1). The annuloplasty ring is sized by measurement of the inter-trigonal distance at the anterior mitral annulus and also the height of the anterior mitral valve leaflet (Fig. 7.2). Typically, the ring is downsized, i.e., a ring two sizes smaller than that measured is used [5, 6]. Such downsizing reduces the septolateral dilatation of the mitral annulus and, hence, increases leaflet coaptation. Newer rings have been designed specifically for functional ischaemic mitral regurgitation, which reduce the septolateral dimension, particularly in the medial part of the posterior annulus and do not require downsizing [7]. A complete rigid or semi-rigid ring is generally recommended in functional ischaemic mitral regurgitation as a higher incidence of recurrent mitral regurgitation has been reported with the use of flexible rings or bands [5, 6].

Good long-term results following undersized mitral annuloplasty for functional ischaemic mitral regurgitation have been associated with: (i) complete coronary artery revascularisation, (ii) use of a complete rigid or semi-rigid ring, (iii) achieving a surface of mitral leaflet coaptation of 8 mm or greater, and (iii) leaving minimal residual mitral regurgitation [5, 8]. Braun et al., for example, reported that at 5 years following mitral annuloplasty combined with CABG in patients with functional ischaemic mitral regurgitation, mean mitral regurgitation grade improved from 3.1 ± 0.6 to 0.8 ± 0.7 ($p < 0.001$) [5, 9]. 84 % had less than moderate mitral regurgitation, 14.6 % had moderate mitral regurgitation, and 1.4 % had moderate-severe mitral regurgitation at 5 years. The mitral leaflet coaptation length was maintained at 8 mm.

However, significant recurrence of mitral regurgitation has been reported in several studies following mitral annuloplasty [10–16]. This has been associated with the following factors:

(i) *Flexible rings or bands* [6, 11, 13–17]. The mitral annulus is dilated both at the anterior annulus and the posterior annulus in functional ischaemic mitral regurgitation with the greatest increase being in the septolateral diameter [1, 3, 18, 19]. The use of a complete rigid or semi-rigid ring, rather than a flexible ring or band, may, therefore, be important to restore mitral annular size and geometry. Moreover, continued left ventricular remodelling has been associated with recurrent mitral regurgitation and the use of a complete rigid or semi-rigid ring may be important to overcome this [12, 20].

(ii) *Failure to undersize* [11–15]. The use of an undersized ring has been recommended to decrease the septolateral dilatation present in functional ischaemic mitral regurgitation and, hence, increase the surface of mitral leaflet coaptation. Studies which have reported good results in functional ischaemic mitral regurgitation have generally used this approach [5, 8].

(iii) *Failure to achieve an adequate surface of mitral leaflet coaptation.* It has been reported that a mitral leaflet coaptation length of at least 8 mm is important to ensure long-term durability of the repair [8, 9].

(iv) *Incomplete coronary artery revascularisation.* The primary cause of functional ischaemic mitral regurgitation is left ventricular dysfunction and dilatation secondary to myocardial ischemia or infarction. Complete coronary artery revascularisation, particularly of viable ischaemic left ventricular segments is, therefore, important to restore left ventricular contractility [21]. Progression of mitral regurgitation has been reported following incomplete coronary artery revascularisation [22].

(v) *Leaving greater than trace mitral regurgitation* [13, 23]. The presence of greater than trace mitral regurgitation at the end of the operation may mean greater severity of the mitral regurgitation during physical activity and, hence, continued left ventricular volume overload and impairment of left ventricular reverse remodelling [24, 25].

(vi) *Excessive dilatation of the left ventricle.* Greater recurrence of mitral regurgitation has been reported with significantly dilated left ventricles (e.g., left ventricular end systolic diameter greater than 51 mm or left ventricular end diastolic diameter greater than 65 mm) [5, 9, 26]. In such patients, it has been suggested that undersized mitral annuloplasty should be combined with additional surgical procedures on the left ventricle such as left ventricular restoration surgery [27], left ventricular infarct plication [28] or external left ventricular constraining devices such as the Coapsys [29].

(vii) *Excessive leaflet tethering.* There are some reports that excessive leaflet tethering is a risk factor for the development of significant recurrent mitral regurgitation (tethering distance greater than 1.1 cm, tethering area greater than 1.6 cm^2) [30, 31]. Such cases may benefit from additional surgical adjuncts to mitral annuloplasty such as papillary muscle relocation [32], papillary muscle sling [33], and secondary chordal cutting [34]. These techniques are discussed in separate chapters. Long-term results of these techniques are currently awaited.

Surgical Operative Technique

Intra-operative trans-oesophageal echocardiographic assessment of the mitral valve is essential to confirm the findings of the pre-operative transthoracic echocardiography. This is usually performed after the induction of general anaesthesia and before the commencement of cardiopulmonary bypass. It is important to ensure that there is no associated structural valve lesions as other etiologies of mitral regurgitation can co-exist with functional ischaemic mitral regurgitation.

As in all mitral valve surgery, optimal setup is very important in ischaemic mitral valve surgery to maximise exposure and visualisation of the mitral valve. This is particularly so in functional ischaemic mitral regurgitation as the left atrium is typically not very enlarged, unlike in degenerative or rheumatic mitral regurgitation. To maximize exposure of the mitral valve, the pericardium should be lifted up on the right side and left free on the left side. This has the effect of rotating the heart upwards and towards the left, bringing the mitral valve into view when the left atrium is opened. A Cosgrove mitral retractor is used. Further visualisation of the mitral valve is enabled by incising the pericardium on top of the superior vena cava (SVC) and perpendicular to it; this allows retraction of the heart upwards when the retractors are placed [35].

The aorta, SVC and IVC are cannulated. An antegrade cardioplegia and a retrograde cardioplegia cannula are inserted. Tapes may be passed around the SVC and IVC. Cardiopulmonary bypass is commenced. A cross clamp is applied. Cardioplegia is delivered antegradely to start with and then every 20 min retrogradely while suction is applied to the aortic root. The venous cannulation lines are placed over on the left side supported by the mitral retractor.

The mitral valve can be approached either through a left atriotomy or a right atriotomy via a trans-septal approach. With a left atriotomy approach, the fat within Sondergaard's grove is dissected with diathermy so as to approach the left atrium more medially and nearer to the mitral valve. Alternatively, an incision is made midway between the inter-atrial septum and the origin of the right superior pulmonary vein, and extended inferiorly along the left atrium towards the left inferior pulmonary vein, ending a few mm inferior to it. The incision is then extended superiorly a few mm beyond the end of the right superior pulmonary vein onto the roof of the left atrium. One or two small mitral retractors are then inserted and lifted up together and towards the left side, opening up the left atrium and exposing the mitral valve. To improve visualisation of the mitral valve further, the incision can be extended superiorly and medially, underneath the SVC and onto the roof of the left atrium [35].

A systematic analysis of the mitral valve is performed. The mitral valve is first inspected. Note is made of any excessive leaflet tissue, leaflet perforations, ruptured chordae or ruptured papillary muscles. The lesion is then determined using a pair of nerve hooks. A reference point, such as P1 or the commissures, is chosen. Each part of the mitral valve leaflet is lifted up in turn and compared to the reference point to determine if there is leaflet prolapse or restriction. Leaflet restriction in functional ischaemic mitral regurgitation is typically difficult to assess in the arrested flaccid heart and is often not apparent. It is important to ensure that there are no associated lesions as these would need to be addressed.

In the absence of any other lesions, an undersized mitral annuloplasty is performed. The mitral annulus is first sized by pulling on the marginal chordae supporting the anterior leaflet with two nerve hooks or a right angled clamp. The ring sizer is then placed over the unfurled anterior leaflet and a sizer is chosen which matches the surface area of the anterior leaflet. If the leaflet restriction is asymmetric and mainly in the P3 area as identified by echocardiography, the Carpentier-McCarthy-Adams IMR ETlogix Annuloplasty Ring (Edwards LifeSciences) is a suitable ring. A ring of the same size as the sizer is used as this ring is already downsized in the P2-P3 area. However, if the leaflet restriction is more symmetrical, as in a more global dilatation of the LV, a symmetrical complete rigid or semi-rigid ring, such as the Carpentier-Edwards Physio or Classic Rings (Edwards LifeSciences), or equivalent, are used, downsized by 2 sizes. For example, if the annulus is sized as 30 mm, a 26 mm ring is used. Undersizing of the annuloplasty ring compensates for the loss of mitral annular function in functional ischaemic mitral regurgitation as discussed in Chap. 2 and increases the coaptation surface area between the anterior and posterior leaflets.

Interrupted non-pledgeted 2/0 ethibond horizontal mattress sutures are placed around the mitral annulus. Unlike in degenerative and rheumatic mitral regurgitation where under-sizing of the annuloplasty ring is not used, the use of an undersized annuloplasty ring in functional ischaemic mitral regurgitation results in increased tension in the annuloplasty ring and care must therefore be taken to ensure that adequate sutures are placed around the mitral annulus, and which are of sufficient length and depth, to avoid ring dehiscence. The sutures can be overlapped if necessary to provide added strength. If the IMR ring is used, this is broader in the P3 region to permit a double row of sutures to be placed. However, care must be taken when using this ring to ensure that the annuloplasty suture positioned at the middle of the P2 scallop is placed in the middle of this ring posteriorly so as not to distort the mitral annulus.

The competency of the mitral valve is tested by injecting water or saline through the valve into the left ventricle. The mitral valve should be able to hold a reasonable pressure of water with no more than trace mitral regurgitation. The final test of the repair is performed using transoesophageal echocardiography when the patient is off cardiopulmonary bypass with a systolic blood pressure above 100 mmHg. There should be no more than trace mitral regurgitation. The left atrium is closed by a single continuous layer of 4/0 polypropylene starting at either end of the incision.

Results of Treatment

Hospital Mortality

The hospital mortality of patients with functional ischaemic mitral regurgitation undergoing mitral annuloplasty combined with CABG in recent series varies from 1.5 to 21 % and may be related to differences in the baseline characteristics of the patients [5, 7, 8, 10, 11, 13, 15, 16, 20, 23, 36–41]. In one study which reported an operative mortality of 21 %, 93 % of patients either had a myocardial infarction within 2 weeks or had unstable angina requiring intravenous heparin and nitrates [10]. Higher operative mortality is also reported for patients with a poor left ventricular ejection fraction (less than 30–40 %) [23, 36–38, 40]. The hospital mortality in the 3 most recent randomised controlled trials of functional ischemic mitral regurgitation was less than 3 % [41–43].

Left Ventricular Reverse Remodelling

Observational studies have long reported significant left ventricular reverse remodelling, improvement in cardiac function and NYHA functional class following concomitant CABG plus mitral valve annuloplasty in functional ischaemic mitral regurgitation. However, most of these studies did not have a control group of patients who only had CABG and so it was not possible to determine how much of these improvements could be attributed to the mitral valve repair and how much was a result of successful coronary artery revascularisation. These findings have now been confirmed in several randomised controlled trials which have recently reported (Table 7.1) [41–43].

Table 7.1 Comparison of left ventricular end systolic volume index (LVESVI) and mitral regurgitation (MR) severity at follow-up in the RIME Trial and the CTSN ischemic mitral regurgitation trials

	LVESVI (ml/m^2)[a]	MR≥2+ (%)
RIME Trial – 1 year results		
CABG	67.4 (−6 %)	50
CABG+MV repair	56.2 (−28 %)	4
p-value	0.002	<0.001
CTSN Moderate MR Trial – 1 year results		
CABG	46.1 (−17 %)	30
CABG+MV repair	49.6 (−16 %)	11
p-value	NS	<0.001
CTSN Severe MR Trial – 1 year results		
CABG+MV repair	54.6 (−11 %)	33
CABG+MV replacement	60.7 (−10 %)	2
p-value	0.18	<0.001
CABG+MV repair (if no recurrent MR)	47.3 (−22 %)	0
CABG+MV repair (if recurrent MR)	64.1 (+5 %)	100
CTSN Severe MR Trial – 2 year results		
CABG+MV repair	52.6 (−15 %)	59
CABG+MV replacement	60.6 (−10 %)	4
p-value	0.19	<0.001
CABG+MV repair (if no recurrent MR)	42.7 (−31 %)[b]	0
CABG+MV repair (if recurrent MR)	62.6 (+2 %)	100

[a]Numbers in parenthesis represent percentage change in LV volumes from baseline
[b]P<0.001 if compared to CABG+MV replacement group

Mean regression of left ventricular volumes and dimensions by up to 28 % have been reported 1–2 years following CABG combined with mitral annuloplasty, provided a durable mitral valve repair is achieved [8, 36, 41, 42]. The reduction in left ventricular volumes appears to be dependent on the success of eliminating the mitral regurgitation. In the Randomised Ischemic Mitral Evaluation (RIME) Trial, left ventricular end systolic volumes decreased by 28 % at 1 year following CABG plus mitral annuloplasty compared to a reduction in 6% in those undergoing isolated CABG [41]. Of note, the freedom from moderate or more mitral regurgitation at 1 year following CABG plus mitral annuloplasty in this study was 96% compared to 50% in those undergoing isolated CABG. Greater reductions in left ventricular dimensions following combined CABG plus mitral valve annuloplasty compared to isolated CABG were also reported in an Italian randomised controlled trial [44]. In the Cardiothoracic Surgical Network (CTSN) moderate ischemic mitral regurgitation trial, left ventricular volumes decreased by 16% at 1 year following CABG plus mitral annuloplasty compared to 17% in those undergoing isolated CABG. The freedom from moderate or more mitral regurgitation following combined CABG plus mitral annuloplasty in this trial was 89% compared to 70% in those undergoing isolated CABG [42]. In the CTSN severe ischemic mitral regurgitation trial, left ventricular volumes decreased by only 11% at 1 year following CABG plus mitral annuloplasty. However, the freedom from moderate or more mitral regurgitation in this trial was only 67% [43]. Of note, in patients who had no recurrent mitral regurgitation at 1 year in this study, left ventricular volumes decreased by 22%, a result similar to that reported in the RIME Trial [41, 43]. Similar results at 2 years were recently reported by the CTSN severe ischemic mitral regurgitation trial. Left ventricular volumes decreased by 15% 2 years after CABG plus mitral valve repair; the freedom from moderate or more mitral regurgitation was only 41%. However, in those with no recurrent mitral regurgitation, left ventricular volumes decreased by 31% at 2 years, as compared to an increase of 2% in those with recurrent mitral regurgitation [45]. A consistent finding in these randomised studies is that significant left ventricular reverse remodelling can be expected if a successful and durable mitral valve repair is achieved at the time of CABG (Table 7.1). However, left ventricular reverse remodelling will not occur if recurrent or persistent mitral regurgitation is present.

The extent of left ventricular reverse remodelling is also dependent on the baseline size of the left ventricle. Bax et al., for example, reported that left ventricular end systolic diameters decreased from 51±10 mm to 43±12 mm ($p<0.001$) 2 years after CABG combined with mitral annuloplasty [8]. Regression of left ventricular size was greater in those in whom the left ventricle was less dilated pre-operatively. Braun et al. reported that a left ventricular end systolic diameter less than 51 mm and a left ventricular end diastolic diameter less than 65 mm were predictive of increased reverse remodelling [5].

Improvement in cardiac function by up to 10% has also been reported following successful mitral annuloplasty combined with CABG. Bonacchi et al. reported an improvement in cardiac index from 2.2±0.4 l/min/m^2 to 2.5±0.3 l/min/m^2 ($p=0.001$) following mitral annuloplasty combined with CABG [40].

Functional Status

An improvement in functional status can be expected if a successful and durable mitral valve repair has been achieved at the time of CABG. In the RIME Trial, peak oxygen consumption, an objective marker of functional capacity, improved by 22% in the CABG plus mitral annuloplasty group compared to a 5% improvement in the isolated CABG group [41]. The median NYHA class was class I in the combined CABG plus mitral annuloplasty group compared to class II in the isolated CABG group ($p=0.03$). Similar results were reported from a randomised trial from Italy where patients who had combined CABG plus mitral annuloplasty had a better NYHA functional class at 3 years [44]. A significant improvement in NYHA class following combined CABG plus mitral annuloplasty was also reported in the CTSN moderate ischemic mitral regurgitation trial although in this trial, a similar improvement was also reported in the isolated CABG group [42]. Similarly, the CTSN severe ischemic mitral regurgitation trial reported significant improvement in NYHA class and quality of life scores 2 years following either mitral valve repair or mitral valve replacement, with the greatest improvement reported in those who did not have recurrent mitral regurgitation [45].

A recent randomised controlled trial from a single Italian centre of 102 patients with moderate functional ischaemic mitral regurgitation who were randomised to either CABG only or concomitant CABG plus mitral annuloplasty reported no difference in survival between the two groups at 3 years (88.8 % ± 3.2 % versus 93.7 % ± 3.1 %) although patients who had concomitant CABG plus mitral valve annuloplasty had a better NYHA functional class (1.6 ± 0.6 versus 0.6 ± 0.8, p < 0.001) and better left ventricular reverse remodelling (LVESD 42 ± 8 mm versus 37 ± 5 mm, p < 0.01) [44].

These findings have also been reported in earlier observational studies with several studies reporting that the majority of patients in NYHA class III and IV pre-operatively were in NYHA class I and II at 1–5 years [8, 16, 20, 36]. Bax et al., for example, reported that NYHA class improved from 3.4 ± 0.8 to 1.3 ± 0.4 (p < 0.01) 2 years after CABG plus mitral annuloplasty with all patients in NYHA class I or II [8].

Survival

In observational studies, the actuarial survival for patients with functional ischaemic mitral regurgitation undergoing mitral annuloplasty combined with CABG is 75–86 % and 60–88 % at 2 years and 5 years respectively. This may be related to the baseline characteristics of the patients and the successful treatment of the mitral regurgitation [5, 8, 16, 20, 37, 40]. The recent CTSN severe ischaemic mitral regurgitation trial reported a 2-year survival of 81 % in the mitral valve repair group and 76.8 % in the mitral valve replacement group [45]. 1-year survival in patients with moderate functional ischaemic mitral regurgitation receiving combined CABG plus mitral valve annuloplasty was 95 % in the RIME Trial and 93 % in the CTSN moderate ischaemic mitral regurgitation trial; 3 year survival was 94 % in an Italian randomised controlled trial [44]. Following isolated CABG in patients with moderate functional ischemic mitral regurgitation, 1-year survival was 94 % in the RIME Trial and 93 % in the CTSN moderate ischaemic mitral regurgitation trial; 3-year survival was 89 % in an Italian randomised trial [41, 42, 44]. It must be emphasised that none of the randomised trials are adequately powered to detect differences in survival in the different randomised groups.

Despite the worse survival of patients with functional ischaemic mitral regurgitation undergoing isolated CABG, it is unclear if performing mitral annuloplasty in addition to CABG improves survival. Observational studies in fact suggest that although mitral valve annuloplasty combined with CABG may reduce the severity of functional ischaemic mitral regurgitation, survival may not actually be improved [46, 47]. Mihaljevic, et al., for example, reported a propensity matched study of 390 patients with severe functional ischaemic mitral regurgitation, 100 of whom underwent CABG only and 290 underwent concomitant CABG plus mitral valve annuloplasty [47]. At a mean follow-up of 5 years, no difference was observed between the two groups in survival (75 % versus 74 %) or NYHA functional class (25 % in NYHA class III/IV versus 23 %). Patients who had concomitant CABG plus mitral valve annuloplasty had lesser degrees of mitral regurgitation at 1 year compared to those who had CABG only (12 % 3–4 + MR versus 48 %, p < 0.001). Complete echocardiographic data was, however, not available at late follow-up but the authors estimate up to 20 % of those who had concomitant CABG plus mitral annuloplasty may have developed significant mitral regurgitation compared to about 50 % in those who underwent CABG only. A meta-analysis of nine non-randomized observational studies involving 2479 patients with severe functional ischaemic mitral regurgitation who underwent either CABG alone or concomitant CABG plus mitral valve annuloplasty reported no difference in late survival between the groups although patients who underwent concomitant CABG plus mitral valve annuloplasty had less residual mitral regurgitation [46].

Durability of Mitral Valve Annuloplasty

The long term durability of mitral valve annuloplasty for functional ischaemic mitral regurgitation has long been a concern with several observational studies reporting a high rate of significant recurrent mitral regurgitation. Mihaljevic, for example, estimates a recurrence rate of up to 20 % at 5 years [47]. A criticism of this study, however, is that there was no standard downsizing of the annuloplasty, and only in 22 % of cases was a rigid complete annuloplasty ring used; a partial flexible band was used in 71 % of cases and suture plication was used in 7 %.

As discussed earlier, several important principles are necessary to help ensure the long term durability of mitral annuloplasty for functional ischaemic mitral regurgitation. These include the use of a complete rigid or semi-rigid annuloplasty ring and not a flexible ring or band, undersizing the annuloplasty ring, achieving an adequate surface of mitral leaflet coaptation of at least 8 mm between the anterior and posterior leaflets, complete coronary artery revascularisation, and ensuring no more than trace mitral regurgitation at the end of the operation [5, 8, 12, 20]. Following these principles, Braun and Dion reported a mean mitral regurgitant grade of 0.8±0.7 at 4 years with 85 % of patients having less than 2+ mitral regurgitation [9]. However, 16 % of survivors had moderate or more mitral regurgitation. Gelsomino et al. reported that 5 years after mitral annuloplasty and CABG, 28 % of patients had moderate mitral regurgitation, 31 % had moderate-severe mitral regurgitation, and 13 % had severe mitral regurgitation [48]. The recurrence of mitral regurgitation developed in most patients after 3 years. Of note, in this study, a complete annuloplasty ring was used, a rigid Classic ring in 52.9 % and a semi-rigid Physio ring in 47.1 %, and there was standard down-sizing of the annuloplasty ring by two sizes. Predictors of recurrent mitral regurgitation in this study was a dilated ventricle (left ventricular end-systolic volume greater than 45 ml), a more spherical left ventricle (sphericity index greater than 0.7), and poorer left ventricular function (left ventricular wall motion score index greater than 1.5). A criticism of this study was that the mean number of coronary artery bypass grafts performed was only 2.2 and it is possible that the patients were under revascularised allowing continued adverse left ventricular remodelling and left ventricular dilatation.

The concern over the long-term durability of mitral annuloplasty for functional ischaemic mitral regurgitation has added to the controversy over the optimal treatment for this condition, particularly if the mitral regurgitation is only of moderate severity. Proponents for concomitant mitral annuloplasty and CABG argue that uncorrected moderate mitral regurgitation will progress and worsen, and will have a significant impact on the ability of the left ventricle to recover and reverse remodel. However, opponents of this strategy argue that if significant numbers of patients are going to develop recurrent moderate or more mitral regurgitation even with mitral annuloplasty, the benefits of this strategy is questionable and needs to be balanced against the slightly increased operative risk of adding mitral annuloplasty to CABG [49].

Which Patient Should Have This Procedure

When deciding on which patient would benefit from combined CABG plus mitral annuloplasty, as compared to isolated CABG only, or mitral annuloplasty plus adjunctive subvalvular repair techniques, or a mitral valve replacement, several factors have to be taken into consideration. These include the severity of the mitral regurgitation, the degree of mitral leaflet tethering, the extent of left ventricular viability, and the size of the left ventricle.

Patients with mild-to-moderate ischemic mitral regurgitation, particularly if the left ventricle is fully viable, do very well with isolated CABG and do not need a concomitant mitral annuloplasty. This has been demonstrated in the CTSN moderate ischemic mitral regurgitation trial where 70 % of patients improved their mitral regurgitation severity with just isolated CABG [42]. When compared to those who had concomitant CABG plus mitral annuloplasty, no differences in left ventricular reverse remodelling were observed. Although left ventricular viability was not assessed in this trial, it is likely that most of the patients had fully viable myocardium as seen by the improvement in mitral regurgitation severity and left ventricular volumes with CABG alone. If large areas of non-viable myocardium are present, concomitant mitral annuloplasty should be considered.

If the mitral regurgitation is more severe with an effective regurgitation orifice area (ERO) between 20 and 40 mm^2, and particularly if there are significant segments of non-viable myocardium, a mitral annuloplasty should be performed in addition to CABG. This has been demonstrated in the RIME Trial which recruited patients with moderate-severe functional ischaemic mitral regurgitation, 75 % of whom had non-viable scarred myocardium. Although the RIME Trial was set up as a trial to assess the best treatment for moderate functional ischaemic mitral regurgitation, a change in the threshold of severity for functional ischemic mitral regurgitation in the guidelines, meant that patients recruited into the RIME Trial can be considered as having moderate-severe functional ischaemic mitral regurgitation according to current guidelines [50]. These patients do much better with a concomitant CABG plus mitral annuloplasty compared to CABG alone, with improvements in functional capacity, symptoms and left ventricular reverse remodelling [41]. Mitral annuloplasty in these patients also have a very good result with a 96 % freedom from moderate or more mitral regurgitation at 1 year. Longer follow-up is obviously needed to ensure that the benefits reported are sustained in the longer term.

In the group of patients with even more severe ischemic mitral regurgitation (ERO greater than 40 mm^2), and particularly if the left ventricle is also very dilated (left ventricular end diastolic diameter greater than 65 mm) with severe leaflet tethering (tethering distance greater than 10 mm), mitral annuloplasty does not appear to give very satisfactory results [9, 45]. This has been demonstrated in the CTSN severe ischemic mitral regurgitation trial where the freedom from moderate or more mitral regurgitation at 2 years was only 41 % [45]. In these patients, additional adjunctive procedures on the subvalvular apparatus should be considered if mitral annuloplasty is to be used, or alternatively, a mitral valve replacement should be considered.

References

1. Kaji S, Nasu M, Yamamuro A, Tanabe K. Annular geometry in patients with chronic ischemic mitral regurgitation. Three dimensional magnetic resonance imaging study. Circulation. 2005;112:I-409–14.
2. Yu H-Y, Su M-Y, Liao T-Y, Peng H-H. Functional mitral regurgitation in chronic ischemic coronary artery disease: analysis of geometric alterations of mitral apparatus with magnetic resonance imaging. J Thorac Cardiovasc Surg. 2004;128:543–51.
3. Ahmad RM, Gillinov M, McCarthy PM, Blackstone EH. Annular geometry and motion in human ischemic mitral regurgitation: novel assessment with three-dimensional echocardiography and computer reconstruction. Ann Thorac Surg. 2004;78:2063–8.
4. Chan KMJ, Amirak E, Zakkar M, Flather M, Pepper JR, Punjabi PP. Ischemic mitral regurgitation: in search of the best treatment for a common condition. Prog Cardiovasc Dis. 2009;51:460–71.
5. Braun J, Bax JJ, Versteegh MIM, Voigt PG. Pre-operative left ventricular dimensions predict reverse remodelling following restrictive mitral annuloplasty in ischemic mitral regurgitation. Eur J Cardiothorac Surg. 2005;27:847–53.
6. Spoor MT, Geltz A, Bolling SF. Flexible versus non-flexible mitral valve rings for congestive heart failure: differential durability of repair. Circulation. 2006;114(1 Suppl):I67–71.
7. Daimon M, Fukuda S, Adams D, McCarthy PM. Mitral valve repair with Carpentier-McCarthy-Adams IMR ETlogix annuloplasty ring for ischemic mitral regurgitation: early echocardiographic results from a multi-center study. Circulation. 2006;114:I588.
8. Bax J, Braun J, Somer S, Klautz R, Holman E. Restrictive annuloplasty and coronary revascularization in ischemic mitral regurgitation results in reverse left ventricular remodelling. Circulation. 2004;110:II-103–8.
9. Braun J, van de Veire NR, Klautz RJM, Versteegh MIM, Holman ER, Westenberg JM, Boersma E, van der Wall EE, Bax JJ, Dion RAE. Restrictive mitral annuloplasty cures ischemic mitral regurgitation and heart failure. Ann Thorac Surg. 2008;85:430–7.
10. Harris KM, Sundt TM, Aeppli D, Sharma T. Can late survival of patients with moderate ischemic mitral regurgitation be impacted by intervention on the valve? Ann Thorac Surg. 2002;74:1468–75.
11. Tahta SA, Oury JH, Maxwell JM, Hiro SP, Duran CMG. Outcome after mitral valve repair for functional ischemic mitral regurgitation. J Heart Valve Dis. 2002;11:11.
12. Hung J, Papakostas L, Tahta SA, Hardy BG. Mechanism of recurrent ischemic mitral regurgitation after annuloplasty. Continued LV remodelling as a moving target. Circulation. 2004;110:II-85–90.
13. Bhudia SK, McCarthy PM, Smedira NG, Lam B-K, Rajeswaran J, Blackstone EH. Edge-to-edge (Alfieri)

mitral repair: results in diverse clinical settings. Ann Thorac Surg. 2004;77:1598–606.

14. McGee EC, Gillinov AM, Blackstone EH, Rajeswaran J, Cohen G. Recurrent mitral regurgitation after annuloplasty for functional ischemic mitral regurgitation. J Thorac Cardiovasc Surg. 2004;128:916–24.
15. Al-Radi OO, Austin PC, Tu JV, David TE, Yau TM. Mitral repair versus replacement for ischemic mitral regurgitation. Ann Thorac Surg. 2005;79:1260–7.
16. Calafiore AM, Di Mauro M, Gallina S, Giammarco GD. Mitral valve surgery for chronic ischemic mitral regurgitation. Ann Thorac Surg. 2004;77:1989–97.
17. Czer LSC, Maurer G, Bolger AF, De Robertis M, Chaux A, Matloff JM. Revascularization alone or combined with suture annuloplasty for ischemic mitral regurgitation: evaluation by color doppler echocardiography. Tex Heart Inst J. 1996;23:270–8.
18. Hueb AC, Jatene FB, Moreira LFP, Pomerantzeff PM. Ventricular remodelling and mitral valve modifications in dilated cardiomyopathy: new insights from anatomic study. J Thorac Cardiovasc Surg. 2002;124.
19. Timek TA, Lai DT, Tibayan F, Liang D. Ischemia in three left ventricular regions: insights into the pathogenesis of acute ischemic mitral regurgitaiton. J Thorac Cardiovasc Surg. 2003;125:559–69.
20. Kang DH, Kim M-J, Kang S-J, Song J-M. Mitral valve repair versus revascularization alone in the treatment of ischemic mitral regurgitation. Circulation. 2006;114:I499.
21. Bax JJ, Visser FC, Poldermans D, Elhendy A. Time course of functional recovery of stunned and hibernating segments after surgical revascularisation. Circulation. 2001;104:I-314–8.
22. Campwala SZ, Bansal RC, Wang N, Razzouk A, Pai RG. Mitral regurgitation progression following isolated coronary artery bypass surgery: frequency, risk factors, and potential prevention strategies. Eur J Cardiothorac Surg. 2006;29:348.
23. Hausmann H, Siniawski H, Hertzer R. Mitral valve reconstruction and replacement for ischemic mitral insufficiency: seven years follow up. J Heart Valve Dis. 1999;8:536–42.
24. Giga V, Ostojic M, Vujisic-Tesic B, Djordjevic-Dikic A. Exercise-induced changes in mitral regurgitation in patients with prior myocardial infarction and left ventricular dysfunction: relation to mitral deformation and left ventricular function and shape. Eur Heart J. 2005;26:1860–5.
25. Lancellotti P, Lebrun F, Pierard LA. Determinants of exercise-induced changes in mitral regurgitation in patients with coronary artery disease and left ventricular dysfunction. J Am Coll Cardiol. 2003;42:1921–8.
26. Ueno T, Sakata R, Iguro Y, Yamamoto H, Ueno M, Ueno T, Matsumoto K. Pre-operative advanced left ventricular remodelling predisposes to recurrence of ischemic mitral regurgitation with less remodelling. J Heart Valve Dis. 2008;17:36–41.
27. Menicanti L, Donato MD, Castelvecchio S, Santambrogio C. Functional ischemic mitral regurgitation in anterior ventricular remodelling: results of surgical ventricular restoration with and without mitral repair. Heart Fail Rev. 2005;9:317–27.
28. Ramadan R, Al-Attar N, Mohammadi S. Left ventricular infarct plication restores mitral function in chronic ischemic mitral regurgitation. J Thorac Cardiovasc Surg. 2005;129:440–2.
29. Mishra YK, Mittal S, Jaguri P, Trehan N. Coapsys mitral annuloplasty for chronic functional ischemic mitral regurgitation: 1-year results. Ann Thorac Surg. 2006;81:42.
30. Kongsaerepong V. Echocardiographic predictors of successful versus unsuccessful mitral valve repair in ischemic mitral regurgitation. Am J Cardiol. 2006; 98:504.
31. Gelsomino S, Lorusso R, Caciolli S, Capecchi I, Rostagno C, Chioccioli M, De Cicco G, Bille G, Stefano P, Gensini GF. Insights on left ventricular and valvular mechanisms of recurrent ischemic mitral regurgitation after restrictive annuloplasty and coronary artery bypass grafting. J Thorac Cardiovasc Surg. 2008;136:507–18.
32. Kron IL, Green GR, Cope JT. Surgical relocation of the posterior papillary muscle in chronic ischemic mitral regurgitation. Ann Thorac Surg. 2002;74: 600–1.
33. Hvass U, Tapia M, Baron F, Pouzet B. Papillary muscle sling: a new functional approach to mitral repair in patients with ischemic left ventricular dysfunction and functional mitral regurgitation. Ann Thorac Surg. 2003;75:809–11.
34. Messas E, Pouzet B, Touchot B, et al. Efficacy of chordal cutting to relieve chronic persistent ischemic mitral regurgitation. Circulation. 2003;108:111–5.
35. Punjabi PP, Chan KMJ. Mitral valve surgery. In: Punjabi PP, editor. Essentials of operative cardiac surgery. Cham: Springer International Publishing; 2015.
36. Vaskelyte J, Stoskute N, Ereminiene E, Zaliunas R, Benetis R. The impact of unrepaired versus repaired mitral regurgitation on functional status of patients with ischemic cardiomyopathy at one year after coronary artery bypass grafting. J Heart Valve Dis. 2006;15:747.
37. Serri K, Bouchard D, Demers P, Coutu M, Pellerin M. Is a good perioperative echocardiographic result predictive of durability in ischemic mitral valve repair? [see comment]. J Thorac Cardiovasc Surg. 2006;131:565.
38. Filsoufi F, Aklog L, Byrne JG, Cohn LH, Adams DH. Current results of combined coronary artery bypass grafting and mitral annuloplasty in patients with moderate ischemic mitral regurgitation. J Heart Valve Dis. 2004;13:747–53.
39. Gillinov AM, Wierup PN, Blackstone EH, Bishay ES. Is repair preferable to replacement for ischemic mitral regurgitation? J Thorac Cardiovasc Surg. 2001;122:1125–41.
40. Bonacchi M, Prifti E, Maiani M, Frati G. Mitral valve surgery simultaneous to coronary revascularization in patients with end-stage ischemic cardiomyopathy. Heart Vessels. 2006;21:20–7.

41. Chan KMJ, Punjabi PP, Flather M, Wage RR, Symmonds K, Roussin I, Rahman-Haley S, Pennell DJ, Kilner PJ, Dreyfus GD, Pepper JR, Investigators R. Coronary artery bypass surgery with or without mitral valve annuloplasty in moderate functional ischemic mitral regurgitation: final results of the randomized ischemic mitral evaluation (RIME) trial. Circulation. 2012;126:2502–10.
42. Smith PK, Puskas JD, Ascheim DD, Voisine P, Gelijns AC, Moskowitz AJ, Hung JW, Parides MK, Ailawadi G, Perrault LP, Acker MA, Arenziano M, Thourani V, Gammie JS, Miller MA, Page P, Overbey JR, Dagenais F, Rose EA, Moquete EG, Jeffries N, Gardner TJ, O'Gara PT, Alexander JH, Michler RE. Surgical treatment of moderate ischemic mitral regurgitation. New Engl J Med. 2014;371:2178–88.
43. Acker MA, Parides MK, Perrault LP, Moskowitz AJ, Gelijns AC, Voisine P, Smith PK, Hung J, Blackstone EH, Puskas JD, Argenziano M, Gammie JS, Mack M, Ascheim DD, Bagiella E, Moquete EG, Ferguson TB, Horvath KA, Geller NL, Miller MA, Woo YJ, D'Alessandro DA, Ailawadi G, Dagenais F, Gardner TJ, O'Gara PT, Michler RE, Kron IL, CTSN. Mitral valve repair versus replacement for severe ischemic mitral regurgitation. New Engl J Med. 2014;370:23–32.
44. Fattouch K, Guccione F, Sampognaro R, Panzarella G, Corrado E, Navarra E, Calvaruso D, Ruvolo G. Efficacy of adding mitral valve annuloplasty to coronary artery bypass grafting in patients with moderate ischemic mitral valve regurgitation: a randomized trial. J Thorac Cardiovasc Surg. 2009;138:278–85.
45. Goldstein D, Moskowitz AJ, Gelijns AC, Ailawadi G, Parides MK, Perrault LP, Voisine P, Dagenais F, Gillinov AM, Thourani V, Argenziano M, Gammie JS, Mack M, Demers P, Atluri P, Rose EA, O'Sullivan K, Williams DL, Bagiella E, Michler RE, Weisel RD, Miller MA, Geller NL, Taddei-Peters WC, Smith PK, Moquete EG, Overbey JR, Kron IL, O'Gara PT, Acker MA, CTSN. Two year outcomes of surgical treatment of severe ischemic mitral regurgitation. New Engl J Med. 2016;374(20):1932–41.
46. Benedetto U, Melina G, Roscitano A, Fiorani B, Capuano F, Sclafani G, Comito C, di Nucci GD, Sinatra R. Does combined mitral valve surgery improve survival when compared to revascularisation alone in patients with ischemic mitral regurgitation? A meta-analysis on 2479 patients. J Cardiovasc Med. 2009;10:109–14.
47. Mihaljevic T, Lam B-K, Razzouk A, Takagaki M, Lauer MS, Gillinov AM, Blackstone EH, Lytle BW. Impact of mitral valve annuloplasty combined with revascularization in patients with functional ischemic mitral regurgitation. J Am Coll Cardiol. 2007;49:2191–201.
48. Gelsomino S, Lorusso R, De Cicco G, Capecchi I, Rostagno C, Caciolli S, Romagnoli S, Broi UG, Stefano P, Gensini GF. Five year echocardiographic results of combined undersized mitral ring annuloplasty and coronary artery bypass grafting for chronic ischaemic mitral regurgitaiton. Eur Heart J. 2008;29: 231–40.
49. Jones RH. Adding mitral valve annuloplasty to surgical revascularisation does not benefit patients with functional ischemic mitral regurgitation. J Am Coll Cardiol. 2007;49:2202–3.
50. Nishimura RA, Otto CM, Bonow RO, Carabello BA, Erwin III JP, Guyton RA, O'Gara PT, Ruiz CE, Skubas NJ, Sorajja P, Sundt III TM, Thomas JD. 2014 AHA/ACC guideline for the management of patients with valvular heart disease: a report of the American College of Cardiology/American Heart Association Task Force on Practice Guidelines. J Am Coll Cardiol. 2014;63:e57–185.

8 Mitral Valve Repair in Non-ischaemic Dilated Cardiomyopathy

K.M. John Chan

Abstract

The role of mitral valve repair for dilated cardiomyopathy is less well established. Observational studies are promising and suggest that it may be beneficial but patient selection needs to be better defined. Longer follow-up is also needed and randomised studies are needed. Important surgical principles must be followed when performing this surgery to ensure long term durability of the valve repair.

Keywords

Dilated cardiomyopathy • Mitral valve repair • Mitral valve annuloplasty • Left ventricular function

Mitral valve repair has been used in patients with dilated cardiomyopathy who have at least moderate mitral regurgitation. Initial observational studies have shown that mitral valve repair in these patients may improve cardiac function and functional status. Survival also appeared to be better compared to historical groups of patients treated by medication alone [1]. These results, however, need to be confirmed in randomised controlled trials. The indications for mitral valve repair in these patients also need to be better defined and predictors of success of surgery need to be better identified. At present, there is no consensus on mitral valve surgery for the treatment of dilated cardiomyopathy.

Principles of Treatment

It is now recognised that the mitral valve is an integral part of the structure of the left ventricle (LV). The mitral valve annulus and papillary muscles contribute significantly to LV function. The reverse is also true and significant impairment of LV function in patients with advanced dilated LV failure can significantly impair mitral valve function such that mitral regurgitation occurs. Dilatation of the LV not only results in dilatation of the mitral annulus but also tethering of the papillary muscles as the ventricular wall

K.M.J. Chan, BM BS, MSc, PhD, FRCS CTh
Department of Cardiothoracic Surgery,
Gleneagles Hospital, Jalan Ampang,
Kuala Lumpur 50450, Malaysia
e-mail: kmjohnchan@yahoo.com

K.M.J. Chan (ed.), *Functional Mitral and Tricuspid Regurgitation*,
DOI 10.1007/978-3-319-43510-7_8

dilates. Both of these lesions result in impaired coaptation of the mitral leaflets with resulting central mitral regurgitation. The anatomy of the mitral valve apparatus with overlap of a large portion of the leaflet surface area in a normal patient means that the left ventricle is often very significantly dilated before functional mitral regurgitation occurs.

The physiological basis for mitral valve annuloplasty in patients with significant mitral regurgitation due to advanced left ventricular failure is to stop the vicious cycle whereby mitral regurgitation begets more mitral regurgitation through volume overload and geometric distortion. Restoring the competency of the mitral valve restores forward flow of blood through the left ventricle and hence increases cardiac output. Both preload and afterload are also reduced as a result. There is also emerging evidence that restoring the size and shape of the mitral annulus in these patients also restores the volume and geometry of the dilated left ventricle. This concept was first proposed by Bolling who suggested that reducing the size of the mitral annulus not only reduces the volume of the dilated left ventricle, but also draws the base of the left ventricle inwards, resulting in the long axis of the left ventricle becoming more ellipsoid from base to apex [2]. This restores the spherical dilated ventricle to a more normal elliptical shape [1, 2]. A reduction in left ventricular volume would reduce left ventricular wall stress and hence improve subendocardial perfusion and oxygenation. Restoring the left ventricle to a more ellipsoid shape would restore the orientation of myofibrils to a more oblique direction optimising its efficiency during ventricular systole.

The technique of mitral annuloplasty has been described in a separate chapter. The mitral annulus is sized and an annuloplasty ring that is at least one size smaller than that measured is implanted. Undersizing is done to achieve leaflet coaptation and to restore the elliptical shape of the left ventricle. An important principle in this type of surgery is to use a rigid complete ring and not a flexible band. This is because the mitral annulus has been shown to dilate in both the anterior and posterior annulus. A smaller ring also achieves better long term results. However, care must be taken to place sufficient number of sutures and of sufficient depth as the sutures and annuloplasty ring are at increased tension due to the undersizing.

Results of Treatment

In Bolling's series of patients with both dilated and ischaemic cardiomyopathy, undersized mitral annuloplasty alone resulted in a reduction in LV end diastolic volume from 281 to 206 mls. This was associated with a marked reduction in the sphericity of the left ventricle. Ejection fraction also improved from 17 to 26 % and cardiac output from 3.3 l/min to 5.2 l/min at 22 months. In-hospital mortality was 2 % and two-year survival was 70 %. NYHA functional class improved from 3.9 to 1.8 and peak oxygen consumption improved from 14.5 to 18.6 ml/kg/min [1]. Bolling's series included patients with both ischaemic and idiopathic dilated cardiomyopathy. All his patients with ischaemic cardiomyopathy had undergone previous coronary artery bypass grafting. None of these patients, however, had regions of hibernating myocardium as determined by a negative dobutamine stress echo test or positron emission tomography. However, in a propensity matched study from the same centre comparing mitral annuloplasty versus medical treatment, Wu, et al., found no differences in survival between the two treatment groups. 30-day mortality was 4.8 % [3].

The results of mitral valve surgery in dilated cardiomyopathy have been reported by several others. Cope, et al., reported an operative mortality of only 3.4 % following undersized mitral annuloplasty in patients with both ischaemic and idiopathic dilated cardiomyopathy [4]. The preoperative ejection fraction was 22.9 %. Although no follow-up data on cardiac function was reported in this study, the mean survival of patients undergoing undersized mitral annuloplasty was 66 months, which is similar to that of patients undergoing heart transplantation (70 months). Bishay, et al., has also recently reported an operative mortality of only 2.3 %

following mitral valve repair in dilated cardiomyopathy with an improvement in NYHA class from 3.8 to 1.2, and ejection fraction from 28 to 36 %. Two and 5 year survival was 86 % and 67 % respectively [5]. Gummert, et al., reported an operative mortality of 6.1 %; 1 and 5 years actuarial survival was 86 % and 66 % respectively [6]. De Bonis, et al., reported an in-hospital mortality of 5.6 % and improvements in LV geometry, ejection fraction and NYHA functional class. Actuarial survival at 6.5 years was 69 % and freedom from recurrence of significant mitral regurgitation was 90 %. Successful atrial fibrillation ablation appeared to improve survival and LV reverse remodelling [7].

Further insights into the role of mitral valve surgery in heart failure was obtained from a subgroup of 102 patients with dilated cardiomyopathy and significant mitral regurgitation in the Acorn Clinical Trial who received mitral valve surgery alone. All of these patients were in NYHA class III or IV, had an ejection fraction of 35 % or less, a left ventricular end diastolic diameter of 60 mm or more, and a six minutes' walk test of 450 m or less. 84 % of the patients received mitral annuloplasty and 16 % had a mitral valve replacement. The overall operative mortality was 1.6 %. The survival at 12 months was 86.5 % and at 24 months was 85.2 %. LV volumes reduced significantly and consistently from baseline to 24 months and ejection fraction improved. Sphericity index also increased consistent with reverse remodelling of the LV into a more ellipsoidal shape from a spherical shape. Mitral regurgitation severity decreased significantly and the mean mitral regurgitation severity was 0.67 at 2 years. Improvements were also shown in NYHA functional class, six minute walk test, and quality of life questionnaires [8]. It should be noted that in this study, 40 % of the patients studied had moderate or less mitral regurgitation.

Several studies have reported on the risk factors for poor outcome in this group of patients. The severity of leaflet tethering and the size of the left ventricle are important risk factors affecting the durability of mitral annuloplasty and LV reverse remodelling. Calafiore, et al., reported that the durability of mitral annuloplasty in dilated cardiomyopathy is reduced when significant leaflet tethering is present (coaptation distance greater than 10 mm) and recommended mitral valve replacement instead of repair in these patients [9]. De Bonis, et al., recommended addition of the edge-to-edge repair to an annuloplasty when the coaptation depth was greater than 10 mm and identified absence of the edge-to-edge repair as a predictor of repair failure [10]. Horii, et al., reported that LV reverse remodelling and improvement in ejection fraction occurred up to 3 years after mitral valve surgery in this group of patients when the LV end-systolic volume index was less than 150 mL/m^2 but not when it was greater than this. 5-year survival was also better in the smaller LV group [11]. A left ventricular end-diastolic diameter of greater than 65 mm has also been reported to be predictive of reduced LV reverse remodelling and survival [12].

Observational studies therefore suggest that undersized mitral annuloplasty can be performed safely in patients with significant mitral regurgitation secondary to dilated cardiomyopathy. Such surgery appears to improve symptoms, cardiac function, LV reverse remodeling and survival compared with historical controls treated by medication alone. These results, however, need to be confirmed in randomised controlled trials. There is also a need to better identify patients who would benefit most from such surgery.

References

1. Bolling SF, Pagani FD, Deeb GM, Bach DS. Intermediate-term outcome of mitral reconstruction in cardiomyopathy. J Thorac Cardiovasc Surg. 1998; 115:381–6.
2. Bolling SF, Deeb M, Brunsting L, Bach DS. Early outcome of mitral valve reconstruction in patients with end stage cardiomyopathy. J Thorac Cardiovasc Surg. 1995;109:676–83.
3. Wu AH, Aaronson KD, Bolling SF, Pagani FF. Impact of mitral valve annuloplasty on mortality risk in patients with mitral regurgitation and left ventricular systolic dysfunction. J Am Coll Cardiol. 2005;45:381–7.
4. Cope JT, Kaza AK, Reade CC, Shockey KS, Kern JA, Tribble CG, Kron IL. A cost comparison of heart transplantation versus alternative operations for cardiomyopathy. Ann Thorac Surg. 2001;72:1298–305.

5. Bishay ES, McCarthy PM, Cosgrove DM, Hoercher KJ, Smedira NG, Mukherjee D, White J, Blackstone E. Mitral valve surgery in patients with severe left ventricular dysfunction. Eur J Cardiothorac Surg. 2000;17:213–21.
6. Gummert JF, Rahmel A, Bucerius J, Onnasch J, Doll N, Walther T, Falk V, Mohr FW. Mitral valve repair in patients with end stage cardiomyopathy: who benefits? Eur J Cardiothorac Surg. 2003;23:1017–22.
7. De Bonis MD, Taramasso M, Verzini A, Ferrara D, Lapenna E, Calabrese MC, Grimaldi A, Alfieri O. Long-term results of mitral repair for functional mitral regurgitation in idiopathic dilated cardiomyopathy. Eur J Cardiothorac Surg. 2012;42:640–6.
8. Acker MA, Bolling SF, Shemin R, Kirklin J, Oh JK, Mann DL, Jessup M, Sabbah HN, Starling RC, Kubo SH, Investigators ATP. Mitral valve surgery in heart failure: insights from the Acorn Clinical Trial. J Thorac Cardiovasc Surg. 2006;132:568–77.
9. Calafiore AM, Gallina S, Di Mauro M, Gaeta F, Iaco AL, D'Alessandro S, Mazzei V, Giammarco GD. Mitral valve procedure in dilated cardiomyopathy: repair or replacement? Ann Thorac Surg. 2001;71:1146–53.
10. De Bonis MD, Lapenna E, Canna GL, Ficarra E, Pagliaro M, Torracca L, Maisano F, Alfieri O. Mitral valve repair for functional mitral regurgitation in end-stage dilated cardiomyopathy. Circulation. 2005;112:I-402–8.
11. Horii T. Left ventricle volume affects the result of mitral valve surgery for idiopathic dilated cardiomyopathy to treat congestive heart failure. Ann Thorac Surg. 2006;82:1349.
12. Braun J, van de Veire NR, Klautz RJM, Versteegh MIM, Holman ER, Westenberg JM, Boersma E, van der Wall EE, Bax JJ, Dion RAE. Restrictive mitral annuloplasty cures ischemic mitral regurgitation and heart failure. Ann Thorac Surg. 2008;85:430–7.

9 Leaflet and Chordal Procedures in Functional Mitral Regurgitation

K.M. John Chan

Abstract

Leaflet and chordal procedures are newer repair techniques in functional ischaemic mitral regurgitation. Early studies with leaflet augmentation and secondary chordal cutting are promising. Long term studies are needed.

Keywords

Functional ischaemic mitral regurgitation • Restricted leaflet motion • Mitral leaflet augmentation • Second order chordal cutting • Edge-to-edge repair

Interventions on the mitral valve leaflets and chordae are less commonly performed procedures in functional mitral regurgitation, performed to increase leaflet coaptation and reduce leaflet tethering. These procedures include leaflet augmentation, edge-to-edge repair and second order chordal cutting. Leaflet augmentation and second order chordal cutting are commonly performed in rheumatic mitral regurgitation, another condition where the lesion is that of restricted leaflet motion. Its use in functional ischaemic mitral regurgitation is showing promise.

K.M.J. Chan, BM BS, MSc, PhD, FRCS CTh
Department of Cardiothoracic Surgery,
Gleneagles Hospital, Jalan Ampang,
Kuala Lumpur 50450, Malaysia
e-mail: kmjohnchan@yahoo.com

Leaflet Augmentation

Experimental studies have shown that mitral leaflet area increases in response to chronic tethering, and that inadequate leaflet enlargement may be a cause of functional mitral regurgitation, whereas if sufficient leaflet enlargement occurs in response to ventricular remodeling, mitral regurgitation would not result [1].

Leaflet augmentation is commonly performed in rheumatic mitral regurgitation to increase the surface area of coaptation in fibrosed, retracted leaflets. It has also been used in chronic functional ischaemic mitral regurgitation [2]. The principle here is to increase the leaflet coaptation surface area to compensate for the leaflet tethering. Leaflet tethering was shown to be improved in one study but not in another, but the increased leaflet surface area from the leaflet augmentation

K.M.J. Chan (ed.), *Functional Mitral and Tricuspid Regurgitation*,
DOI 10.1007/978-3-319-43510-7_9

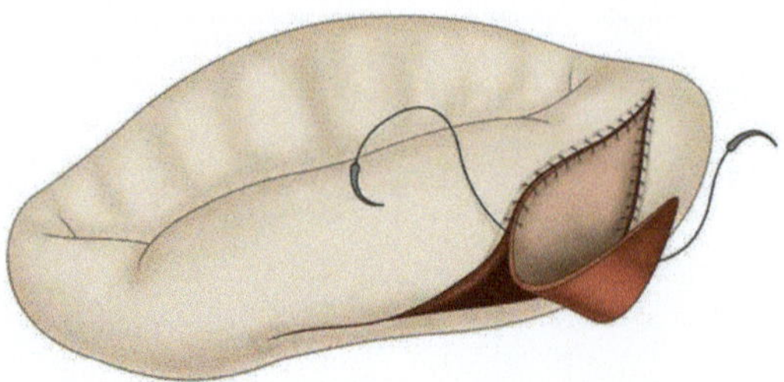

Fig. 9.1 Posterior leaflet augmentation for functional ischaemic mitral regurgitation (From de Varennes et al. [2])

was more than sufficient to reduce the mitral regurgitation in either case [3, 4].

Autologous or bovine pericardium can be used. The posterior leaflet is detached from its base from the middle of P2 all the way to the posterior commissure. Annuloplasty sutures are then applied around the annulus. The pericardial patch is rinsed thoroughly and cut in an oblong fashion with a height of 1 cm and a length of 3.5 to 4.5 cm. The patch is sutured to the edge of the posterior leaflet defect and the posterior mitral annulus using 5/0 polytetrafluoroethylene suture (W.L. Gore and Associates, Flagstaff, Arizona) or equivalent (Fig. 9.1) [2]. The annuloplasty is then sized using the inter-commissural distance and the exact surface area of the anterior leaflet. No downsizing is needed as the leaflet surface area has been increased. The posterior leaflet is effectively increased in height by about 1 cm in the area of P3 and the medial half of P2.

Early results are good using this technique with Varennes, et al, reporting freedom from moderate or more mitral regurgitation of 90 % at 2 years, and 90 % of patients were in NYHA class I [2]. Long term results are awaited.

Second Order Chordal Cutting

This technique was first proposed by Messas, et al, and popularized by Borger, et al. [5, 6] Secondary chords attach to the basal and mid body of the mitral leaflet and typically restrict leaflet motion in chronic functional ischemic mitral regurgitation, particularly of the anterior leaflet, leading to the so called "seagull wing". This bend in the anterior leaflet represents abnormal tethering by the basal chordae. Experimentally, cutting secondary chords relieved leaflet tethering and improved leaflet coaptation, reducing mitral regurgitation [5]. There is, however, some concern that cutting secondary chords may affect local haemodynamics, shear stress distribution, and left ventricular function [7, 8].

Borger, et al, describe cutting all secondary chords arising from the papillary muscle causing leaflet restriction, usually the posteromedial papillary muscle [6]. The chords are cut at their insertion to the anterior and posterior leaflets. An undersized annuloplasty ring is then implanted.

Follow-up echocardiography in Borger's series revealed trivial or mild mitral regurgitation in 97 % of patients at 2 years. Long term results are awaited [6].

Edge-to-Edge Leaflet Repair

The edge-to-edge leaflet repair, first described by Alfieri, is used in many mitral valve lesions [9]. A suture is used to join the edges of the anterior and posterior leaflets creating a double orifice mitral valve. A mitral annuloplasty ring is implanted to improve long term durability. Recently, Bhudia, et al, reported that at 2 years, 24 % of patients who had undergone this procedure for functional ischemic mitral regurgitation had developed recurrent moderate-severe mitral regurgitation, and 23 % had moderate mitral regurgitation [10]. The authors recommended against the use of this technique in functional ischemic mitral regurgitation.

References

1. Chaput M, Handschumacher MD, Tournoux F, Hua L, Guerrero JL, Vlahakes GJ, Levine RA. Mitral leaflet adaptation to ventricular remodelling: occurrence and adequacy in patients with functional mitral regurgitation. Circulation. 2008;118:845–52.
2. de Varennes B, Chaturvedi R, Sidhu S, Cote AV, Shan WLP, Goyer C, Hatzakorzian R, Buithieu J, Sniderman A. Initial results of posterior leaflet extension for severe type IIIb ischemic mitral regurgitation. Circulation. 2009;119:2837–43.

3. Langer F, Rodriguez F, Cheng A, Ortiz S, Nguyen TC, Zasio MK, Liang D, Daughters GT, Ingels NB, Miller DC. Posterior mitral leaflet extension: an adjunctive repair option for ischemic mitral regurgitation? J Thorac Cardiovasc Surg. 2006;131:868–77.
4. Robb JD, Minakawa M, Koomalsingh KJ, Shuto T, Jassar AS, Ratcliffe SJ, Gorman RC, Gorman JH. Posterior leaflet augmentation improves leaflet tethering in repair of ischemic mitral regurgitation. Eur J Cardiothorac Surg. 2011;40:1501–7.
5. Messas E, Pouzet B, Touchot B, et al. Efficacy of chordal cutting to relieve chronic persistent ischemic mitral regurgitation. Circulation. 2003;108:111–5.
6. Borger MA. Chronic ischemic mitral regurgitation: repair, replace or rethink? Ann Thorac Surg. 2006;81:1153.
7. Rodriguez F, Langer F, Harrington KB. Importance of mitral valve second order chordae for left ventricular geometry, wall thickening mechanics, and global systolic function. Circulation. 2004;110: 115–22.
8. Xiong F, Yeo JH, Chong CK, Chua YL, Lim KH, Ooi ET, Goetz WA. Transection of anterior mitral basal stay chords alters left ventricular outflow dynamics and wall shear stress. J Heart Valve Dis. 2008;17: 54–61.
9. Alfieri O, Maisano F, De Bonis M. The double orifice technique in mitral valve repair: a simple solution for complex problems. J Thorac Cardiovasc Surg. 2001;122:674–81.
10. Bhudia SK, McCarthy PM, Smedira NG, Lam B-K, Rajeswaran J, Blackstone EH. Edge-to-edge (Alfieri) mitral repair: results in diverse clinical settings. Ann Thorac Surg. 2004;77:1598–606.

Subvalvular Techniques for Ischemic Mitral Regurgitation

10

Daniel P. Mulloy and Irving L. Kron

Abstract

Surgical treatment of ischemic mitral regurgitation with reduction ring annuloplasty is the current standard of practice, yet recurrence in a third of patients limits the benefit of this approach. In an effort to improve outcomes, attention has turned to understanding the contribution of leaflet tethering in this disease process. Subvalvular techniques to alleviate leaflet restriction have been shown to be safe, and in the appropriate patient population decrease recurrence of ischemic mitral regurgitation when combined with reduction annuloplasty. We describe our preferred technique of posterior papillary muscle repositioning. Further understanding of the preoperative parameters that predict recurrence, and deployment of concomitant subvalvular repair techniques in this subset of patients will be the next important breakthrough in the surgical treatment of ischemic mitral regurgitation.

Keywords

Heart failure • Ischemic mitral regurgitation • Mitral repair • Tricuspid repair • Cardiomyopathy

Pathophysiology

The term functional mitral regurgitation is used to describe mitral regurgitation in the absence of any "organic" lesions of the mitral valve. It includes mitral regurgitation (MR) that results from dilated cardiomyopathy and also mitral regurgitation caused by ischemic dysfunction of the ventricle and subvalvular apparatus. Using the Carpentier pathophysiologic triad ischemic MR has an *etiology* of known coronary artery stenosis with

D.P. Mulloy, MD (✉)
Division of Thoracic and Cardiovascular Surgery, University of Virginia Health System, PO Box 800679, Charlottesville, VA 22908, USA
e-mail: DPM7G@hscmail.mcc.virginia.edu

I.L. Kron, MD
Division of Thoracic and Cardiovascular Surgery, University of Virginia, Charlottesville, VA, USA

K.M.J. Chan (ed.), *Functional Mitral and Tricuspid Regurgitation*,
DOI 10.1007/978-3-319-43510-7_10

evidence of prior myocardial infarction with regional or global left ventricular dysfunction. The primary l*esion* causing regurgitation in this setting is tethering of the mitral valve leaflets often combined with some degree of annular dilation. The resulting *dysfunction* in the case of chronic ischemic MR is most frequently Carpentier type IIIb dysfunction caused by restricted leaflet motion which occurs in response to ventricular remodeling after myocardial infarction. Carpentier type I dysfunction, or MR resulting from annular dilation with a lack of leaflet coaptation despite normal leaflet motion, may occur in the setting of basal infarction but accounts for less than 10% of ischemic MR cases and should be easily repairable with a reduction ring annuloplasty. Carpentier type II dysfunction, or leaflet prolapse, may occur with complete or partial rupture of the posteromedial papillary muscle but is rare in the current era of percutaneous early revascularization for myocardial infarction.

The normal mitral valve function involves a complex interaction among the valve leaflets, annulus, subvalvular apparatus, and left ventricle. In ischemic mitral regurgitation, the leaflets are spared but each of the other components of the normally functioning mitral valve are differentially affected. Annular dilation and distortion is present, dilation and increased sphericity of the ventricle occurs, and with these changes the papillary muscles of the subvalvular apparatus are displaced. All of these changes combine to cause leaflet tethering and therefore poor coaptation, creating a regurgitant valve. It is commonly and accurately stated that ischemic mitral regurgitation is a disease of ventricle, not a disease of the valve, and understanding it in this manner is necessary when pursuing effective and durable repair techniques.

Breaking down the changes in the valve components that lead to the final common pathway of Carpentier IIIb MR caused by leaflet tethering we can start with the most important changes which occur in the left ventricle. Myocardial ischemia or infarction with remodeling leads to regional distortion and ultimately poor leaflet coaptation. Watanabe and colleagues have shown that in patients with inferior infarction, tethering was more localized in the medial posterior leaflet, while anterior infarction results in more widespread tethering of both leaflets [1]. This observation confirms the crucial role that regional ventricular geometry and function play in the pathophysiology of ischemic MR and helps explain why some patients with only mildly impaired LV function develop severe ischemic MR. Indeed, the geometry of ventricle as it remodels in response to ischemia and infarction seems to be more important determinant of ischemic MR than the LV volume or ejection fraction.

Annular dilation is common in chronic ischemic MR however the degree of annular dilation does not necessarily correlate with the degree of MR. Some patients have severe MR with very little annular dilation while others with significant annular dilation have only mild regurgitation. Several studies have noted that the degree of septolateral (SL) dilation seems more important in the pathophysiology of ischemic MR than the commisure-commisure (CC) dilation [2, 3]. In severe cases of ischemic MR the SL dimension can approach the CC dimension which results in a circular annulus instead of the usual elliptical one. Most often, the majority of the dilation occurs in the posterior annulus, particularly in the region of the posterior commissure [4, 5].

When examining the role of the subvalvular apparatus, it is clear that papillary muscle displacement plays a critical role in the development of ischemic MR. On the contrary, papillary muscle dysfunction itself does not seem to significantly contribute to ischemic MR [6, 7]. Carpentier and colleagues demonstrated in sheep studies in the 1980s that formaldehyde injection in the posterior papillary muscle did not produce MR [8]. Instead, MR could only be produced by extending formaldehyde injection into the adjacent myocardium resulting in regional wall motion abnormality. The pattern of papillary muscle displacement necessary to yield ischemic MR is complex and involves displacement of the muscle tips posterolaterally and apically away from the anterior annulus and away from each other. The tethering distance has been shown experimentally to correlate with the severity of ischemic MR [9]. Displacement of both papillary muscles is likely necessary to induce severe MR but particularly displacement of the posteromedial muscle usually predominates.

The combination of regional LV dysfunction and sphericity, annular dilation, and papillary muscle displacement all create a tethering force that leads to apical tenting of the mitral valve leaflets and Carpentier IIIb MR. Tethering of the primary chordae leads to restricted motion of the free margins of the leaflets which prevents them from rising to the plane of the annulus during systole with resultant poor coaptation and regurgitation. In addition, tethering of the secondary chordae can result in deformation of the body of the leaflet which also contributes to impaired coaptation.

Therapeutic targets for correction of ischemic MR include the coronary arteries, mitral annulus, subvalvular apparatus, valve leaflets, and the ventricle itself. Any surgery for ischemic MR should include full coronary artery revascularization. To date, the most common surgical treatment for ischemic MR involves coronary revascularization and a reduction ring annuloplasty which restores leaflet coaptation but fails to address the underlying tethering component in the pathophysiology of ischemic MR. This failure may explain why about a third of patients develop recurrent MR within a year of successful reduction annuloplasty. The remainder of this chapter will focus on surgical approaches to management of the subvalvular apparatus via varying techniques of papillary muscle relocation and several techniques of chordal modification in an effort to obtain a more durable correction of ischemic MR that is more resistant to continued ventricular remodeling and tethering. In rare cases, a simultaneous ventricular remodeling procedure such as a Dor operation may be indicated or necessary but this will be discussed elsewhere.

Principles of Treatment

To determine which patients are appropriate candidates for mitral valve repair with the employment of adjunctive subvalvular techniques, a thorough understanding of the latest data on ischemic MR is necessary. Traditional mitral valve repair for ischemic MR involves revascularization of ischemic myocardium along with a reduction ring annuloplasty as first described by Bolling and Bach in 1995 [10]. This repair technique is simple and has demonstrated a large degree of success over the past two decades but as alluded to earlier, this approach addresses the annulus only and ignores the underlying contributions of ventricular dysfunction and changes in geometry of the subvalvular apparatus to the development of ischemic mitral regurgitation. Not surprisingly, the rates of recurrent MR after reduction ring annuloplasty have been shown to be higher than 30 %.

As mentioned previously, results from the recent Cardiothoracic Surgical Trials Network (CTSN) randomized study on mitral valve repair versus replacement for severe ischemic MR [11] suggest that this approach alone is inadequate for some patients. In this trial, 251 patients with severe ischemic MR were randomized to mitral valve repair or chordal-sparing mitral valve replacement with a primary endpoint on left ventricular end-systolic volume index (LVESVI) and secondary endpoints of major adverse cardiac and cerebrovascular events, mortality, degree of residual MR, functional status, and quality of life. The vast majority of mitral valve repairs in this trial were done with reduction ring annuloplasty of 1–2 sizes. At 1 year, there was no significant difference between repair and replacement in either the primary or any secondary outcome. Notably, the rate of recurrent moderate or severe MR at 1 year in the repair group was 32.6 % vs. only 2.3 % in the replacement group ($P<0.001$). Of those undergoing repair, the LVESVI was 64.1 ± 23.9 ml/m^2 in those with recurrent MR versus 47.3 ± 23.0 ml/m^2 in those without recurrent MR ($P<0.001$) suggesting that if a durable repair can be achieved, there likely remains an advantage to repair over replacement.

In order to further investigate the question of whether failure of mitral valve repair can be predicted by certain preoperative characteristics, the CTSN investigators have performed a recent posthoc analysis of the 116 patients who were randomized to and received mitral valve repair in the Severe MR trial with 2-year follow-up [12]. Logistic regression was used to determine baseline echocardiographic and clinical characteristics that predict failure of repair or death and a predictive model based on 10 factors (age; gender; race; body mass index; NYHA class; effective regurgitant orifice; basal aneurysm/dyskinesia; and history of coronary artery bypass grafting, percutaneous coronary intervention, or ventricular arrhythmias) was developed with a favorable area under the receiver operating characteristic curve of 0.82. Those patients who suffered from recurrent moderate/severe MR or who died were older, had a lower frequency of NYHA class III or IV, and had a higher frequency of basal aneurysm/dyskinesis. Of the ten variables, the standout predictor of recurrent moderate or severe MR, or death, was basal aneurysm/dyskinesia; reflecting a severe form of preoperative LV ischemic remodeling with the abnormalities of papillary muscle displacement, leaflet tethering, and annular dilation. It stands to reason that in these patients with preoperative basal aneurysm/dyskinesia, mitral repair with a downsized annuloplasty ring alone is insufficient and that either upfront replacement or additional subvalvular repair techniques are necessary for a durable result.

Techniques of Repair

No large randomized study exists to confirm the benefit of subvalvular techniques for repair of ischemic MR however multiple smaller studies support the adoption of various subvalvular techniques. Papillary muscle relocation to alleviate leaflet restriction was first reported one decade ago [13]. The original technique consisted of passing a prolene suture through the posterior papillary muscle and then through the mitral annulus immediately posterior to the right fibrous trigone prior to reduction annuloplasty. In the initial study, echocardiographic follow-up revealed restoration of a more physiologic configuration of the relocated posterior papillary muscle and no patient had recurrence of MR 2 months after repair. There were no mortalities and relocation of the papillary muscle, easily visualized through a standard left atriotomy, was demonstrated to be a safe and simple additional procedure. However, this technique requires a fibrotic posterior papillary muscle.

These encouraging initial results prompted further revisions in the technique of papillary muscle relocation, including a sling to anchor the bases of the papillary muscle together [14] and direct approximation of the tips of the two papillary muscles together [15]. Years after papillary muscle relocation, the majority of patients in these studies remain free from recurrent mitral regurgitation with evidence of reversal in left ventricular remodeling and improvement in both ejection fraction and New York Heart Association functional class. One recent study highlighted the importance of papillary muscle approximation in limiting further posterior leaflet tethering following reduction ring annuloplasty. Often reduction annuloplasty can worsen posterior leaflet tethering but Manabe et al. demonstrated decreased posterior leaflet restriction with papillary muscle approximation [16].

In 2013, results of the first retrospective study directly comparing outcomes after reduction annuloplasty alone versus concomitant papillary muscle relocation were published [17]. In this study, both papillary muscles were reapproximated to the mitral annulus using a CV-4 Gore-Tex suture placed through the head of each papillary muscle and tied to the ipsilateral mitral annulus. Postoperatively, patients who underwent this combined procedure had significantly decreased mean tenting area and coaptation depth as well as decreased left ventricular end systolic and diastolic diameter over a mean follow-up of 32 months. Recurrent mitral regurgitation was significantly decreased with the addition of papillary muscle relocation. There were no differences in early or late mortality and patients who underwent papillary muscle relocation had a decreased incidence of late cardiac events.

Concomitant procedures involving the chordae tendinae have also been reported in attempts to mitigate leaflet restriction. Chordal cutting has been met with resistance due to the potential for disruption of the valvular-ventricular continuity and concern for progressive left ventricular modeling. However, these procedures target the secondary chordae and leave the basal and marginal chordae intact. In one recent study, addition of bileaflet secondary chordal cutting to reduction annuloplasty resulted in increased leaflet mobility which significantly decreased the severity of recurrent MR [18]. Importantly, reversal in left ventricular remodeling was also observed without adverse effect on left ventricular function.

Severity of distal anterior leaflet tethering, mediated by secondary chordae, has been found to be a risk factor for recurrent mitral regurgitation after reduction annuloplasty. This tenting effect results in the characteristic seagull sign of the anterior leaflet in ischemic mitral regurgitation, and the angle between the two segments of the anterior leaflet is known as the bending angle. One group recently stratified patients with excessive tethering of the anterior leaflet, as measured by a bending angle less than 145°, to undergo concomitant cutting of all secondary chordae to the anterior leaflet from both papillary muscles [19]. Compared with patients who underwent reduction annuloplasty alone, patients who underwent chordal cutting had significantly decreased recurrent or persistent mitral regurgitation and improved New York Heart Association functional class at a mean follow-up of 33 months. There were no deaths attributable to cardiovascular causes, and ejection fraction increased to a more significant degree after chordal cutting.

To preserve all aspects of the subvalvular apparatus, chordal reimplantation has been reported as an alternative procedure to chordal cutting. In a recent retrospective study, patients with chronic ischemic mitral regurgitation and severe leaflet restriction underwent detachment and reimplantation of secondary chordae to a primary position along the anterior mitral leaflet [20]. In addition to this cut-and-transfer technique, these patients underwent posterior papillary muscle relocation and a subset underwent infarct plication of the lateral left ventricular wall, maneuvers both intended to realign the displaced subvalvular apparatus to a more physiologic configuration under the mitral valve. The majority of patients were free of recurrent mitral regurgitation at 1 year, with echocardiographic and clinical findings revealing a significant improvement in ejection fraction and New York Heart Association functional class at follow-up. Based on these results, chordal procedures represent a valid option in our current armamentarium of concomitant subvalvular techniques in the treatment of ischemic mitral regurgitation.

Surgical Operative Technique

Our preferred subvalvular technique for repair of ischemic mitral regurgitation is well established and has been previously described [13, 21, 22]. This type of repair is appropriate for treatment of Carpentier IIIb MR and we have achieved excellent durable results utilizing these techniques. After standard preoperative preparation, intraoperative transesophageal echocardiography is performed to carefully assess the mechanism of MR. We typically repair greater than 2+ MR and this determination should be made based on the preoperative surface echo rather than in the operating room when afterload reduction may mask clinically significant MR. Conduit harvesting for coronary artery bypass is performed and cardiopulmonary bypass is established using standard aortic and bicaval cannulation with antegrade and retrograde cardioplegia. Distal coronary anastomoses are performed first before turning attention to the mitral valve. Caval tapes are placed and elevated to help facilitate exposure of the mitral valve which is obtained through a standard left atriotomy utilizing a Cosgrove self-retaining retractor.

Systematic valve inspection is performed to confirm the echocardiographic findings. In the typical case of A3/P3 regurgitation due to posteromedial papillary muscle tethering, we proceed with posterior papillary muscle relocation. First, circumferential mitral annular horizontal mattress stitches are placed and the mitral valve is sized using the inter-trigonal distance. We typically downsize by 1 to 2 sizes which generally results in a 26- or 28-mm semi-rigid complete annuloplasty ring. The annular stiches are passed through the sewing ring at appropriate intervals to produce an even annular reduction and the ring is lowered onto the annulus and sutures tied. The valve is re-tested and if significant residual MR is detected then the tethering of the posterior papillary muscle and dysfunction of the subvalvular apparatus must be addressed.

A 3-0 polypropylene suture is placed through the fibrotic papillary muscle and the two ends are then passed through the annulus behind the previously placed ring in the area posterior to the right fibrous trigone. The suture is tied over a felt pledget and adjusted to restore the posterior papillary muscle to a more anatomic position. This adjustment correlates to the degree of tethering visualized on intraoperative transthoracic echocardiography. Prior to locking the suture, valve function is again tested with the saline test to assure no residual regurgitation and necessary adjustments are made. The atriotomy is then close as standard, deairing measures are performed and any proximal coronary conduit anastomoses are completed. Further deairing, removal of the aortic cross-clamp, and weaning from bypass are performed per routine. Transesophageal echocardiography is used to confirm adequacy of the repair. MR $<1+$ is deemed acceptable but MR $\geq 1+$ necessitates further repair or valve replacement.

Patient Selection

The next step in subvalvular repair techniques is to more accurately determine those patients who will derive maximal benefit from these techniques. In a report published last year, a subset of patients undergoing reduction annuloplasty for ischemic MR was selected to undergo a concomitant subvalvular procedure [23]. Patients with significant left ventricular dilatation and increased tethering angles of the anterior and posterior mitral leaflets were selected to undergo papillary muscle approximation and suspension as well as left ventricular restoration. One year after surgery, bileaflet tethering angles were significantly increased in the group that did not undergo subvalvular repair and recurrent MR occurred only in this group. These results suggest that incorporating subvalvular techniques into repair in patients with left ventricular dilation and leaflet tethering impedes further left ventricular remodeling, papillary muscle displacement, leaflet tethering, and recurrent MR. Nevertheless, we have not perfected the identification of those patients who will depend on concomitant subvalvular procedures for a durable repair.

The recent efforts of the CTSN investigators to develop a risk model for prediction of recurrent MR after repair of ischemic MR offers a step in the right direction toward evidence-based treatment of ischemic MR and deployment of select subvalvular repair techniques in the setting of predicted failure of reduction annuloplasty alone. As described previously, the standout predictor of recurrent MR or death in this model, was basal aneurysm/dyskinesia. While the presence of a basal aneurysm/dyskinesia is a helpful predictor of repair failure using reduction annuloplasty alone, it is likely just a reflection of a severe form of preoperative LV ischemic remodeling with accompanying papillary muscle displacement, leaflet tethering, and annular dilation. As of yet, no data exists to completely predict repair failure for ischemic MR. Similarly, defined preoperative characteristics that guide which adjunctive subvalvular techniques are most appropriate in a given patient have not been fully elucidated. Our understanding of this complex pathophysiology has improved, as well as our ability to safely perform complex subvalvular repair maneuvers, but the systematic and appropriate deployment of these valuable techniques must be further investigated through rigorous collaborative investigation.

Conclusion

We have discussed the pathophysiology of ischemic mitral regurgitation and the principles of treatment with particular attention to techniques addressing the subvalvular apparatus. What must be understood beyond all else is that ischemic MR is a disease of the ventricle, not of the valve, and must be treated as such. With this in mind, it should not be surprising that the rate of recurrent mitral regurgitation after simple reduction annuloplasty for ischemic MR is high. The ventricle continues to remodel after ring annuloplasty with further displacement of the papillary muscles and subsequent leaflet tethering and regurgitation. To correct this problem, the underlying dysfunction in each patient must be addressed. We have detailed a technique of posterior papillary muscle repositioning that we have found to be particularly effective in treating patients with typical Carpentier IIIb ischemic MR but this technique is not intended as a cure-all. Additional subvalvular adjunctive repair techniques such as chordal cutting and papillary muscle reapproximation are promising. Despite this promise, there is poor data to direct which technique to employ and only an early understanding of which patients may benefit from these approaches. Determination of those patients whose outcomes depend on these concomitant techniques of subvalvular repair will be the next important breakthrough in the surgical treatment of ischemic mitral regurgitation.

References

1. Watanabe N, Ogasawara Y, Yamaura Y, et al. Geometric differences of the mitral valve tenting between anterior and inferior myocardial infarction with significant ischemic mitral regurgitation. J Am Soc Echocardiogr. 2006;19:71–5.
2. Kaji S, Nasu M, Yamamuro A, et al. Anular geometry in patients with cronic ischemic mitral regurgitation: three dimensional magnetic resonance imaging study. Circulation. 2005;112:1409–14.
3. Timek TA, Lai DT, Liang D, et al. Effects of paracommisusural septal-lateral anular cinching on acute ischemic mitral regurgitation. Circulation. 2004;110:1179–84.
4. Hueb AC, Jatene FB, Moreira LF, et al. Ventricular remodeling and mitral valve modifications in dilated cardiomyopathy: new insights from anatomic study. J Thorac Cardiovasc Surg. 2002;124:1216–24.
5. Ahmad RM, Gillinov AM, McCarthy PM, et al. Anular geometry and motion in human ischemic mitral regurgitation: novel assessment with three dimensional echocardiography and computer reconstruction. Ann Thorac Surg. 2004;78:2063–8.
6. Timek TA, Lai DT, Tibayan F, et al. Ischemia in three left ventricular regions: Insights into the pathogenesis of acute ischemic mitral regurgitation. J Thorac Cardiovasc Surg. 2003;125:559–69.
7. Green GR, Dagum P, Glasson JR, et al. Mitral anular dilatation and papillary muscle dislocation without mitral regurgitation in sheep. Circulation. 2002;106:127–32.
8. Carpentier A. Ischemic mitral valve insufficiency. In: Carpentier A, Starr A, editors. Surgery of the mitral valve and the left atrium. Paris: Masson; 1990. p. 60.
9. Dagum P, Timk TA, Green GR, et al. Coordinate-free analysis of mitral valve dynamics in normal and ischemic hearts. Circulation. 2000;102:1162–9.
10. Bolling SF, Deeb GM, Brunsting LA, Back DS. Early outcome of mitral valve reconstruction in patients with end-stage cardiomyopathy. J Thorac Cardiovasc Surg. 1995;109:767–82.
11. Acker MA, Parides MK, Perrault LP, et al. Mitral-valve repair versus replacement for severe ischemic mitral regurgitation. N Engl J Med. 2014;370:23–32.
12. Kron IL, Hung J, Overbey JR, et al. Predicting recurrent mitral regurgitation after mitral valve repair for severe ischemic mitral regurgitation. J Thorac Cardiovasc Surg. 2015;149:752–61.
13. Kron IL, Green GR, Cope JT. Surgical reolocation of the posterior papillary muscle in chronic ischemic mitral regurgitation. Ann Thorac Surg. 2002;74:600–1.
14. Hvass U, Joudinaud T. The papillary muscle sling for ischemic mitral regurgitation. J Thorac Cardiovasc Surg. 2010;139:418–23.
15. Rama A, Praschker L, Barreda E, et al. Papillary muscle approximation for functional ischemic mitral regurgitation. Ann Thorac Surg. 2007;84:2130–1.
16. Manabe S, Shimokawa T, Fukui T, et al. Impact of papillary muscle approximation on mitral valve configutation in the surgical correction of ischemic mitral regurgitation. Thorac Cardiovasc Surg. 2012;60:269–74.
17. Fattouch K, Lancelloti P, Castrovinci S, et al. Papillary muscle relocation in conjuction with valve annuloplasty improves repair results in severe ischemic mitral regurgitation. J Thorac Cardiovasc Surg. 2012;143:1352–5.
18. Szymanski C, Bel A, Cohen I, et al. Comprehensive annular and subvalvular repair of chronic ischemic mitral regurgitation improves long-term results with the least ventricular remodeling. Circulation. 2012;126:2720–7.
19. Calafiore A, Refaie R, Iaco A, et al. Chordal cutting is ischemic mitral regurgitation: a propensity-matched study. J Thorac Cardiovasc Surg. 2014;148(1):41–6.
20. Cappabianca G, Bichi S, Patrini D, et al. Cut-and-transfer technique for ischemic mitral regurgitation and severe tethering of mitral leaflets. Ann Thorac Surg. 2013;96:1607–13.
21. Peller BB, Kron IL. Suture relocation of the posterior papillary muscle in ischemic mitral regurgitation. Op Tech Thorac Cardiovasc Surg. 2005;5:113–22.
22. LaPar DJ, Kron IL. Repair techniques for ischemic mitral regurgitation. Op Tech Thorac Cardiovasc Surg. 2012;8:204–12.
23. Yamaguchi K, Adachi K, Yuri K, et al. Reduction of mitral valve leaflet tethering by procedures targeting the subvalvular apparatus in addition to mitral annuloplasty. Circ J. 2013;77:1461–5.

11 Suture Annuloplasty for Ischemic Mitral Valve Repair

Rimantas Benetis

Abstract

Mitral valve suture annuloplasty has been in use for a long time although it is less commonly used in ischemic mitral regurgitation. It does, however, have advantages over other repair techniques and may be suitable in ischemic mitral regurgitation for selected patients. As in other repair techniques, important principles must be followed to ensure long term durability of the repair.

Keywords

Ischemic mitral regurgitation • Suture annuloplasty • Mitral valve repair • Mitral valve repair techniques • Durability of repair

Abbreviations

AV	Atrioventricular
AVR	Aortic valve replacement
CABG	Coronary artery bypass grafting
IMR	Ischemic mitral regurgitation
LA	Left atrium
LV	Left ventricle
LVEDD	LV end diastolic diameter
LVEDDI	LVEDD index
LVEF	LV Ejection fraction
LVESD	LV end systolic diameter
LVESDI	LVESD index
MI	Myocardial infarction
MR	Mitral regurgitation
MV	Mitral valve
NYHA	New York heart association
PTFE	Polytetrafluoroethylene
TEE	Transesophageal echocardiography

R. Benetis
Department of Cardiac Surgery, Hospital of Lithuanian University of Health Sciences, Kaunas Clinics, Eiveniu 2, Kaunas 50009, Lithuania
e-mail: Rimantas.Benetis@kaunoklinikos.lt

Despite the latest achievements in early coronary artery revascularization (angioplasty, coronary stenting, coronary artery bypass grafting sugery) of stenotic or occluded coronary arteries due to chronic or acute coronary syndromes, so preventing and reducing myocardial damage, ischemic

K.M.J. Chan (ed.), *Functional Mitral and Tricuspid Regurgitation*,
DOI 10.1007/978-3-319-43510-7_11

mitral regurgitation (IMR) is still an important clinical problem. However, the incidence of IMR during the last decade in an era of early invasive cardiology intervention is decreasing.

Several studies found that the most important factor improving early and late survival in IMR is effective surgical revascularization of ischemic myocardium. And some conclude that although mitral valve repair appears to be more effective at reducing functional IMR, coronary artery bypass grafting surgery (CABG) alone may be a preferable treatment option for patients with moderate mitral regurgitation (MR) and high operative risk factors such as an advanced patient age [1–3]. Others did show, that CABG alone does not resolve IMR, nor improve early and/or late postoperative outcomes [4, 5].

Therefore, management of IMR, both by coronary revascularization alone or combined with mitral valve repair remains controversial. The American College of Cardiology (ACC)/ American Heart Association (AHA) and European Society of Cardiology (ESC) guidelines recommend mitral valve repair in moderate or severe IMR cases but not as a Class I, Level of Evidence A recommendation [6, 7]. For chronic moderate-severe IMR, repair/replacement is reasonable for patients who are undergoing CABG or aortic valve replacement (AVR) (class IIa recommendation) and for the patients with severe NYHA class (III-IV, stage D) symptoms and stage B patients who are undergoing other cardiac surgery (class IIb recommendations). If one follows the above recommendations, the question remains about durability of mitral valve repair. Recent North American prospective, randomized studies and some others raised a question whether mitral valve repair is beneficial in the long term because of increased mortality/morbidity and recurrence of mitral regurgitation (MR).

Mitral valve replacement with a tissue heart valve prosthesis may resolve the issue of IMR recurrence [8]. However, early postoperative survival might be better in ring annuloplasty group compared to replacement [9]. On the other hand, MR recurrence may reach up to 30% of cases within 1–2 years after surgery and may impair early mid-term and late survival of patients, and have an impact onto quality of life. Rigid, full ring annuloplasty (or a special shape and design annuloplasty ring designed for IMR) generally is accepted as a standard technique to resolve IMR problems. However, there are positive and negative sides of rigid annuloplasty techniques, in certain cases restrictive annuloplasty may induce functional mitral stenosis [10].

Ischemic MR is primarily a ventricular problem due to LV dilatation and dysfunction, that leads to both anterior and posterior leaflet tethering towards the apex. Severity of LV derangements after myocardial infarction do not mirror the degree of IMR. Secondly, changes occur with the size, shape and function of the mitral valve annulus and especially of LV basal segment motion contributing to IMR. It have been suggested that rigid annuloplasty ring may further impair mobility and function of LV basal segments, further increase tethering of mitral valve leaflets, increasing tension onto both commissures and subsequently onto both papillary muscles and in that way impair LV segmental function. This may further impair general LV systolic and diastolic function and subsequently postoperative clinical outcomes.

Indications for Suture Annuloplasty

As an alternative, mitral valve suture annuloplasty has been used with success in congenital, degenerative and ischemic MR cases. Several authors described and promoted different suture annuloplasty techniques (De Vega type, Panneth, Fratter), using different suture material. Polypropylene, PTFE, polyester braided sutures have been used. Polypropylene suture annuloplasty have been analyzed in a degenerative MR subset of patients [11]. The group have discovered week points of this suture material with ruptures and loosening of the suture within 8 years of the postoperative period. Others have used Goretex (PTFE) No. 2 suture with similar success and failure rates, because of suture material failure postoperatively. Much less is known about Polyester braided sutures. The main concern regarding suture annuloplasty remains durability of the results because of suture failures, annulus disruption and mitral valve annulus stability. Nevertheless, suture annuloplasty, if it is properly applied in selected groups of patients, may be easy and fast to perform, and give safe and durable results. Suture annuloplasty interferes least with the mitral valve annulus diameter, and the size and shape of the anterior leaflet; it also does not increase tethering of both commissural areas and the posterior mitral valve leaflet.

Paneth type suture annuloplasty effectively reduces septal-lateral and intercommisural annular diameters but does not reduce annular systolic shortening. It also does not have the additional effect on annular fixation and does not have impact onto both anterior and posterior leaflet mobility or excursions [12]. However, one must be aware of the anatomical and histological features of the mitral valve annulus. It appears, that a minority of the population have solid, well-defined mitral valve annulus. In the vast majority, the mitral valve annulus is present as an incomplete ring with only constant fibrous tissue in the trigones; the intertrigonal area although not ideally constant, remains stable in a majority of IMR patients [13]. Therefore, the fibrous trigones serving as an anchoring areas for suture annuloplasty.

Surgical Technique

With IMR, the majority of patients can be successfully treated using posterior mitral valve suture annuloplasty when the IMR is due to mitral valve annulus flattening and dilatation. In general, the same criteria applies when we select patients for rigid ring annuloplasty. The technique itself consists of a typical direct posterior left atriotomy or trans-septal approach. As a suture material, we use 2-0 Ethibond (Ethicon, Johnson & Johnson) suture with 3×1×6 mm pledgets. The suture line around the posteromedial commissure starts from the right fibrous trigone (Fig. 11.1). The first needle passes through the fibrous trigone to the mitral valve annulus, slightly into the LV base and then back to the annulus and 1 to 2 mm into the atrial side. The second needle/suture follows parallel to the first one but more to the atrial side, taking care of the coronary vessels within the atrio-ventricular grove (Fig. 11.2). The length of one step (bite) is approximately 7–9 mm. Then both needles are passed through the pledget, which is positioned perpendicular to the annulus, before repeating the next step: passing needle again into annulus, LV base and back to the annulus, and atrial site close to the annulus.

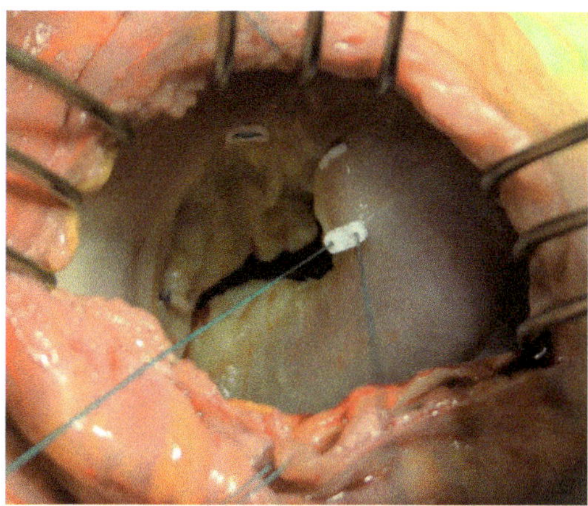

Fig. 11.1 Annuloplasty suture starts at the right fibrous trigone and a single bite (step) involves 7–9 mm of mitral valve annulus, and pledgets are positioned at the commissures, posterior leaflet identations and in the midportion of P2

All the pledgets are placed perpendicular to the mitral valve annulus except at the two trigones in order to avoid suture "waves" that can lead to suture straightening and loosening with subsequent annulus dilatation under volume loaded LV conditions. After the suture reaches the left fibrous trigone, the last pledget is oriented parallel to the annulus, and the suture tied. The posterior annulus is adjusted to the mitral valve anterior leaflet surface area size. This maneuver can be performed also using commercially available heart valve sizers (Fig. 11.3). By pulling the double Ethibond suture, one plicates the posterior annulus, and the perpendicular position of the pledgets allows this maneuver to be performed without excess tension on the mitral valve annulus at the suture insertion site. Also, the pledgets will disappear within the wrinkles of the atrial endocardium without distorting or deforming the mitral valve

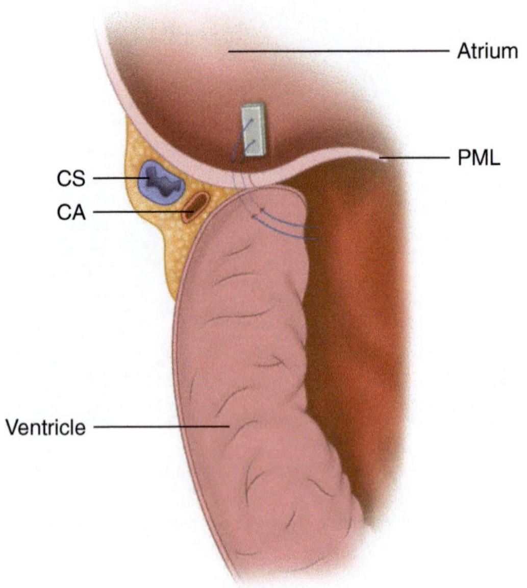

Fig. 11.2 Line diagram showing the direction of needle placement avoiding the coronary vessels in the atrioventricular groove. *Abbreviations*: atrium-left atrial wall, ventricle-left ventricular wall base, *PML* posterior mitral valve leaflet, *CS* coronary sinus, *CA* coronary artery

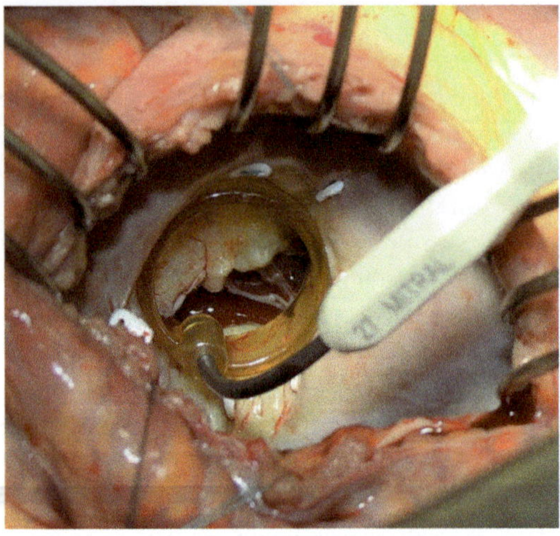

Fig. 11.3 Sizing of the MV annulus with heart valve sizer

posterior annulus and leaving minimum amount of prosthetic material within the left atrium (Fig. 11.4). Also, it should be noted that the preferred positions of the pledgets are: both commissures, the clefts between P1-P2 and P2-P3 and the central part of the P2 scallop (Fig. 11.5).

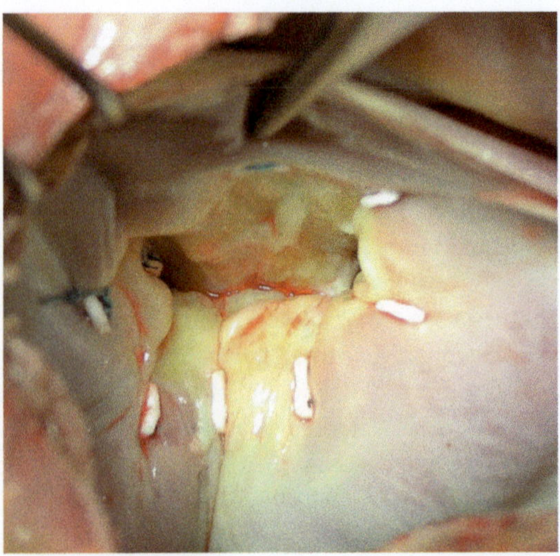

Fig. 11.4 Mitral valve view after suture annuloplasty is completed. Note: the shape of the mitral valve annulus is round and the pledgets disappear with endocardial folds

The positioning of the pledgets, regardless of the degree of posterior annulus diameter reduction, does not affect the shape and surface of posterior mitral valve leaflet (Fig. 11.6).

The placement of annuloplasty sutures within the annulus, towards the LV, and the second suture close to the first one, within the atrioventricular grove, does not present a higher risk of catching coronary vessels at any place of the mitral valve annulus. In the left fibrous trigone area, care has to be taken during suture placement because the aortic valve cusps are in the vicinity. Keeping the anterior mitral valve annulus free from any type of annuloplasty preserves the anterior mitral valve leaflet movement towards the posterior annulus during the beginning of LV systole. Such a double suture purse string annuloplasty can be easily controlled by performing hydraulic/water test before atrial closure and absolutely obligatory transesophageal echocardiography (TEE) after aortic cross clamp is released and the heart starts beating.

What might be unfavorable clinical situations for suture annuloplasty? In fact, the same TEE characteristics which are unfavorable for ring annuloplasty: MV leaflet coaptation depth $\geq$ 1 cm,

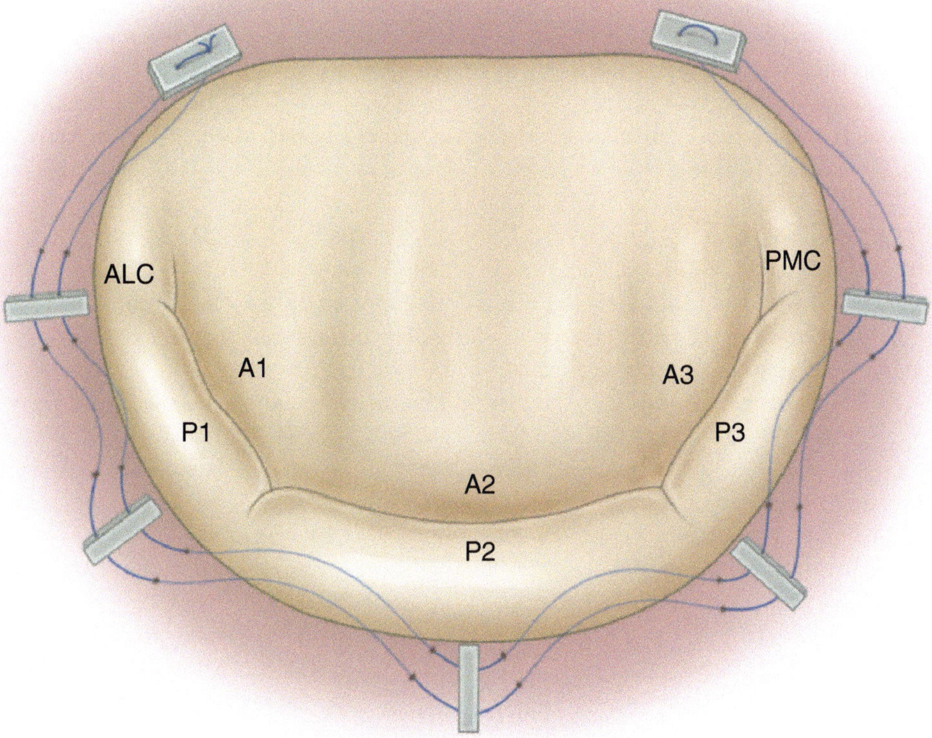

Fig. 11.5 Line diagram showing the placement of pledgets and sutures for suture annuloplasty. Note that the first and last pledgets are placed at the fibrous trigones and are oriented parallel to the mitral annulus, all other pledgets in between are orientated perpendicular to the mitral annulus and are positioned at the commissures, at the clefts between P1 and P2, between P2 and P3 and in the middle of the P2 scallop. *Abbreviations*: *ALC* anterolateral commissure, *PMC* posteromedial commissure, *A1-A2-A3* anterior mitral valve leaflet scallops, *P1-P2-P3* posterior mitral valve leaflet scallops

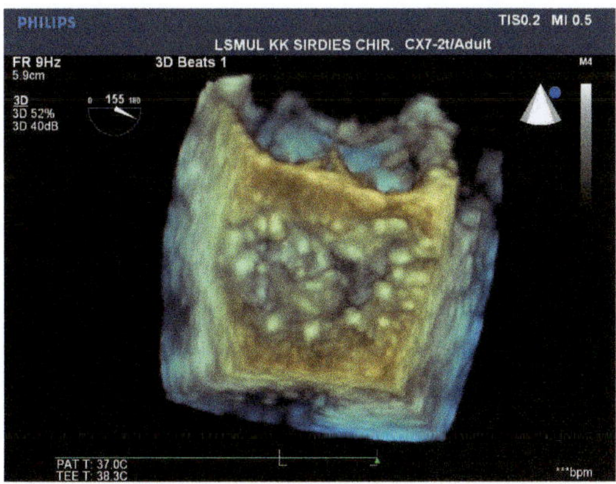

Fig. 11.6 3D echocardiographic image of suture annulo plasty. Note: No deformities and immobilization of the anterior mitral valve leaflet base

mitral valve tenting area >2.5–3 cm^2, high posterior leaflet tethering (postero-lateral angle >45°), interpapillary muscle distance >20 mm, posterior papillary muscle-right fibrous trigone distance >40 mm, basal lateral LV aneurysm (between mitral valve annulus and papillary muscle), global LV remodeling (LVEDD > 65 mm, LVESD > 51 mm, ESV > 140 ml), and systolic sphericity index > 0.7 [14].

Results

From our own series, we have analyzed 361 patients out of 518 in whom during the period of 1998–2011 we have performed suture annuloplasty along with CABG. The mean age of patients was 66.6 ± 9.4 years, mean NYHA class 2.8 ± 0.6, mean IMR grade 2.7 ± 0.5, mean LVEF 34.6 ± 10.7 %, mean LVEDDI 29.4 ± 4.8 mm/m^2. One year mortality (including hospital mortality) was 13.6 %. Late mortality was 9.3 %.

At a mean follow-up of 43.2 months, LVEDDI increased by at least 10 % in 22.6 % of patients, and in 77.4 %, LVEDDI increased by less than 10 % or remained the same. Mild and/or trivial MR was observed in 85.5 % of patients, and in 14.5 % increased up to moderate/severe. There were stable changes in mitral valve annulus septolateral diameter within a group of patients without MR recurrence. Mitral valve septal-lateral diameters reduced from 38.09 ± 4.62 mm preoperatively to 23.92 ± 3.65 mm early postoperatively, and remained at a mean of 27.22 ± 4.26 mm 43.18 months after surgery. And in a group of patients with MR recurrence (IMR ≥ moderate), mean septal-lateral diameter reduced from 43.5 ± 5.32 mm preoperatively to 30.0 ± 6.25 mm early postoperatively, and remained at 30.6 ± 2.41 mm 43.18 months postoperatively.

However, not only mitral valve annulus diameter have played a role in IMR recurrence. We have found that in patients with mild to moderate MR, LVEDD was significantly higher in MV recurrence group (52.61 ± 5.04 mm vs 47.38 ± 2.82 mm, $p = 0.014$), LA diameter 45.29 ± 1.77 mm vs 38.92 ± 2.85, $p < 0.001$) and regional wall contraction index 1.76 ± 0.33 vs 1.51 ± 0.13, $p = 0.032$ (Table 11.1). While in a group of patients with mild MR, only LVEF was important with a p value < 0.05 in a MR recurrence group 38.24 ± 8.9 % vs 46.94 ± 4.76 % (Table 11.2).

When the factors of further negative LV remodeling following CABG + MV repair after 1 year postoperatively have been analyzed, only LVEDDI ($p < 0.001$), LVEDSI ($p = 0.003$), preoperative tricuspid regurgitation ($p = 0.042$) and early postoperative residual MR ($p = 0.033$) were identified as risk factors. Multivariate ANOVA analysis revealed that if LVEDDI before surgery is less than 25 mm/m^2, the probability for LVEDDI to diminish or to stay at the same range is 84,6 % higher than in the case of preoperative LVEDDI ≥ 25 mm/m^2 and the same applies to other above mentioned predictive variables. On the other hand the most predictive factors correlating with recurrent MR following ischemic MV repair have been found as follows: LVEDDI ($p = 0.037$), LV wall motion score index ($p = 0.042$), high preoperative MR grade ($p = 0.013$) and increased preoperative systolic pulmonary artery pressure ($p = 0.04$), while no correlations have been found between MR recurrence and patient age, NYHA class, number of involved coronary arteries, multiple MI in the past and/or surgical technique: ring or suture annuloplasty [15].

For the surgeons dealing with all the spectrum of clinical situations in patients with IMR, it is important to have as many surgical techniques as possible, not only dealing with LV restoration, subvalvular procedures, but also sometimes simple suture annuloplasty techniques to correct MV annulus size in a selected group of patients. This technique is fast and easily reproducible, which is very important in complex cardiac surgery procedures and provides comparable results to rigid ring annuloplasty.

Table 11.1 Echocardiographic changes in patients with moderate/severe MR

Echocardiographic parameters	MR progressed	MR did not change	p
Left ventricular end diastolic diameter, mm	52.61 ± 5.04	47.38 ± 2.82	0.014
Left ventricular end diastolic diameter index, mm/m^2	26.21 ± 2.27	25.35 ± 1.04	0.379
Left ventricle ejection fraction, %	39 ± 7.63	42.42 ± 3.96	0.279
Left atrium size, mm	45.29 ± 1.77	38.92 ± 2.85	<0.001
Pulmonary artery mean gradient, mmHg	22.69 ± 6.83	25.38 ± 3.36	0.642
Region wall contraction	1.76 ± 0.34	1.51 ± 0.13	0.032

Table 11.2 Echocardiographic changes in patients with mild MR

Echocardiographic parameters	MR progressed	MR did not change
Left ventricular end diastolic diameter, mm	49.55±4.97	49.19±5.43
Left ventricular end diastolic diameter index, mm/m^2	24.8±2.1	24.13±1.95
Left ventricle ejection fraction, percentage	38.24±8.9	46.94±4.76*
Left atrium, mm	41.19±3.75	39.13±2.97
Pulmonary artery mean gradient, mmHg	27.69±6.69	27.07±9.09
Region wall contraction	1.74±0.22	1.66±0.21

* $p < 0.05$

References

1. Kang DH, Kim M-J, Kang S-J, Song J-M. Mitral valve repair versus revascularization alone in the treatment of ischemic mitral regurgitation. Circulation. 2006;114:I499.
2. Mallidi HR, Pelletier MP, Jennifer L, Nimesh D, Sever J. Late outcomes in patients with uncorrected mild to moderate mitral regurgitation at the time of isolated coronary artery bypass grafting. J Thorac Cardiovasc Surg. 2004;127:636–44.
3. Mihaljevic T, Lam B-K, Razzouk A, Takagaki M, Lauer MS, Gillinov AM, Blackstone EH, Lytle BW. Impact of mitral valve annuloplasty combined with revascularization in patients with functional ischemic mitral regurgitation. J Am Coll Cardiol. 2007;49:2191–201.
4. Fattouch K, Guccione F, Sampognaro R, Panzarella G, Corrado E, Navarra E, Calvaruso D, Ruvolo G. Efficacy of adding mitral valve annuloplasty to coronary artery bypass grafting in patients with moderate ischemic mitral valve regurgitation: a randomized trial. J Thorac Cardiovasc Surg. 2009;138:278–85.
5. Chan KMJ, Punjabi PP, Flather M, Wage RR, Symmonds K, Roussin I, Rahman-Haley S, Pennell DJ, Kilner PJ, Dreyfus GD, Pepper JR, Investigators R. Coronary artery bypass surgery with or without mitral valve annuloplasty in moderate functional ischemic mitral regurgitation: final results of the randomized ischemic mitral evaluation (RIME) trial. Circulation. 2012;126:2502–10.
6. Nishimura RA, Otto CM, Bonow RO, Carabello BA, Erwin JP, Guyton RA, O'Gara PT, Ruiz CE, Skubas NJ, Sorajja P, Sundt TM, Thomas JD. 2014 AHA/ACC guideline for the management of patients with valvular heart disease. J Am Coll Cardiol. 2014;63:e57–185.
7. Vahanian A, Alfieri O, Andreotti F, Antunes MJ, Baron-Esquivias G, Baumgartner H, Borger MA, Carrel TP, De Bonis M, Evangelista A, Falk V, Iung B, Lancellotti P, Pierard LA, Price S, Schafers H-J, Schuler G, Stepinska J, Swedberg K, Takkenberg J, Oppel UOV, Windecker S, Zamorano JL, Zembala M. ESC/EACTS guidelines on the management of valvular heart disease (version 2012). Eur Heart J. 2012;33:2451–96.
8. Acker MA, Parides MK, Perrault LP, Moskowitz AJ, Gelijns AC, Voisine P, Smith PK, Hung JW, Blackstone EH, Puskas JD, Argenziano M, Gammie JS, Mack M, Ascheim DD, Bagiella E, Moquete EG, Ferguson TB, Horvath KA, Geller NL, Miller MA, Woo YJ, D'Alessandro DA, Ailawadi G, Dagenais F, Gardner TJ, O'Gara PT, Michler RE, Kron IL. Mitral valve repair versus replacement for severe ischemic mitral regurgitation. N Engl J Med. 2014;370:23–32.
9. Vassileva CM, Boley T, Markwell S, Hazelrigg S. Meta-analysis of short term and long term survival following repair versus replacement for ischemic mitral regurgitation. Eur J Cardiothorac Surg. 2011;39:295–303.
10. Magne J, Senechal M, Mathieu P, Dumesnil JG, Dagenais F, Pibarot P. Restrictive annuloplasty for ischemic mitral regurgitation may induce functional mitral stenosis. J Am Coll Cardiol. 2008;51:1692–701.
11. Aybek T, Risteski P, Miskovic A, Simon A, Dogan S, Abdel-Rahman U, Moritz A. Seven years' experience with suture annuloplasty for mitral valve repair. J Thorac Cardiovasc Surg. 2006;131:99–106.
12. Tibayan FA, Rodriguez F, Liang D, Daughters GT, Ingels NB, Miller C. Paneth suture annuloplasty abolishes acute ischemic mitral regurgitation but preserves annular and leaflet dynamics. Circulation. 2003;108:II-128–33.
13. Angelini A, Ho SY, Anderson RH, Davies MJ, Becker AE. A histological study of the atrioventricular junction in hearts with normal and prolapsed leaflets of the mitral valve. Br Heart J. 1988;59:712–6.
14. Lancellotti P, Marwick T, Pierard LA. How to manage ischaemic mitral regurgitation. Heart. 2008;94:1497–502.
15. Mikuckaite L, Vaskelyte J, Radauskaite G, Zailunas R, Benetis R. Left ventricular remodeling following ischemic mitral valve repair: predictive factors. Scand Cardiovasc J. 2009;43(1):57–62.

Mitral Valve Replacement for Functional Mitral Regurgitation

12

Arminder S. Jassar and Michael A. Acker

Abstract

Functional mitral regurgitation (FMR) is defined as mitral regurgitation in absence of any primary leaflet pathology. FMR occurs in the setting of an abnormal and dilated left ventricle and apically displaced papillary muscles, with leaflet malcoaptation occurring either as a result of annular dilation or leaflet tethering, or both. FMR can either be ischemic, where adverse LV remodeling is caused by coronary artery disease and myocardial infarction, or non-ischemic due to idiopathic or dilated cardiomyopathy. Thus, in FMR, mitral regurgitation is only one component of the disease pathophysiology, and the treatment of MR is not curative of the underlying disease pathology. The current mainstay of treatment of FMR is undersized ring annuloplasty that treats only the annular dilation but does little to improve leaflet tethering. As such, mitral valve repair for FMR is far less durable than repair of myxomatous mitral regurgitation and is associated with significant rate of recurrent MR. Thus, in patients whom limited repair durability and FMR recurrence is expected, mitral valve replacement (MVR) with a prosthetic valve may be a better choice than MV repair. In this chapter, we discuss indications, techniques, results, and evidence based decision making for mitral valve replacement for severe FMR

Keywords

Functional mitral regurgitation • Ischemic mitral regurgitation • Mitral valve replacement • Prosthetic mitral valve

A.S. Jassar, MBBS (✉)
Division of Cardiovascular Surgery,
Hospital of the University of Pennsylvania,
3400 Spruce Street, 6 Silverstein Pavilion,
Philadelphia, PA 19104, USA
e-mail: ASJassar@gmail.com

M.A. Acker
Division of Cardiovascular Surgery, Penn Medicine
Heart and Vascular Center, Philadelphia, PA, USA

Department of Surgery, Hospital of the University
of Pennsylvania, Perelman School of Medicine
of the University of Pennsylvania, 3400 Spruce
Street, Philadelphia, PA 19104, USA

K.M.J. Chan (ed.), *Functional Mitral and Tricuspid Regurgitation*,
DOI 10.1007/978-3-319-43510-7_12

Principles of Treatment

Functional mitral regurgitation (FMR) is defined as mitral regurgitation (MR) in absence of any primary leaflet pathology. FMR occurs in the setting of an abnormal and dilated left ventricle and apically displaced papillary muscles, with leaflet malcoaptation occurring either as a result of annular dilation (type I dysfunction) or leaflet tethering (type IIIb dysfunction), or both. FMR can either be ischemic, where adverse LV remodeling is caused by coronary artery disease and myocardial infarction, or non-ischemic due to idiopathic or dilated cardiomyopathy. Thus, in FMR, mitral regurgitation is only one component of the disease pathophysiology, and the treatment of MR is not curative. The current mainstay of treatment of FMR is undersized ring annuloplasty that treats only the annular dilation but does little to improve leaflet tethering. As such, mitral valve repair for FMR is far less durable than repair of myxomatous mitral regurgitation and is associated with significant rate of recurrent MR [1, 2]. Presence of MR after myocardial infarction increases mortality risk in direct relation to the degree of MR [3]. Thus, in patients whom limited repair durability and FMR recurrence is expected, mitral valve replacement (MVR) with a prosthetic valve may be a better choice than MV repair.

Echocardiography remains the mainstay for assessment of FMR and is useful to establish MR etiology and assess global LV function. Quantification of FMR is more challenging than for MR due to leaflet prolapse because the regurgitant orifice and the resultant MR jet in FMR is often non-circular and asymmetric, and can be underestimated by standard flow convergence methods of grading MR severity. Recently, 3D-echocardiography has been utilized for characterizing regional patterns of leaflet tethering and direct assessment of severity of FMR [4–6]. Adjunct studies (nuclear stress test, PET scan, Cardiac MR, cardiac catheterization) may help assess myocardial viability and influence management of FMR.

Choice of valve intervention (repair vs. replacement) and prosthetic valve type (bioprosthetic vs. mechanical) should be a shared decision process between the surgeon and the patient with full disclosure of recurrence risk, risks of anticoagulant therapy and the potential need for reoperation, and must take into account the patient's preference. A mechanical prosthesis is reasonable in patients <60 years of age who do not have a contraindication to anticoagulation. A bioprosthesis is recommended in patients of any age for whom anticoagulant therapy is contraindicated, or cannot be managed appropriately, or is not desired. A bioprosthesis is reasonable in patients >70 years of age. Either a bioprosthetic or mechanical valve is reasonable in patients between 60 and 70 years of age [7]. These recommendations are based on the risk of anticoagulation with mechanical prostheses and limited durability and need for redo replacement with bioprosthetic valves. However, recent studies have reported low operative mortality (~5 %) for redo-MVR and have suggested use of bioprosthetic valves even in younger patients [8, 9].

Surgical Operative Technique and Perioperative Care

Preoperative Work-Up

All patients should have a detailed history and physical examination, chest x-ray, and echocardiography. Standard laboratory tests (CBC, serum chemistry, liver function tests, coagulation profile, blood typing and cross matching) are performed. Additional testing (e.g., liver ultrasound, carotid duplex) is performed to further characterize any abnormalities that may be discovered. In diabetic patients, hemoglobin A_{1C} levels are measured to determine efficacy of glycemic control. Coronary angiography is performed to detect presence of coronary artery disease. Right heart catheterization is useful to assess cardiac output and degree of pulmonary hypertension. For reoperative patients, chest computed tomography is performed to assess relationship of aorta, right ventricle, and any patent bypass grafts to the sternum. Dental clearance should be obtained prior to valve replacement surgery. Patient's medication list should be carefully reviewed; most medications should be continued until the day before the operation, with some exceptions. ACE inhibitors should be stopped 48 h before surgery to prevent intraoperative vasodilation and hypotension. It is advisable to discontinue Plavix for 5–7 days before surgery whenever possible. Patients taking warfarin should stop taking this medication for 2–3 days prior to operation, and bridge therapy with either subcutaneous low molecular weight or intravenous heparin may be considered in select patients with high risk of thromboembolic events (e.g., previous mechanical valve).

Anesthesia and Monitoring

In the operating room, general anesthesia is induced and endotracheal intubation is performed. Arterial line, pulmonary artery catheter and urinary catheter are placed. External defibrillator pads are applied for redo operations and for minimally invasive approaches. Intraoperative TEE is performed in every patient to assess overall cardiac function and presence of any other concomitant pathology. Intraoperative TEE is a great tool for evaluating mechanism, etiology and anatomic pathology of FMR, however it is not reliable to assess MR severity due to altered physiologic loading conditions under general anesthesia. Intraoperative TEE is also critical to assess prosthetic valve function, presence of any paravalvular leaks, to assess cardiac function and guide de-airing of the heart after MV implantation.

Surgical Approaches

Median Sternotomy

Median sternotomy is the traditional approach to mitral valve operations, and is suitable for all patients including patients undergoing redo operations and those undergoing concomitant cardiac procedures. Patient is placed supine with arms tucked by their side and a shoulder roll placed behind their back. Small skin sparing incisions can be performed with excellent visualization of the mitral valve. Pericardium is opened in midline to expose the heart; no pleural space is entered. This incision is the most versatile and provides complete access to all cardiac structures.

Right Anterolateral Thoracotomy

This incision is performed for cosmetic reasons, and is preferred by some surgeons for redo operations. It is generally contraindicated in cases of previous right chest surgery because dense pulmonary adhesions may be encountered, and in patients with severe COPD where single lung ventilation may be poorly tolerated. Although some concomitant procedures (e.g., Tricuspid valve repair or replacement, MAZE procedure) can be performed using this approach, it is not suitable when other procedures such as CABG or AVR may be indicated. Double lumen endotracheal tube is placed to provide single lung ventilation to the left lung. Patient is positioned supine with a bump under the right chest to elevate it by about 30°. Arms can be left at the patient's side while ensuring access to the right axilla. External defibrillator pads are placed prior to incision. In redo operations, placing epicardial pacing wires can be challenging and a swan ganz catheter with transvenous pacing capablity may be utilized. After right lung is deflated, right pleural cavity is entered via the fourth intercostal space. Pericardium is entered anterior to the Phrenic nerve to expose the heart.

Minimally Invasive Approaches: Partial Sternotomy, Video Assisted and Robotic Approaches

Lower hemisternotomy incision can be used for mitral and tricuspid valve procedures. A small skin incision is made inferior to the manubrium and the sternotomy is extended from the xiphoid process up to the second intercostal space and teed off to the right side. Care must be taken to avoid injury to the right internal mammary artery during this process.

The video assisted and robotic approaches use the right chest to access the mitral valve, usually through a small (4–5 cm) incision in the fourth intercostal space. Alternate cannulation and cross clamp strategies (discussed below) are often necessary for conduct of the operation through these approaches.

Cardiopulmonary Bypass and Myocardial Protection

Sternotomy/Partial Sternotomy: Arterial cannulation for cardiopulmonary bypass is established via the ascending aorta. Venous drainage is established by cannulating the superior and the inferior vena cava (SVC, IVC). Retrograde cardioplegia catheter is placed into the coronary sinus. A catheter is placed in the ascending aorta to deliver antegrade cardioplegia. Initial cardiac arrest is attained with antegrade cardioplegia (1 L of high potassium cardioplegia) after aorta is cross clamped. Intermittent retrograde cardioplegia is given during the procedure using either a low potassium cardioplegia solution or with cold blood. Mild systemic hypothermia is maintained at 30–32 °C.

Alternate Cannulation Strategies

Alternate approaches to establishing cardiopulmonary bypass are necessary for minimally invasive and robotic approaches. Arterial cannulation is generally established via the femoral artery, although right axillary artery can be used as well. Bi-caval venous drainage is achieved by cannulating the internal jugular vein with a 16 Fr cannula, and cannulating the right atrium using a long venous drainage cannula introduced through the femoral vein. Aortic occlusion can be obtained either by inflating an intra-arterial balloon in the ascending aorta (Endoballoon) or by directly clamping the ascending aorta using the Chitwood clamp [10]. Antegrade cardioplegia is delivered either through a port of the endoballoon or through a catheter directly placed in the ascending aorta if a Chitwood clamp is used. A retrograde cardioplegia catheter can be placed under echocardiographic guidance via the internal jugular vein if necessary.

In patients where aortic cross clamping is not possible (adhesions, porcelain aorta), the operation can be performed on a fibrillating heart without aortic cross clamping.

Exposure of the Mitral Valve

Surgical exposure of the mitral valve is traditionally obtained by developing the interatrial groove of Sondergaard and entering the left atrium anterior to the right pulmonary veins, close to the interatrial septum (Fig. 12.1). The incision is carried from in front of the SVC superiorly and to a point midway between the right inferior pulmonary vein and the IVC inferiorly. Care must be taken not to make the incision too close to the pulmonary veins to avoid narrowing during closure. If the right atrium is inadvertently entered, it can be closed with a running prolene suture. Blades of a self-retaining Cosgrove retractor are placed to retract the left atrial walls anteriorly to expose the mitral valve. Once the left atrium is open, a flexible cardiotomy suction is placed into the dependent pulmonary veins to drain the pulmonary venous return and maintain a bloodless field.

Alternatively, in some cases of previous aortic valve replacement, or in some reoperative mitral valve operations with significant adhesions between the right atrium and the pericardium, a trans-septal approach can be utilized. This involves making a longitudinal right atriotomy and entering the left atrium by incising the fossa ovalis. After the prosthetic valve is implanted, the interatrial septum is closed using a running 3-0 prolene stuture or with a pericardial patch.

In cases where the exposure of mitral valve is difficult, additional maneuvers may be necessary for better visualization. Circumferential dissection can be carried out around the SVC and the IVC to extend the left atrial incision both cephalad and caudad and allow better retraction of the left atrium. The SVC can also be divided circumferentially to enhance left atrial retraction and expose the mitral valve. SVC is then re-anastomosed in an end to end fashion using a running 5-0 prolene suture. The mitral valve exposure can also be enhanced by making an additional incision perpendicular to the left atrial incision and extending into the right atrium and the septum through the fossa ovalis.

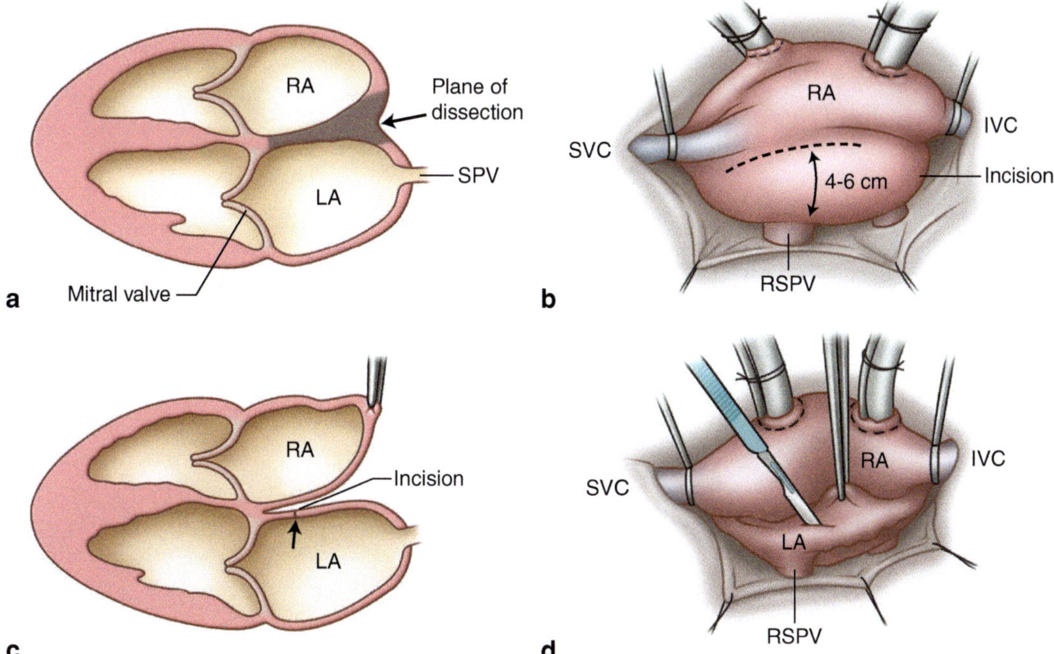

Fig. 12.1 Schematic of approach to the mitral valve through the Sondergaard's groove. The Sondergaards groove is developed to separate the right atrium from the left atrium (**a**). The left atrium is entered 4–6 cm in front of the pulmonary veins, close to the mitral valve (**b**–**d**). *IVC* inferior vena cava, *LA* left atrium, *RA* right atrium, *RSPV* right superior vena cava, *SPV* superior pulmonary cava, *SVC* superior vena cava (From Cohn [34])

Mitral Valve Implantation

Mitral valve replacement should be a total chordal sparing replacement; non-chordal sparing mitral replacement should be completely abandoned. Several studies comparing no chordal sparing techniques, partial or complete chordal sparing mitral valve replacement have demonstrated that left ventricular volume and function are much better preserved with complete chordal sparing techniques [11–13].

Several techniques have been described for total chordal preservation during MVR for functional MR, including anterior flip-over, in which a C-shaped curved incision is placed in the anterior leaflet 2–3 mm away from the anterior annulus and extended from anterolateral to posteromedial commissures and the entire anterior leaflet apparatus is moved posteriorly (Fig. 12.2a, b). A second method of achieving chordal preservation is to separate the anterior leaflet from the annulus as described above, but then resect the center of the anterior leaflet and affix the remaining portions of the anterior leaflet to the anterior and posterior commissures using a prolene suture (Fig. 12.2c, d). The sutures for MVR are placed around the posterior annulus, and incorporating the posterior leaflet, thus placing both the chordal apparatus and leaflets posterior to the mitral valve prosthesis. This is critically important for mechanical valves because any loose native leaflet tissue may impede opening of prosthetic valve leaflets.

MV prosthesis can be affixed to the mitral annulus using either a running or an interrupted technique. We prefer the interrupted technique where pledgeted 0-Ticron stitches are placed circumferentially in a horizontal mattress configuration. The pledgets are typically placed on the atrial side and the suture is passed from the atrium to the ventricle then passed either around or through the leading leaflet edge to allow for an intra-annular placement of the MV prosthesis. First suture is placed in the midportion of the posterior annulus;

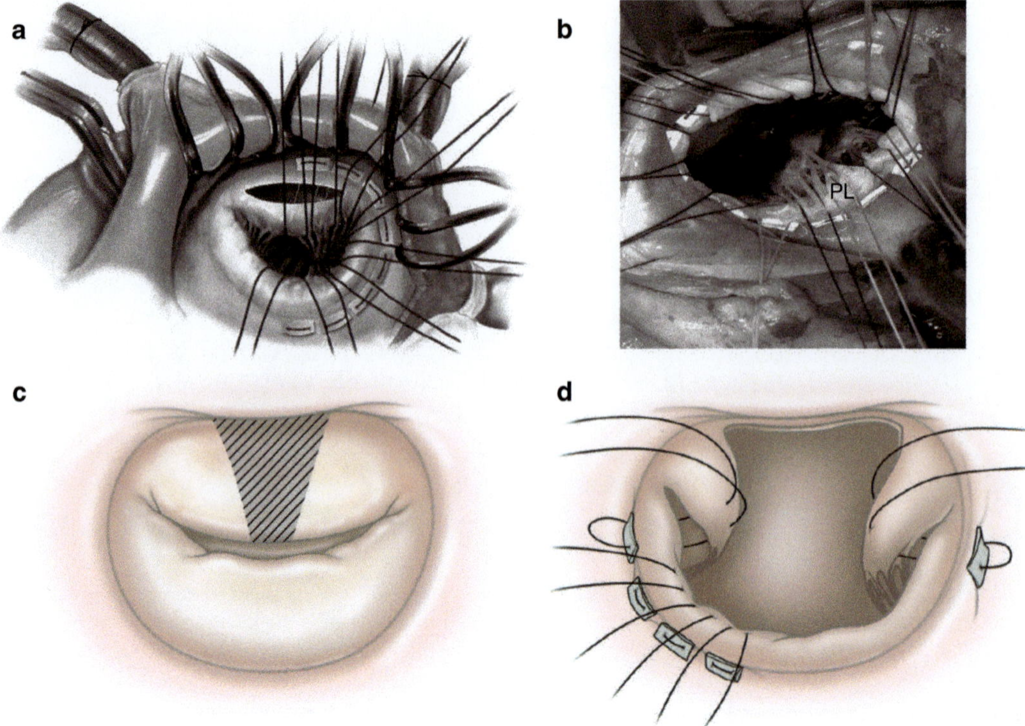

Fig. 12.2 Techniques of chordal preservation for mitral valve replacement. A flap is cut from the central portion of the anterior leaflet and is flipped to the posterior annulus (**a**, **b**). Alternatively, the central portion of the anterior leaflet is resected (*Shaded area* in **c**). The remnants are anchored to the anterior and posterior commissure and incorporated in the annular stitches (**c**, **d**). *PL* posterior leaflet (Figures 12.2a, b Courtesy of Dr. Steven Bolling, University of Michigan, Ann Arbor, Michigan)

the strings of this suture can then be used to retract and expose the annulus to facilitate placement of the next stitch. Sutures are, placed in this fashion, first towards the posterior trigone, then towards the anterior trigone, and finally around the anterior annulus. Several important structures lie in close proximity to the mitral valve and their location must be kept in mind as sutures are being placed (Fig. 12.3). The circumflex artery lies adjacent to the posterior annulus and comes closest to annulus in the region of the anterior commissure of the mitral valve. The coronary sinus lies close to the posteromedial aspect of the mitral annulus. The left- non coronary commissure of the aortic valve lies behind the midpoint of the anterior mitral valve leaflet. The conduction system lies close to the posteromedial trigone. These structures can be damaged if excessively deep sutures are placed during mitral valve replacement.

Valve sizing for IMR should be prudent and not "oversized". With modern mitral valve prostheses there should not be a worry of stenosis. Overly large bulky valves may impair LV dynamics and interventricular conduction, in these already poor LVs. Also, if concomitant aortic valve replacement is planned, oversizing of the mitral prosthesis may necessitate undersizing of the aortic prosthesis and result in patient prosthesis mismatch. Once appropriate valve is chosen, individual sutures are passed through the sewing ring while maintaining proper suture orientation. Attention must be paid to orienting the valve properly to avoid LV outflow tract obstruction, especially by the strut posts of the bioprosthetic valves. This can be avoided by aligning one of the valve posts with the native anterior commissure and allow the valve posts to straddle the LVOT. This is not an issue with mechanical

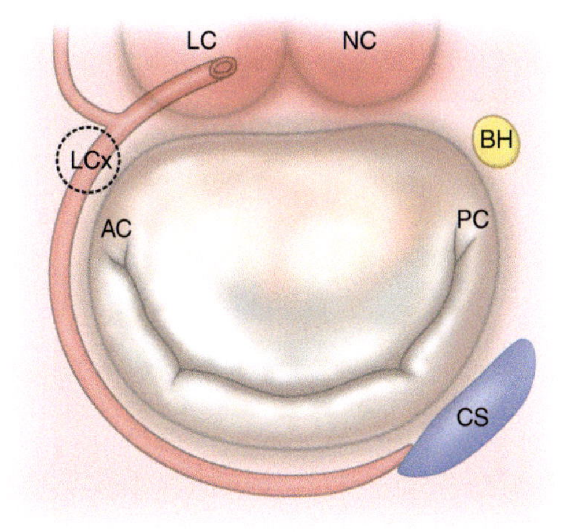

Fig. 12.3 Structures at risk of injury during placement of annular stitches for mitral valve replacement. *AC* anterior commissure, *BH* bundle of his, *CS* coronary sinus, *LC* left coronary sinus of the aortic valve, *LCx* left circumflex artery, *NC* non coronary sinus of the aortic valve, *PC* posterior commissure

valves due to their lower profile as compared to bioprosthetic valves. The exact orientation of a mechanical valve is not important as long as the leaflets open and close without obstruction. Once all the sutures are passed through the valve sowing ring, the valve is lowered to the annulus and sutures are tied. During this step, it is crucial to ensure that none of the suture strings are looped around the valve posts, as this will result in improper seating of the valve on to the annulus and significant paravalvular MR.

Presence of mitral annular calcification (MAC) can make the procedure very challenging and even perilous. Surgical approach must be modified to avoid catastrophic complications. In presence of severe MAC, we place the sutures in a non-everting fashion from the ventricular to the atrial side, thus reducing the stress on the annulus as the sutures are tied down. Aggressive debridement of annular calcification can result in injury to the circumflex artery or even disruption of the atrioventricular groove. We debride the calcium only to the minimum extent necessary to allow sutures to be placed around the annulus. Ultrasonic tissue ablation can be used to facilitate annular debridement in a controlled fashion.

After the sutures are tied, the prosthetic valve is checked for proper function. For bioprosthetic valves, this can be done by instillation of saline into the left ventricle and checking proper leaflet apposition. For mechanical valves, the leaflets are held in the open position and inspection of the subvalvular structures is conducted circumferentially. Any tissue that may restrict leaflet opening must be resected. A metal hook is used to check the suture line on the sowing ring to detect any gaps. If any gaps are found, extra stitches can be placed to reef up atrial tissue to prevent paravalvular leaks.

Completion of Procedure and Weaning from Bypass

After satisfactory valve inspection, left atrium is closed. To achieve this, pledgeted 3-0 prolene sutures are placed at either end of the atriotomy incision and run towards the middle. Once in the middle, they are snared and a left ventricular suction catheter is placed through the prosthetic valve under direct vision, and brought out through the atriotomy incision. The heart is de-aired, and aortic cross clamp is removed. Temporary atrial and ventricular epicardial pacing wires are placed. The LV vent is removed once adequate LV ejection is achieved. TEE is performed to ensure complete de-airing and proper valve functioning. Once heart is de-aired, and adequate cardiac function is observed, patient is weaned from bypass, and protamine is administered. All cannulae are removed, hemostasis is ensured, and chest is closed after placement of drainage catheters. In patients with depressed cardiac function and concomitant coronary artery disease, intra-aortic balloon pump placement may be necessary.

Concomitant Procedures

If concomitant CABG is planned, the distal anastomoses are performed prior to mitral valve replacement. Adequate hemostasis must be achieved at distal anastomotic sites as they may not be accessible after mitral valve implantation because aggressive lifting or manipulation of the heart is avoided after MVR as it may result in ventricular perforation by a valve strut, especially in the setting of calcified annuli. This order also allows delivery of cardioplegia through the vein grafts.

If patient also needs AVR at the time of mitral surgery, this is generally performed after the MVR. Many surgeons open the aorta, resect leaflets and debride the aortic annulus in preparation for AVR, before directing attention to the mitral valve, and then return to implant the aortic valve after the MVR has been completed. In absence of significant aortic regurgitation, this approach can sometimes be modified to leave the aortic valve in situ till after the MVR to give a robust dose of antegrade cardioplegia after MVR before opening the aorta. Tricuspid valve repairs are performed after the mitral and the aortic valves have been replaced.

Postoperative Care

Inotropic support is generally necessary to maintain adequate perfusion, but should be weaned as feasible. Once the bleeding has subsided, anticoagulation is initiated. Anticoagulation is recommended for both bioprosthetic (short-term) and mechanical prosthetic valves. We generally bridge with intravenous heparin while awaiting for therapeutic INR level (2.5–3.5).

Results

Operative mortality for mitral valve replacement has decreased significantly in recent years. A recent study by Acker et al. [1] reported risk of mortality and stroke after MVR for ischemic mitral regurgitation to be 4 % and 3.2 % respectively at 30 days and 14.3 % and 4.0 % respectively at 1 year. There was reduction in heart failure symptoms in 61.2 % of patients, and improvement in physical health in 18.4 % of patients at 1 year. A subset of patients remain in heart failure due to presence of depressed LV function prior to the operation. Chikwe et al. [9] studied survival and outcomes after bioprosthetic and mechanical mitral valve replacement in patients 50–69 years of age and reported 4–5 % risk of mortality, 2 % risk of stroke, 4–6 % risk of bleeding, 10–13 % incidence of atrial fibrillation, 4 % risk of acute kidney injury and 16–21 % risk of respiratory failure within 30 days of MVR. Actuarial 15 year survival was 57.5 % in the patients who received mechanical prosthetic and 59.9 % in patients who received a bioprosthetic valve. While risk of reoperation was lower in patients who received a mechanical prosthetic (5 % vs 11.1 %), risk of bleeding (14.9 % vs 9 %) and risk of stroke (14 % vs. 6.8 %) was higher as compared to patients who received a bioprosthetic valve. Similar to their results, Ribeiro et al [14] found no difference in long term survival between valve prosthesis types. These authors reported a 10 and 20 year survival of 74.2 % and 69.3 % after replacement with mechanical prosthetic and 71 % and 56.6 % with biologic valve prosthesis respectively. The probabilities of remaining free of reoperation at 10 years after surgery was higher using a mechanical substitute (92.7 %) than after surgery with a bioprosthesis (86.4 %). However, in this series the probability of remaining free of bleeding events at 10 years after surgery was similar when using a mechanical substitute (91.0 %) or a bioprosthesis (94.0 %, $p=0.267$). Based on these observations these authors have suggested that implantation of bioprosthetic valves may be reasonable even in younger patients.

The incidence of thromboembolism is about 1.5–3 % per patient year after MVR and is thought to be similar between currently used mechanical and bioprosthetic valves. Patients with large left atrium with intra-atrial clot or chronic atrial fibrillation are at a higher risk of thromboembolic complications. As long as effective anticoagulation is maintained, thrombosis of mechanical valves is relatively uncommon. Patients who present with mechanical valve thrombosis may need surgery if other methods fail or if patient is in shock because of MV obstruction. Generally, this can be treated with removing the clot from the valve, and does not require re-replacement of the valve as long as there is no concern for infection and the leaflets are functioning normally.

Incidence of paravalvular leak is about 0–1.5 % per patient year and is more common with mechanical valves. Patients may present with anemia due to hemolysis or symptoms of recurrent heart failure due to MR. At surgery, if the site of leak is identified, it is generally possible to close the defect with additional pledgeted sutures in that area.

Prosthetic mitral valve endocarditis is a serious complication and can present with fevers, embolic complications, septicemia or signs of heart failure due to valve dysfunction. It may be associated with valve vegetations and annular abscesses. Incidence of endocarditis is similar after biologic or mechanical prosthetic valves. Surgery is indicated for persistent sepsis, heart failure, significant paravalvular leak, large vegetations, or occurrence of embolic phenomenon. Optimal timing of surgery is debated, but early surgery is generally recommended, except in presence of recent intracranial hemorrhage. The cornerstone of surgical intervention is removal of all infected tissue and debridement back to healthy tissue that will hold suture. Sometimes this may require pericardial patch reconstruction of the mitral valve annulus. In cases of large mobile vegetations, the heart should be minimally manipulated during dissection and cannulation to decrease risk of embolism.

Which Patient Should Have This Procedure?

Current AHA/ACC guidelines recommend that MV surgery is reasonable for patients with chronic severe FMR who are undergoing CABG or AVR. Both European and U.S. guidelines stipulate that mitral valve surgery can be considered for patients with severe functional mitral regurgitation who remain significantly symptomatic despite optimal medical therapy, including cardiac resynchronization when indicated [7, 15]. The guidelines provide no recommendation for offering MV replacement vs MV repair. The treatment choice is controversial since there is the perception that MV repair is associated with lower short term as well as longer term morbidity and mortality as compared to replacement [16–19].

However, some recent studies have disputed these findings. Lorusso et al. [20] in a propensity matched comparison between mitral valve repair and replacement demonstrated similar 30-day mortality between mitral valve repair (3.3 %) or replacement (5.3 %, $p = 0.32$). Eight-year survival was 81.6 % ± 2.8 % and 79.6 % ± 4.8 % ($p = 0.42$) in the repair and replacement group respectively. Actual freedom from all-cause reoperation and valve-related reoperation were 64.3 % ± 4.3 % versus 80 % ± 4.1 %, and 71.3 % ± 3.5 % versus 85.5 % ± 3.9 in mitral valve repair and mitral valve replacement, respectively ($p < 0.001$). At follow-up, recurrence of mitral valve regurgitation after mitral valve repair was 25 %. Left ventricular function was comparable in the 2 groups postoperatively (36.9 % vs 38.5 %, $p = 0.66$). MV repair was the strongest multivariable predictor of the need for valve-related reoperation (HR 2.9, $p < 0.001$). Similarly, a recent multicenter randomized trial by the CTS Network comparing MV repair and replacement for patients with severe ischemic MR demonstrated no difference in 30 day or 1 year mortality, composite end point of major cardiac or neurological adverse event or reduction in indexed left ventricular volumes between the two therapies. The MV repair group had a much higher rate of recurrent MR as compared to the MVR group (32.6 % vs. 2.3 %). In patients who underwent repair, the degree of LV reverse remodeling was much higher in the absence of recurrent MR (LVESVI = 47.3 ± 23.0 ml per square meter) as compared to patients who had recurrent MR (LVESVI = 64.1 ± 23.9 ml per square meter) [1]. These findings suggest that patients who have recurrent MR had no reduction in their LVESVI after the operation.

Several observational studies have identified predictors of recurrent ischemic MR after MV repair. These factors fall into two categories: echocardiographic parameters of the extent of MV leaflet tethering and indices of adverse LV remodeling/dilatation. The former include anterior and posterior leaflet angles, leaflet tethering length, and leaflet tenting area [21–24]. LV size and function and the qualitative degree of MR have also been identified as key independent determinants of recurrent MR [25–28]. In the CTSN trial [2], leaflet tethering was determined to be the cause of recurrent IMR; however, none of the preoperative echocardiographic measures of MV tethering were independently predictive of recurrent IMR. The strongest (and only independent) predictor of recurrent MR in the repair group was the presence of basal aneurysm/dyskinesis. A recent study using 3D-echocardiography demonstrated significantly higher global and regional leaflet tethering preoperatively in patients who developed recurrent IMR as compared with patients with no recurrent IMR, especially towards the posterior commissure (segments P2 and A3-P3). Multivariate logistic regression analysis revealed preoperative P3 tethering angle as an independent predictor of IMR recurrence with an optimal cut-off value of 29.9° (AUC 0.92, 95% CI 0.84–1.00, $P<0.001$) [29]. These findings confirm the complex 3D pathologic anatomy of IMR and its variability between patients and within different regions of mitral valve, and suggest superiority of 3D – echocardiography to better characterize IMR and to identify patients at a higher risk of recurrent MR after MV repair.

Based on these observations, we believe that the presence of basal aneurysm/dyskinesis, echocardiographic evidence of significant leaflet tethering, and/or moderate to severe LV dilatation (LVEDD > 70 mm) favor the use of chordal sparing mitral valve replacement over mitral valve repair for treatment of medically refractory severe ischemic MR. In the absence of either basal aneurysm/dyskinesis, the echocardiographic evidence of significant leaflet tethering, or moderate to severe LV dilatation (LVEDD >70 mm), MV repair using an undersized, complete, rigid ring may be reasonable. More complex mitral repair operations that specifically address leaflet tethering have shown promising results [30–33], but remain investigational and incompletely validated.

Although the debate over superiority of MV repair vs replacement for FMR continues, MVR has been established as a safe and acceptable treatment strategy for patients with this complex disease pathology. Long term follow up of the randomized MV repair and replacement patients will be important to determine the clinical consequences of recurrent MR as well as prosthetic valve deterioration/complications. Current recommendations will need to be modified to reflect this new evidence as it becomes available.

References

1. Acker MA, Parides MK, Perrault LP, et al. Mitral-valve repair versus replacement for severe ischemic mitral regurgitation. N Engl J Med. 2014;370(1):23–32.
2. Kron IL, Hung J, Overbey JR, et al. Predicting recurrent mitral regurgitation after mitral valve repair for severe ischemic mitral regurgitation. J Thorac Cardiovasc Surg. 2015;149(3):752–61, e751.
3. Grigioni F, Enriquez-Sarano M, Zehr KJ, Bailey KR, Tajik AJ. Ischemic mitral regurgitation: long-term outcome and prognostic implications with quantitative Doppler assessment. Circulation. 2001;103(13):1759–64.
4. Vergnat M, Jassar AS, Jackson BM, et al. Ischemic mitral regurgitation: a quantitative three-dimensional echocardiographic analysis. Ann Thorac Surg. 2011;91(1):157–64.
5. Zeng X, Levine RA, Hua L, et al. Diagnostic value of vena contracta area in the quantification of mitral regurgitation severity by color Doppler 3D echocardiography. Circ Cardiovasc Imaging. 2011;4(5):506–13.
6. Zeng X, Nunes MC, Dent J, et al. Asymmetric versus symmetric tethering patterns in ischemic mitral regurgitation: geometric differences from three-dimensional transesophageal echocardiography. J Am Soc Echocardiogr. 2014;27(4):367–75.
7. Nishimura RA, Otto CM, Bonow RO, et al. 2014 AHA/ACC guideline for the management of patients with valvular heart disease: a report of the American College of Cardiology/American Heart Association Task Force on Practice Guidelines. Circulation. 2014;129(23):e521–643.
8. Potter DD, Sundt 3rd TM, Zehr KJ, et al. Risk of repeat mitral valve replacement for failed mitral valve prostheses. Ann Thorac Surg. 2004;78(1):67–72; discussion 67–72.
9. Chikwe J, Chiang YP, Egorova NN, Itagaki S, Adams DH. Survival and outcomes following bioprosthetic vs mechanical mitral valve replacement in patients aged 50 to 69 years. JAMA. 2015;313(14):1435–42.
10. Atluri P, Goldstone AB, Fox J, Szeto WY, Hargrove WC. Port access cardiac operations can be safely performed with either endoaortic balloon or Chitwood clamp. Ann Thorac Surg. 2014;98(5):1579–83; discussion 1583–1574.

11. Yun KL, Sintek CF, Miller DC, et al. Randomized trial comparing partial versus complete chordal-sparing mitral valve replacement: effects on left ventricular volume and function. J Thorac Cardiovasc Surg. 2002;123(4):707–14.
12. Ucak A, Ugur M, Onan B, et al. Conventional versus complete chordal-sparing mitral valve replacement: effects on left ventricular function and end-systolic stress. Acta Cardiol. 2011;66(5):627–34.
13. Chowdhury UK, Kumar AS, Airan B, et al. Mitral valve replacement with and without chordal preservation in a rheumatic population: serial echocardiographic assessment of left ventricular size and function. Ann Thorac Surg. 2005;79(6):1926–33.
14. Ribeiro AH, Wender OC, de Almeida AS, Soares LE, Picon PD. Comparison of clinical outcomes in patients undergoing mitral valve replacement with mechanical or biological substitutes: a 20 years cohort. BMC Cardiovasc Disord. 2014;14:146.
15. Vahanian A, Alfieri O, Andreotti F, et al. Guidelines on the management of valvular heart disease (version 2012). Eur Heart J. 2012;33(19):2451–96.
16. Reece TB, Tribble CG, Ellman PI, et al. Mitral repair is superior to replacement when associated with coronary artery disease. Ann Surg. 2004;239(5):671–5; discussion 675–677.
17. Thourani VH, Weintraub WS, Guyton RA, et al. Outcomes and long-term survival for patients undergoing mitral valve repair versus replacement: effect of age and concomitant coronary artery bypass grafting. Circulation. 2003;108(3):298–304.
18. Micovic S, Milacic P, Otasevic P, et al. Comparison of valve annuloplasty and replacement for ischemic mitral valve incompetence. Heart Surg Forum. 2008;11(6):E340–5.
19. Milano CA, Daneshmand MA, Rankin JS, et al. Survival prognosis and surgical management of ischemic mitral regurgitation. Ann Thorac Surg. 2008; 86(3):735–44.
20. Lorusso R, Gelsomino S, Vizzardi E, et al. Mitral valve repair or replacement for ischemic mitral regurgitation? The Italian Study on the Treatment of Ischemic Mitral Regurgitation (ISTIMIR). J Thorac Cardiovasc Surg. 2013;145(1):128–39; discussion 137–128.
21. Magne J, Pibarot P, Dumesnil JG, Senechal M. Continued global left ventricular remodeling is not the sole mechanism responsible for the late recurrence of ischemic mitral regurgitation after restrictive annuloplasty. J Am Soc Echocardiogr. 2009;22(11): 1256–64.
22. Lee AP, Acker M, Kubo SH, et al. Mechanisms of recurrent functional mitral regurgitation after mitral valve repair in nonischemic dilated cardiomyopathy: importance of distal anterior leaflet tethering. Circulation. 2009;119(19):2606–14.
23. Gelsomino S, Lorusso R, De Cicco G, et al. Five-year echocardiographic results of combined undersized mitral ring annuloplasty and coronary artery bypass grafting for chronic ischaemic mitral regurgitation. Eur Heart J. 2008;29(2):231–40.
24. Onorati F, Rubino AS, Marturano D, et al. Midterm clinical and echocardiographic results and predictors of mitral regurgitation recurrence following restrictive annuloplasty for ischemic cardiomyopathy. J Thorac Cardiovasc Surg. 2009;138(3):654–62.
25. Crabtree TD, Bailey MS, Moon MR, et al. Recurrent mitral regurgitation and risk factors for early and late mortality after mitral valve repair for functional ischemic mitral regurgitation. Ann Thorac Surg. 2008;85(5):1537–42; discussion 1542–1533.
26. Ueno T, Sakata R, Iguro Y, Yamamoto H, Ueno M, Matsumoto K. Preoperative advanced left ventricular remodeling predisposes to recurrence of ischemic mitral regurgitation with less reverse remodeling. J Heart Valve Dis. 2008;17(1):36–41.
27. De Bonis M, Lapenna E, Verzini A, et al. Recurrence of mitral regurgitation parallels the absence of left ventricular reverse remodeling after mitral repair in advanced dilated cardiomyopathy. Ann Thorac Surg. 2008;85(3):932–9.
28. Lee LS, Kwon MH, Cevasco M, et al. Postoperative recurrence of mitral regurgitation after annuloplasty for functional mitral regurgitation. Ann Thorac Surg. 2012;94(4):1211–6; discussion 1216–1217.
29. Bouma W, Lai EK, Levack MM, et al. Preoperative three-dimensional valve analysis predicts recurrent ischemic mitral regurgitation after mitral annuloplasty. Ann Thorac Surg. 2016;101(2):567–75.
30. Szymanski C, Bel A, Cohen I, et al. Comprehensive annular and subvalvular repair of chronic ischemic mitral regurgitation improves long-term results with the least ventricular remodeling. Circulation. 2012; 126(23):2720–7.
31. Bouma W, van der Horst IC, Wijdh-den Hamer IJ, et al. Chronic ischaemic mitral regurgitation. Current treatment results and new mechanism-based surgical approaches. Eur J Cardiothorac Surg. 2010;37(1): 170–85.
32. Borger MA, Murphy PM, Alam A, et al. Initial results of the chordal-cutting operation for ischemic mitral regurgitation. J Thorac Cardiovasc Surg. 2007;133(6): 1483–92.
33. Magne J, Senechal M, Dumesnil JG, Pibarot P. Ischemic mitral regurgitation: a complex multifaceted disease. Cardiology. 2009;112(4):244–59.
34. Cohn L. Cardiac surgery in the adult. 4th ed. New York/Toronto: McGraw-Hill Education; 2012.

Addressing the Left Ventricle in Functional Mitral Regurgitation

13

Serenella Castelvecchio, Andrea Garatti, and Lorenzo Menicanti

Abstract

Functional ischemic mitral regurgitation may occur as part of the complex process of left ventricular remodeling and affects the prognosis unfavourably. Chronic ischemic MR occurs in approximately 30 % of patients followed up after a myocardial infarction and in 50 % of those with post-infarct congestive heart failure. The treatment of ischemic mitral regurgitation is still debated. Medical management alleviates symptoms but does not alter the progression of the disease. The matter of surgery for ischemic mitral regurgitation, in terms of whether, when and how it should be corrected is still considerably controversial. Surgery is recommended for moderate-to-severe or severe mitral regurgitation in patients with symptoms or evidence of left ventricular dysfunction. Myocardial revascularization paired to valve surgery can be performed to treat the underlying coronary artery disease. Surgical Ventricular Reconstruction offers either the possibility to repair the mitral valve through the left ventricular opening or the potential of improving mitral functioning by reducing left ventricular volumes and rebuilding a more normal geometry.

This chapter will discuss the principles of treatment for ischemic mitral regurgitation according to the different phenotypes of left ventricular remodelling, the surgical techniques and the results, focusing on which patients may have greater benefit to the best of our knowledge.

Keywords

Myocardial infarction • Left ventricular remodeling • Ischemic mitral regurgitation • Surgical ventricular reconstruction

S. Castelvecchio, MD, FESC (✉)
Division of Cardiac Surgery, I.R.C.C.S. Policlinico San Donato, Piazza E. Malan 1, San Donato Milanese, Milan 20097, Italy
e-mail: serenella.castelvecchio@grupposandonato.it

A. Garatti, MD • L. Menicanti, MD, FECTS
Department of Cardiac Surgery, I.R.C.C.S., Policlinico San Donato, Milan, Italy

K.M.J. Chan (ed.), *Functional Mitral and Tricuspid Regurgitation*,
DOI 10.1007/978-3-319-43510-7_13

Introduction

Functional mitral regurgitation (MR) broadly indicates abnormal function of normal mitral leaflets in the context of impaired left ventricular function; it typically occurs in globally dilated and hypokinetic ventricles or with segmental damage that affects valve closure. Functional ischemic MR is caused by changes in ventricular structure and function related ultimately to ischemia [1]; it is predominantly postinfarction MR and occurs as part of the complex process of left ventricular (LV) remodeling (Fig. 13.1). Despite advances in coronary reperfusion, MR remains common following an acute MI, occurring in up to 30% of patients [2, 3] and in 50% of those with congestive heart failure [4], adversely affecting the prognosis, even when mild [5].

Although the knowledge of the mechanisms underlying ischemic mitral regurgitation has improved over half a century, many aspects remain controversial, leaving the therapeutic strategies perplexing in their diversity and not fully effective. Indeed, chronic ischemic MR is a "complex and dynamic disease", involving coronary arteries, mitral annulus, subvalvular apparatus and ventricle, in which the large number of geometric and hemodynamic variables and the complex interaction between each other carries the risk of a suboptimal result when treated.

From Ischemic LV Remodeling to Mitral Regurgitation: In Search of the Target Lesion

LV remodeling is a complex, dynamic and time-dependent process, which may occur in different clinical conditions, including MI, leading to chamber dilatation, altered configuration and increased wall stress [6]. It begins within the first few hours after an MI and results from fibrotic repair of the necrotic area with scar formation, elongation, and thinning of the infarcted zone. LV volumes increase, a response that is sometimes considered adaptive, associated with stroke volume augmentation in an effort to maintain a normal cardiac output as the ejection fraction declines. However, beyond this early stage, the remodeling process is driven predominantly by

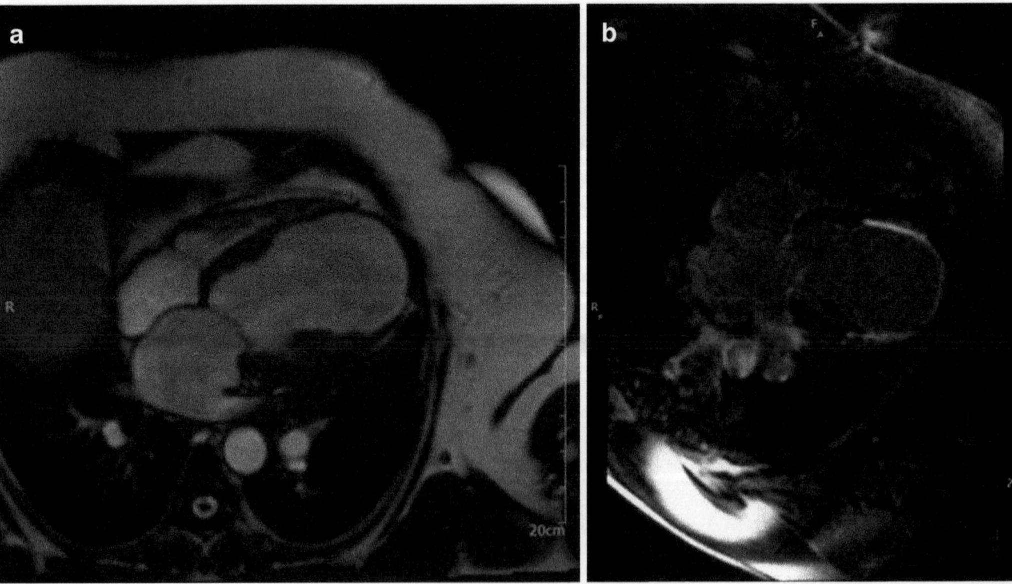

Fig. 13.1 Left ventricular remodeling. Contrast-enhanced cardiac Magnetic Resonance. (**a**) *Left panel*: LV chamber appears dilated and distorted. (**b**) *Right panel*: late gadolinium enhancement images showing extensive antero-apical ventricular remodeling in 2-chamber view surrounded by transmural fibrosis

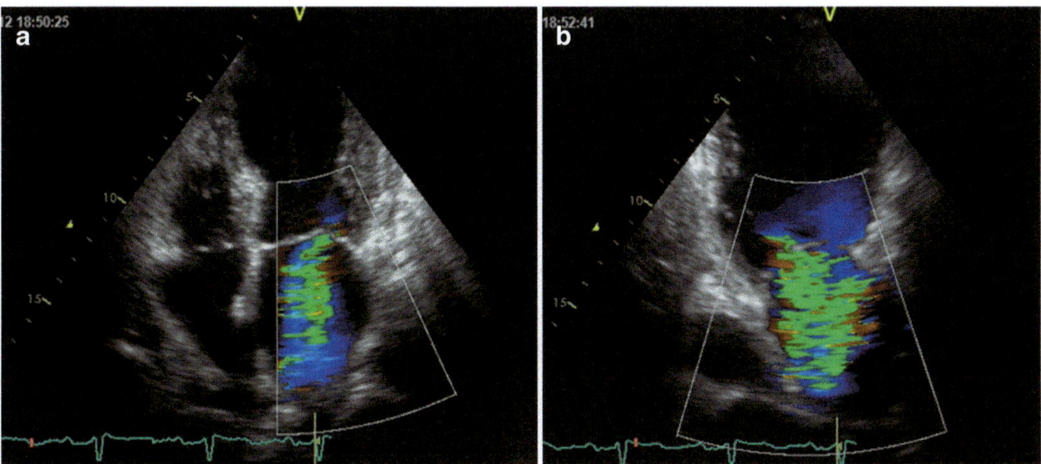

Fig. 13.2 Ischemic mitral regurgitation. Apical 4- (**a**) and 2-chamber (**b**) view showing ischemic MR

eccentric hypertrophy of the non-infarcted remote regions, resulting in increased wall stress, chamber enlargement and geometric distortion [7]. These changes, along with a decline in performance of hypertrophied myocyte, increased neurohormonal activation, collagen synthesis, fibrosis and remodeling of the extracellular matrix within the non-infarcted zone, result in a progressive decline in ventricular performance [8]. At the same time, the papillary muscle (PM) displacement, which may occur as a consequence of the LV dilatation, results in leaflet tethering of the mitral valve at closure with lack of a proper coaptation, in turn leading to secondary MR (Fig. 13.2). In addition, ventricular dilatation results in annular enlargement, which further increases valve incompetence. Indeed, after the first description by Burch et al. [9] in 1963 supporting the central role of PM dysfunction as the basic mechanism of ischemic MR, a large number of experimental and clinical studies have reported contrary results. Large-animal models have shown that both left ventricular dilation and posterior PM infarction were necessary for the development of MR [10]. A retrospective study by Okayama et al. [11] in patients with single-vessel coronary disease using cardiac magnetic resonance (CMR) to quantify PM infarction and MR found an association between the presence of delayed enhancement (DE) in PM and MR, specifically in patients with large infarctions and bilateral PM enhancement. Other studies, however, have underlined a weaker role for PMs in ischemic MR. Dog models of ischemic MR showed that when PM was selectively infarcted, it did not produce MR, whereas larger infarctions encompassing the PM and adjacent myocardium did produce MR [12]. In the same study by Okayama et al. [11], patients with single vessel right coronary artery disease as well as PM infarction had less MR than patients who had no PM infarction.

One of the latest studies seems to have elegantly reconciled this old debate to better clarify the role of papillary muscles compared to that of the adjacent remodeled LV wall. In a large prospective cohort of 153 patients with first ST-segment elevation MI without intrinsic mitral valve disease, Chinitz et al. [13] evaluated the incidence and severity of ischemic MR as well as coronary and ventricular anatomy using a multimodality imaging (echocardiography to quantify MR, angiography to identify the culprit coronary lesions, and a high resolution DE-CMR sequence to define the extent of PM infarction – partial vs. complete – and ventricular infarction). The results showed that neither complete nor partial PM infarction necessarily led to the development of MR. However, the amount of infarcted myocardium was significantly associated with the development of ischemic MR, even after a multivariate analysis,

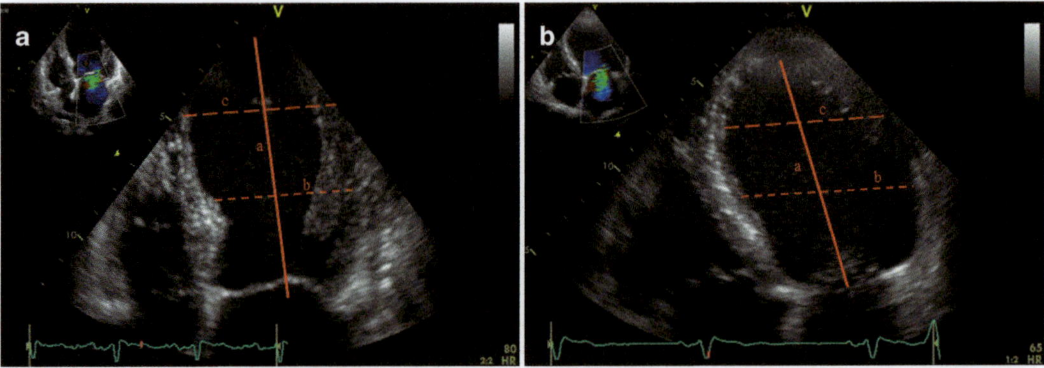

Fig. 13.3 (**a**) *Left panel*: the LV apex is primarily involved after an anterior MI. As a consequence, the conicity index (CI, obtained from the apical – *c* – to short axis ratio – *b*) is significantly greater in the anterior remodeling compared to posterior remodeling group. (**b**) *Right panel*: a previous inferior MI induces a regional remodeling of the basal and mid segments of the inferopostero-lateral wall, with a significant increase in LV transverse diameters and consequently in the sphericity index (SI, obtained from the short – *b* -to long axis ratio – *a*)

confirming the role of the underlying ventricular infarction and adverse remodeling as the primary culprit for the development and progression of chronic ischemic MR. Furthermore, once established, ischemic MR, can itself worsen the remodeling process, altering LV loading conditions, increasing diastolic wall stress (which can worsen eccentric hypertrophy with further LV dilatation and dysfunction) and end-systolic wall stress in patients with chronic MR because of induced LV remodeling, with decreased contractility and increased end-systolic volume, driving a vicious circle in which MR begets more MR [14]. Having said that, it is still unclear if the volume overload created by MR adds a greater pathologic burden to an already adverse condition or, simply, the worse prognosis is related to a poorer LV function and functional MR is merely an indicator of this bad condition.

Ischemic Mitral Regurgitation According Different Phenotypes of LV Remodeling

Usually, ischemic MR occurs in nearly 50–60 % of patients with previous inferior MI due to a bulging of the inferior and posterior LV basal and midventricular segments underlying the PMs [3, 15, 16]. However, clinical studies, including one of the most recent from Levine and co-workers, outlined the importance of anteroapical MI causing MR despite the absence of inferobasal wall motion abnormalities [17]. In this case, mitral regurgitation grade correlated most strongly with tethering length due to the displacement of the papillary muscles.

Recently, our group addressed the differences between anterior and posterior remodeling in patients with previous MI undergoing surgical ventricular reconstruction (SVR) [18]. From a morphological point of view, post-infarction remodeling occurred at different LV levels in the two study groups (A, anterior versus P, posterior). The LV apex is primarily involved after an anterior MI (Fig. 13.3, left panel), as we previously reported [19]. As a consequence, the conicity index (obtained from the apical to short axis ratio) was significantly greater in the anterior remodeling group (A) compared to posterior (P). Conversely, a previous inferior MI determined a regional remodeling of the basal and mid segments of the infero-postero-lateral wall (Fig. 13.3, right panel), with a significant increase in LV transverse diameters and consequently in the sphericity index (obtained from the short to long axis ratio). LV basal involvement in posterior dilatation causes lateral displacement of the posteromedial PM leading to a significant increase in the interpapillary distance in Group P compared to Group A. As a consequence, patients in group P presented with a higher incidence of severe MR (55% vs 25%, respectively, p=0.01), which determined higher LV mass, larger left atrium dimensions, higher pulmonary artery pressure and higher rate of right ventricular dysfunction. After analyzing the data according to the presence or not of moderate to severe MR in the two different patterns of LV remodeling, we observed that in posterior remodeling the main geometrical change associated with severe MR was ***an increase in the interpapillary distance***, without significant difference in the tenting area. On the contrary in anterior remodeling, MR occurs mainly in the setting of global LV dilatation, with tethering of both mitral valve leaflets due to apical displacement of PMs; hence, ***increased mitral tenting area*** was the major determinant of severe MR, without a concomitant significant increase in interpapillary distance. Furthermore, when Cox Regression analysis was applied separately to the two study groups, severe preoperative MR remained a significant independent predictor of long-term mortality in Group A but not in Group P. We speculated that, behind the above mentioned geometrical assumptions, in patients with previous anterior MI, MR occurs mainly in the setting of global LV dilatation and severe dysfunction, reflecting a more advanced stage of disease.

This is also consistent with the fact that, in the group A, patients with severe MR showed worsened right ventricular function compared to patients with mild MR. This phenomenon was not observed in the group P even though in both groups, patients with severe MR showed a similar increase in systolic pulmonary artery pressure.

Surgical Operative techniques

The Rationale to Perform Surgical Ventricular Reconstruction to Reverse LV Remodeling

Surgical Ventricular Reconstruction (SVR) of the LV chamber has been introduced as an optional therapeutic strategy aiming to reduce LV volumes through the exclusion of the scar tissue from the LV cavity, thereby reducing the ventricle size to a more physiological volume, reshaping the distorted chamber and improving cardiac function through a reduction of LV wall stress in accordance with the principle of Laplace's law. Since LV wall stress is directly proportional to LV internal radius and pressure, and inversely proportional to wall thickness, any intervention to optimize this relationship would be beneficial either in terms of improving wall compliance and reducing filling pressure, or as wall stress is a crucial determinant of afterload, in terms of enhancing contractile performance of the LV by increasing the extent and velocity of systolic fiber shortening [20]. Furthermore, SVR of failing ventricles is usually combined with myocardial revascularization with the aim of treating the underlying coronary artery disease, although in recent years the percentage of patients with ischemic LV dysfunction without significant coronary disease has increased due previous percutaneous coronary interventions (PCI). Lastly, SVR offers either the possibility to repair the mitral valve through the LV opening or the potential of improving mitral functioning by improving the LV [21, 22].

SVR Technique

The operation is performed under cardiac arrest, with antegrade cold crystalloid cardioplegia. A complete myocardial revascularization is performed first, when indicated, with particular attention to revascularize the proximal left anterior descending segment, to preserve the upper part of the septum. For this purpose, a left internal mammary artery is almost always placed on the left anterior descending artery. Revascularization is completed, when indicated, through sequential saphenous vein coronary bypass grafting on other diseased coronary arteries.

After completion of coronary grafting, the ventricle is opened with an incision parallel to the left anterior descending artery, starting at the middle scarred region and ending at the apex. The cavity is carefully inspected and any thrombus is removed if present. The surgeon identifies the transitional zone between scarred and non-scarred tissue, driven by cardiac magnetic

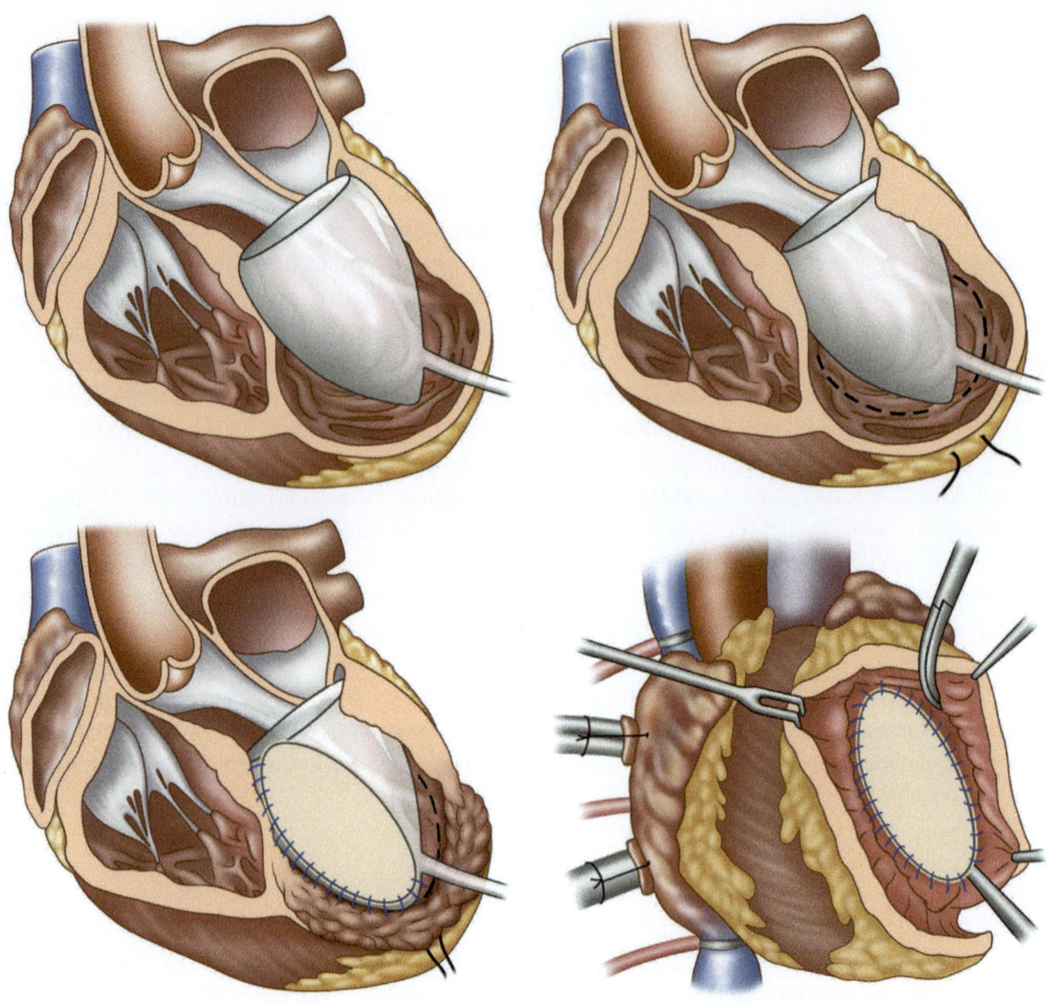

Fig. 13.4 SVR procedure for anterior remodeling (schematic). *Upper panel*: The mannequin is inside the ventricle (*on the left*); the circular suture follows the curvature of the mannequin to re-shape the ventricle in an elliptical way (*on the right*). *Lower panel*: The patch is used to close the ventricular opening

resonance with late gadolinium enhancement (LGE), when previously performed, or alternatively by echocardiographic analysis. After that, a pre-shaped mannequin is inserted into the LV chamber and inflated with saline (Fig. 13.4, *upper panel on the left*). The mannequin is useful to optimize the size and shape of the new LV, particularly when the ventricle is not very enlarged (to reduce the risk of a too small residual cavity), or when the transitional zone between scarred and non-scarred tissue is not clearly demarcated, as occurs in akinetic remodeling. Furthermore, the mannequin is useful in giving the surgeon the correct position of the apex and in maintaining the long axis of the ventricle in a physiologic range (7.5/8.5), reducing thereby the risk of sphericalization of the new ventricle. The size of the device is defined by multiplying the body surface area of the patient by 50 ml. The exclusion of dyskinetic or akinetic LV free wall is performed through an endoventricular circular suture passed in the tissue of the transitional zone (Fig. 13.4, *upper panel on the right*). The conical shape of the mannequin guides the orientation of the plane of the endoventricular circular suture at the transitional zone, obliquely towards the aortic flow tract, mainly in rebuilding the new apex. The reconstruction of the apex may be difficult when

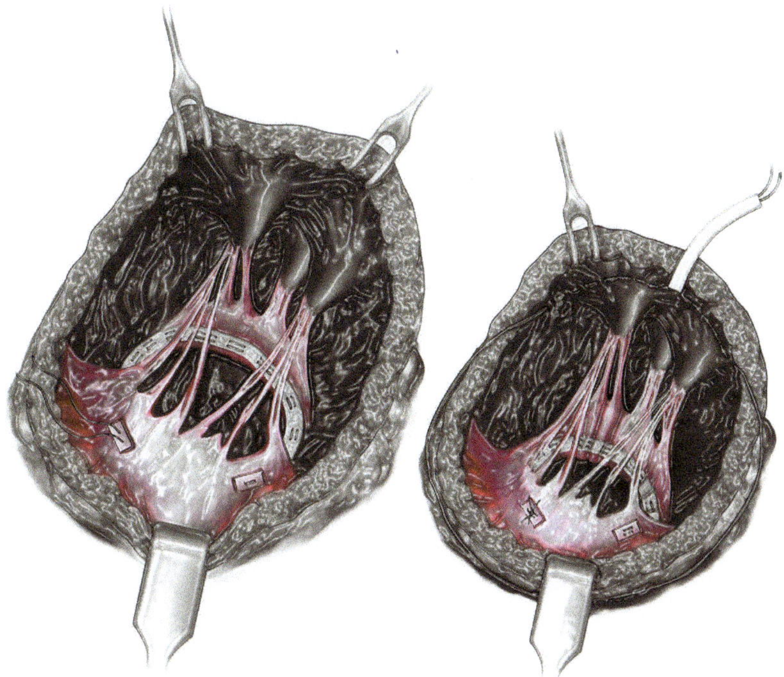

Fig. 13.5 Mitral valve repair. Mitral valve is repaired through the ventricular opening with a double arm stitch running from one trigone to the other one

the apical and inferior regions are severely dilated and scarred; in this case, a plication of the distal inferior wall is performed before patch suturing, thus placing the apex in a more superior position leaving a small portion of scar. The mannequin is removed before the closure of the ventricle and the opening is closed with a direct suture (simple stiches) if it is less than 3 cm large or with an elliptical, synthetic patch if greater than 3 cm to avoid distortion of the cavity (Fig. 13.4, *lower panel on the left*). In the first case, a second stratum with the excluded tissue is sutured on the first suture to avoid bleeding. If the closure is performed by using a patch (usually a Dacron patch), a few millimeters of border is left when sewing the patch in an everting way (Fig. 13.4, *lower panel on the right*). This technique assures a good hemostasis and makes it easier to put some additional stiches, if needed. The position of the patch is crucial in determining the residual shape of the new ventricle. To this aim, the surgeon pays attention to positioning the patch with an oblique orientation, toward the aortic outflow tract. In this way we avoid obtaining a box-like shape of the ventricle that may occur when the orientation of the patch is almost parallel to the mitral valve. More recently, the growing number of PCI has changed the pattern of LV remodeling in that the classical, dyskinetic aneurysm has almost disappeared and there is an increased incidence of a more diffuse akinetic remodeling. In the latter case, the use of the mannequin is crucial in determining the final result. The LV cavity is restored using the mannequin as a cast and the wall is closed with a running suture over the mannequin without a suture on the transitional zone. The final shape is more elliptical because the surgeon starts the suture in a higher position close to the aortic valve.

Mitral Valve Repair When indicated, the mitral valve is repaired through the ventricular opening with a double arm stitch running from one trigone to the other one, embedding the two arms in the posterior anulus of the mitral valve (Fig. 13.5). To avoid tears of the posterior left of the mitral valve (as has previously occurred), the suture is reinforced with a Teflon strip. After that, the

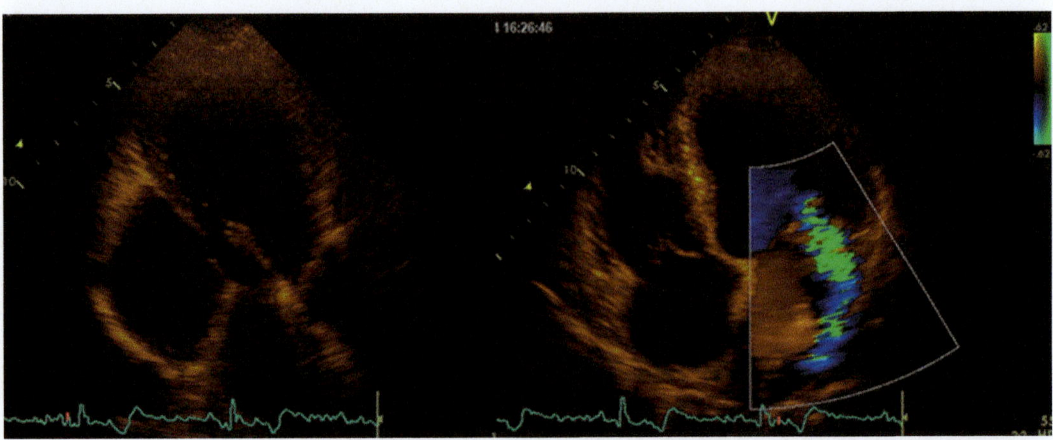

Fig. 13.6 Posterior remodeling. The classic posterior aneurysm with a bulging of the inferior wall and a well-defined neck

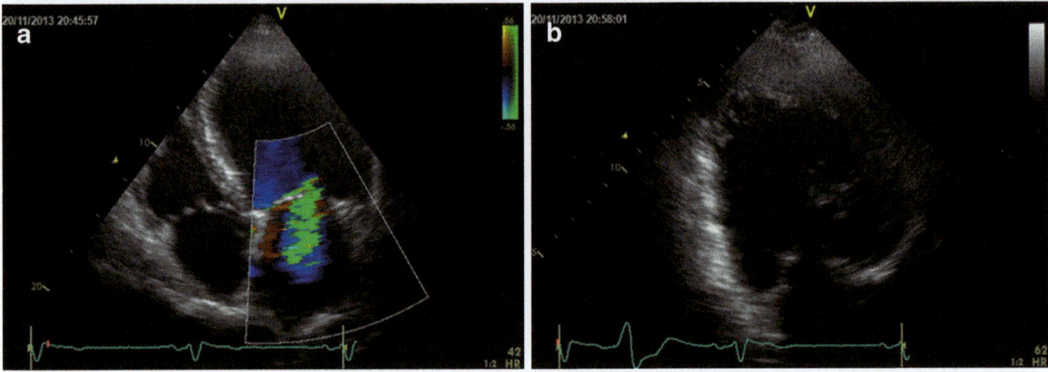

Fig. 13.7 Posterior remodeling. Global LV dilatation (**a**) with scar tissue at the inferior and posterior region (**b**)

suture is tied to undersize the mitral orifice. A Hegar sizer no. 26 is used to size the mitral annulus. Alternatively, a restrictive mitral annuloplasty with a ring implantation may be performed in selected patients, when the LV opening is not big enough to have a good exposition of the mitral valve.

Tailored Approaches The surgical procedure as described above is usually performed to reverse LV remodeling after an anterior MI. However, the procedure may be tailored to approach different patterns of post-infarction LV remodeling, varying from the classic posterior aneurysm with a bulging of the inferior wall and a well-defined neck (Fig. 13.6), to a global LV dilatation with regional wall dysfunction at the inferior and posterior region, according to the site of coronary occlusion (Fig. 13.7). Surgery for the posterior aneurysm generally involves a patch to close the neck of the aneurysm. Otherwise, the treatment of global dilatation of the infero-posterior wall is more complex and varies according to the relationship between the site of the scar and the dilatation (with or without involvement of the posterior septum) with respect to the papillary muscles. After an inferior MI, there are two possibilities: a – the dilatation is mainly between the two papillary muscles (Fig. 13.8) or b – the dilatation is between the posteromedial papillary muscle and the septum, which is deeply involved (Fig. 13.9). We use two techniques for LV dilatation after an inferior MI. The first involves opening the scarred wall at the level of the scar or at the

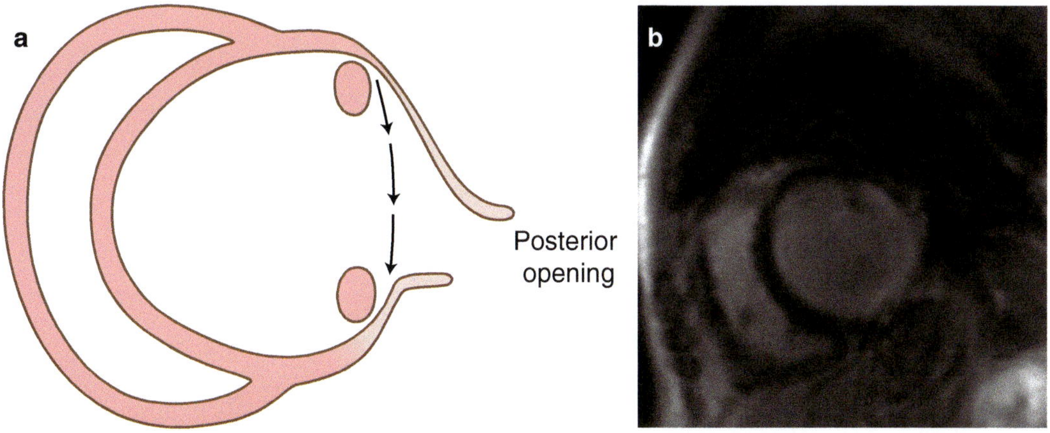

Fig. 13.8 The dilatation is mainly between the two papillary muscles: (**a**) schematic; (**b**) as observed after contrast-enhanced cardiac magnetic resonance

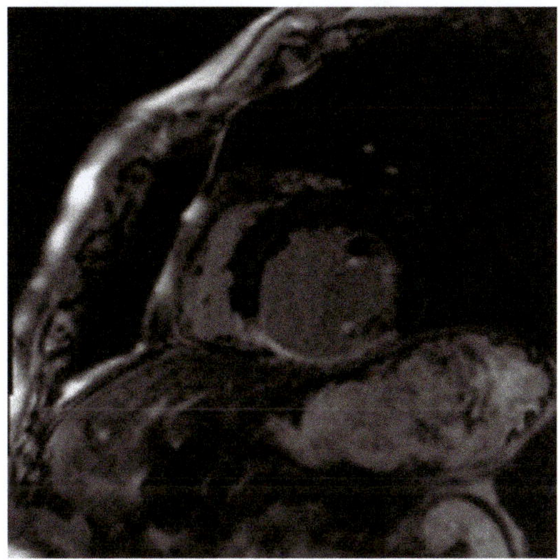

Fig. 13.9 The dilatation is between the posteromedial papillary muscle and the septum, which appears involved

level of the collapsed area, parallel to the posterior descending artery (Fig. 13.10, *on the left panel*). A continuous 2/0 Prolene suture is performed to obtain the re-approximation of the two papillary muscles and the exclusion of the entire dilated zone. The suture is started at the beginning of the dilatation (sometimes just at the level of the mitral annulus) and continues toward the apex. According to the second technique, the wall is opened and the continuous suture is brought behind the posteromedial papillary muscle, bringing the posterior wall against the septum.

Results

The matter of functional chronic ischemic MR in terms of whether, when and how it should be corrected is one of the most common and controversial dilemmas faced by cardiac surgeons in the daily practice [23]. Certainly, the existing body of mostly retrospective and scarce literature has not contributed to general agreement. Authors advocating MV repair refer to the well-established negative impact that ischemic MR has on survival in patients undergoing CABG alone [24, 25], for whom the presence of even mild degrees of ischemic MR is thought to increase long-term mortality. Clinicians supporting the role of the LV ventricle in causing ischemic MR argue in favour of CABG alone which should theoretically improve regional wall motion abnormalities, papillary muscle function, and stimulate reverse LV remodeling avoiding the incremental perioperative morbidity and mortality with which adjunctive MV repair has been historically associated [26]. Not surprisingly, some retrospective studies show that CABG alone improves both ischemic MR and functional status in the short term [27, 28], whereas others show that MR is not reversed [29] and may progress further [30] with negative impact on survival [29]. Recently, Gelsomino and co-workers [31] showed that anterior mitral leaflet tethering is a powerful predictor of MR recurrence after undersized mitral ring annuloplasty,

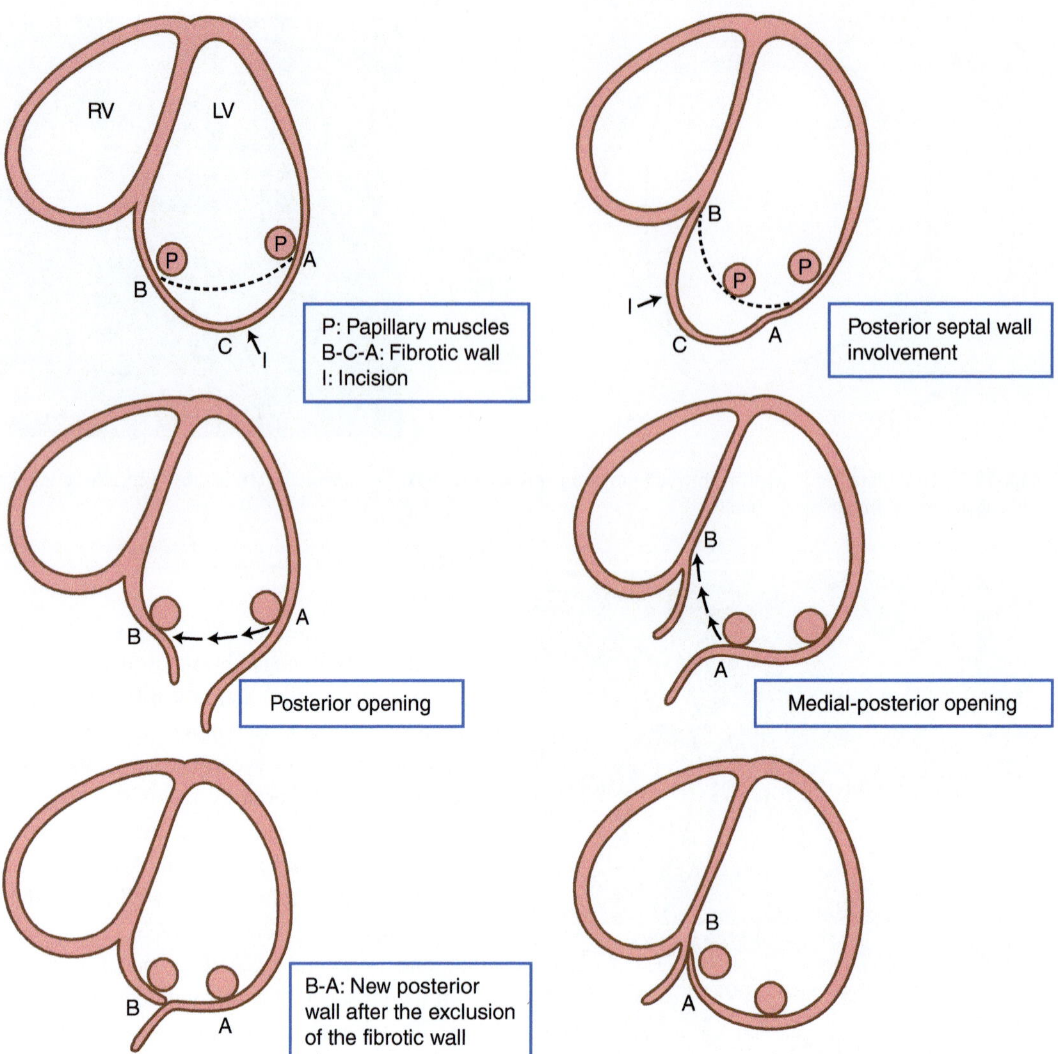

Fig. 13.10 SVR procedure for posterior remodeling (schematic). The picture shows the two different techniques, from *top to bottom* on *the left* (which is applied when the dilatation occurs mainly between the two papillary muscles) and from *top to bottom* on *the right* (which is applied when the dilatation occurs between the posteromedial papillary muscle and the septum)

suggesting the need for concomitant or alternative surgery addressing the leaflet tethering (i.e., papillary muscle repositioning). In this regard, LV reconstruction has the advantage of addressing both the ventricle and mitral apparatus.

In 2002 we reported our initial experience on a small group of patients undergoing complete coronary revascularization, SVR and mitral valve repair for *moderate or severe MR* [32]. The mitral valve was repaired through the LV cavity without a prosthetic ring. Postoperative MR was absent or minimal in 84 % of patients; only one patient experienced severe MR a few days after surgery, requiring MV replacement. The follow-up analysis showed a cumulative survival of 63 % at 30-months.

Later, we addressed the effectiveness of SVR on unrepaired mild ischemic mitral regurgitation, showing that SVR improves mitral functioning by improving geometrical abnormalities [22]. Overall mid-term survival, including early mortality, was 93 % at 1 year and 88 % at 3 years, higher than it would be expected in patients with post-infarction remodelled ventricles and depressed LV function, suggesting that mitral repair in conjunction with SVR would be unnecessary in such patients.

Most recently, we re-analysed the data from our database, which comes from a prospective registry in which follow-up is carried out every 6 months. From January 2001 to October 2014, 175 patients out of 626 (28 %) heart failure patients undergoing SVR had associated MV repair. CABG was performed in 86 % of patients. The mean follow-up for death from any cause was 42 ± 37 months and was 100 % complete. In this latter population, the actuarial survival rate of the whole population, including operative mortality (25/175, 14,3 %), was 72 % ± 4 %, 65 % ± 4 %, and 45 % ± 6 % at 3, 5 and 8 years, respectively [33].

Although the comparison between populations of different studies is always difficult because of differences in baseline characteristics, our findings deserve some considerations. The operative mortality is relatively high but not disproportionally when compared to mortality associated with *CABG plus MV surgery* in previous reports (10,8 % by Schurr et al. [34]; 12 % by Kang et al. [35]). Surprisingly, possibly due to the large number of participating centers with different experience, Deja and colleagues, addressing the matter of MV surgery in the STICH hypothesis 1 population (among 104 patients assigned to CABG with moderate to severe MR, 91 underwent CABG and *49 received an adjunctive concomitant mitral valve procedure*), showed a significantly higher operative mortality in patients treated with CABG only compared to patients treated with CABG plus an added MV repair (14,3 % vs 2 %, p=0.046) [36]. Overall, it seems that it is not MV surgery *per se* which increase the operative risk rather the ischemic MV regurgitation in patients with LV dysfunction carries a higher risk regardless of treatment. In this regard, our results are not a cause of concern, especially if the relative "higher price to pay" early is compensated by a late benefit. Indeed, the observational data from the STICH trial indicate that adding MV repair to CABG in patients with LV dysfunction and moderate to severe MR may improve survival compared with CABG alone or MED alone (50 % of mortality risk at 5 years in the latter). Compared with these data, our results, coming from a larger population with a longer follow-up, show that combining MV repair with SVR added to CABG in the majority may further improve survival at 5 year (59 % in the STICH population vs 65 % in our series).

The Black Hole Beyond Repair: The Issue of Durability

LV *adverse* remodeling is a dynamic process as well as LV *reverse* remodeling, both evolving over time, the latter depending on the completeness of revascularization, the residual shape of the LV (in case of performing SVR), the decision to repair or not the mitral valve (left to the surgeon at the time of surgery), the technique to repair (with or without a prosthetic ring and type of ring) and the complex interaction between each other.

Accordingly, the rate of recurrence of MR after MV repair surgery is significantly high, extremely variable among different series, and poorly predictable. Recently, Kron and coworkers reported a particularly high rate of recurrence (ranging from 25.5 % at 6 months up to 39 % at 24 months) coming from the Cardiothoracic Surgical Trials Network [37]. The authors identified basal aneurysm/dyskinesis as one of the mechanisms of mitral valve annuloplasty failure, at least in this population, calling the need for different repair techniques. In 2002, the same Author described the direct relocation of the posterior papillary muscle tip in a small group of patients with previous inferior MI, not severely dilated ventricles (<6 cm in end-systolic diameter) and regional left ventricular (LV) geometric changes causing MR. In patients with dilated left ventricles (> 6 cm end-systolic diameter), the Dor procedure, relocating the papillary muscle base, was advocated [38]. In this regard, our surgical approach of the left ventricle, as described above, and tailored according to different phenotypes of LV remodeling, has the advantage to act on different mechanisms, although with different results. Preliminary data from the echocardiographic

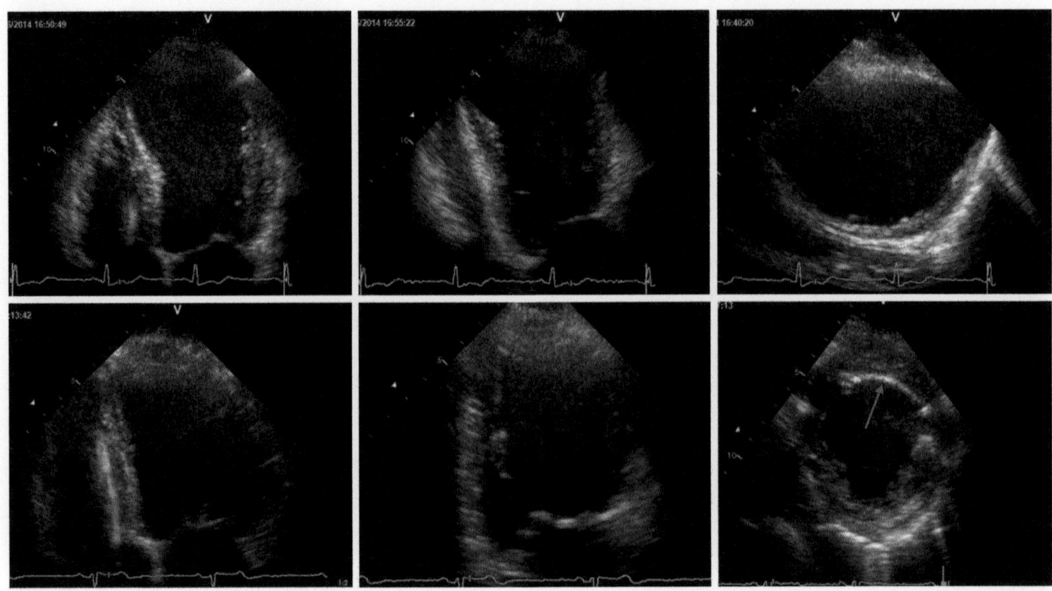

Fig. 13.11 Changes in LV geometry *Upper panel*: LV anterior remodeling before SVR. The LV geometry is altered and the apex is widely dilated, without significant MR; SI is within the normal range, conversely the CI is increased SId = 0.53 CId = 1.10 SIs = 0.49 CIs = 1.22 *Lower panel*: After SVR, the apex has been rebuilt excluding the scar tissue and shortening inevitably the longitudinal diameter; SI increased although not disproportionally, while CI decreased, as expected after reshaping of the apex. The *red arrow* indicates the Dacron patch used to close the LV cavity SId = 0.67 CId = 0.87 SIs = 0.63 CIs = 0.86

follow-up of 114 patients who underwent MV repair combined with SVR at our Institution (overall actuarial survival free from recurrence of 84 % ± 4 % and 63 % ± 7 % at 1 and 5 years, respectively) show that, both anterior remodeling (OR = 3.7, p = 0.05) and end-diastolic diameter (OR 1.08 per mm, p = 0.009) are independent predictors of recurrence, but not posterior remodeling (including basal aneurysm/dyskinesis) (unpublished data). The reason can probably be ascribed to the fact that the surgical technique reduces the short axis in the posterior remodeling, while acting mostly on the longitudinal axis in the anterior remodeling leading to an increase of the sphericity (Fig. 13.11) and a higher rate of recurrence. Recently, Oh and colleagues claimed that the significant increase in sphericity index observed after SVR in the STICH hypothesis 2 population was accompanied by a worsening of diastolic function and less improvement in mitral regurgitation [39]. The increase in sphericity index was ascribed to the amputation of the apex as result of SVR, which is not exactly the aim of this procedure. Rather, the apex should be reshaped (if distorted) while the surgeon must be aware to preserve the length of the ventricle (Fig. 13.12).

Which Patient Should Have This Procedure: A Complex Surgery for Complex Patients

Ischemic MR is a complex disease which adversely affect the prognosis of patients with post-infarction LV remodeling. While the therapeutic strategy remains controversial, a greater focus must be placed on understanding the complex interaction between the ventricle, in terms of geometry and function, and valve functioning. According to our knowledge, the reconstruction of the left ventricle should be considered in selected HF patients with a baseline LVESVI $\geq$ 60 ml/m^2 and a scar either in the antero-septal wall or in the infero-lateral wall.

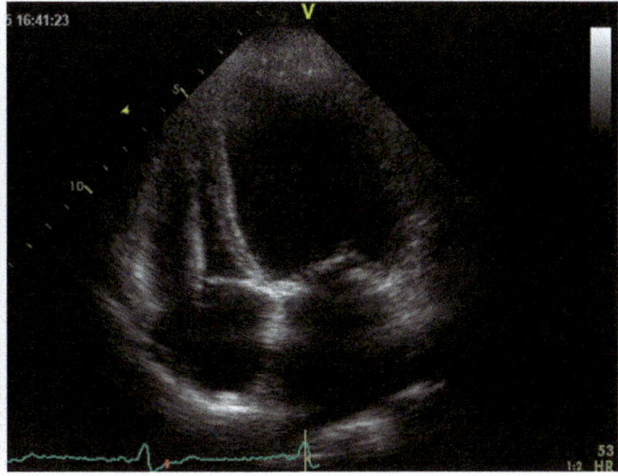

Fig. 13.12 Changes in LV geometry. LV anterior remodeling before SVR: the LV geometry is quite preserved; in this case, it has been possible to preserve the longitudinal diameter without changes in SI. No patch has been used to close the cavity SId = 0.76 SId = 0.76 SIs = 0.67 SIs = 0.68

Mitral valve repair is indicated in presence of moderate to severe MR or even mild if the mitral annulus is greater than 40 mm. When the internal diameter is greater than 65 mm, it is probably reasonable to consider to replace the valve in patients with anterior remodeling. In the presence of posterior remodeling, MV replacement is not advised because the LV reconstruction, addressing mainly the internal diameter, produces a greater shortening of the short axis compared to the long one, fixing the mitral valve in a stable way.

References

1. Levine RA, Schwammenthal E. Ischemic mitral regurgitation on the threshold of a solution: from paradoxes to unifying concepts. Circulation. 2005;2(112):745–58.
2. Lamas GA, Mitchell GF, Flaker GC, Smith Jr SC, Gersh BJ, Basta L, et al. Clinical significance of mitral regurgitation after acute myocardial infarction. Survival and Ventricular Enlargement Investigators. Circulation. 1997;96:827–33.
3. Kumanohoso T, Otsuji Y, Yoshifuku S, Matsukida K, Koriyama C, Kisanuki A, et al. Mechanism of higher incidence of ischemic mitral regurgitation in patients with inferior myocardial infarction: quantitative analysis of left ventricular and mitral valve geometry in 103 patients with prior myocardial infarction. J Thorac Cardiovasc Surg. 2003;125:135–43.
4. Trichon BH, Felker GM, Shaw LK, Cabell CH, O'Connor CM. Relation of frequency and severity of mitral regurgitation to survival among patients with left ventricular systolic dysfunction and heart failure. Am J Cardiol. 2003;91:538–43.
5. Grigioni F, Enriquez-Sarano M, Zehr KJ, Bailey KR, Tajik AJ. Ischemic mitral regurgitation: long-term outcome and prognostic implications with quantitative Doppler assessment. Circulation. 2001;103:1759–64.
6. Konstam MA, Kramer DG, Patel AR, Maron MS, Udelson JE. Left ventricular remodeling in heart failure. Current concepts in clinical significance and assessment. JACC Cardiovasc Imaging. 2011;4:98–108.
7. Pfeffer MA, Braunwald E. Ventricular remodeling after myocardial infarction. Experimental observations and clinical implications. Circulation. 1990;81:1161–72.
8. Braunwald E. Biomarkers in heart failure. N Engl J Med. 2008;15(358):2148–59.
9. Burch GE, Depasquale NP, Phillips JH. Clinical manifestations of papillary muscle dysfunction. Arch Intern Med. 1963;112:112–7.
10. Llaneras MR, Nance ML, Streicher JT, Lima JA, Savino JS, Bogen DK, et al. Large animal model of ischemic mitral regurgitation. Ann Thorac Surg. 1994;57:432–9.
11. Okayama S, Uemura S, Soeda T, Onoue K, Somekawa S, Ishigami K, et al. Clinical significance of papillary muscle late enhancement detected via cardiac magnetic resonance imaging in patients with single old myocardial infarction. Int J Cardiol. 2011;146:73–9.
12. Mittal AK, Langston Jr M, Cohn KE, Selzer A, Kerth WJ. Combined papillary muscle and left ventricular wall dysfunction as a cause of mitral regurgitation. An experimental study. Circulation. 1971;44:174–80.
13. Chinitz JS, Chen D, Goyal P, Wilson S, Islam F, Nguyen T, et al. Mitral apparatus assessment by delayed enhancement CMR: relative impact of infarct

distribution on mitral regurgitation. JACC Cardiovasc Imaging. 2013;6:220–34.

14. Beeri R, Yosefy C, Guerrero JL, Nesta F, Abedat S, Chaput M, et al. Mitral regurgitation augments post-myocardial infarction remodeling failure of hypertrophic compensation. J Am Coll Cardiol. 2008;51:476–86.
15. Sabbah HN, Rosman H, Kono T, Alam M, Khaja F, Goldstein S. On the mechanism of functional mitral regurgitation. Am J Cardiol. 1993;72:1074–6.
16. Gaasch WH, Zile MR. Left ventricular structural remodeling in health and disease: with special emphasis on volume, mass, and geometry. J Am Coll Cardiol. 2011;18(58):1733–40.
17. Yosefy C, Beeri R, Guerrero JL, Vaturi M, Scherrer-Crosbie M, Handschumacher MD, et al. Mitral regurgitation after anteroapical myocardial infarction: new mechanistic insights. Circulation. 2011;123:1529–36.
18. Garatti A, Castelvecchio S, Bandera F, Guazzi M, Menicanti L. Surgical ventricular restoration: is there any difference in outcome between anterior and posterior remodeling? Ann Thorac Surg. 2015;99:552–9.
19. Di Donato M, Dabic P, Castelvecchio S, Santambrogio C, Brankovic J, Collarini L, et al.; RESTORE Group. Left ventricular geometry in normal and post-anterior myocardial infarction patients: sphericity index and 'new' conicity index comparisons. Eur J Cardiothorac Surg. 2006;29 Suppl 1:S225–30.
20. Di Donato M, Sabatier M, Toso A, Barletta G, Baroni M, et al. Regional myocardial performance of non-ischaemic zones remote from anterior wall left ventricular aneurysm. Effects of aneurysmectomy. Eur Heart J. 1995;16:1285–92.
21. Menicanti L, Di Donato M, Frigiola A, Buckberg G, Santambrogio C, Ranucci M, et al. RESTORE Group. Ischemic mitral regurgitation: intraventricular papillary muscle imbrication without mitral ring during left ventricular restoration. J Thorac Cardiovasc Surg. 2002;123:1041–50.
22. Di Donato M, Castelvecchio S, Brankovic E, Santambrogio C, Montericcio V, Menicanti L. Effectiveness of surgical ventricular restoration in patients with dilated ischemic cardiomyopathy and unrepaired mild mitral regurgitation. J Thorac Cardiovasc Surg. 2007;134:1548–53.
23. Bouma W, van der Horst IC, Wijdh-den Hamer IJ, Erasmus ME, Zijlstra F, Mariani MA, et al. Chronic ischaemic mitral regurgitation. Current treatment results and new mechanism-based surgical approaches. Eur J Cardiothorac Surg. 2010;37:170–85.
24. Dion R. Ischemic mitral regurgitation: when and how should it be corrected? J Heart Valve Dis. 1993;2:536–43.
25. Chen FY, Adams DH, Aranki SF, Collins Jr JJ, Couper GS, Rizzo RJ. Mitral valve repair in cardiomyopathy. Circulation. 1998;98:II124–7.
26. Tolis Jr GA, Korkolis DP, Kopf GS, Elefteriades JA. Revascularization alone (without mitral valve repair) suffices in patients with advanced ischemic cardiomyopathy and mild-to-moderate mitral regurgitation. Ann Thorac Surg. 2002;74:1476–80.
27. Balu V, Hershowitz S, Zaki Masud AR, Bhayana JN, Dean DC. Mitral regurgitation in coronary artery disease. Chest. 1982;81:550–5.
28. Aronson D, Goldsher N, Zukermann R, Kapeliovich M, Lessick J, Mutlak D, et al. Ischemic mitral regurgitation and risk of heart failure after myocardial infarction. Arch Intern Med. 2006;166:2362–8.
29. Lam BK, Gillinov AM, Blackstone EH, Rajeswaran J, Yuh B, Bhudia SK, et al. Importance of moderate ischemic mitral regurgitation. Ann Thorac Surg. 2005;79:462–70; discussion 470.
30. Campwala SZ, Bansal RC, Wang N, Razzouk A, Pai RG. Mitral regurgitation progression following isolated coronary artery bypass surgery: frequency, risk factors, and potential prevention strategies. Eur J Cardiothorac Surg. 2006;29:348–53.
31. Gelsomino S, van Garsse L, Lucà F, Lorusso R, Cheriex E, Rao CM, et al. Impact of preoperative anterior leaflet tethering on the recurrence of ischemic mitral regurgitation and the lack of left ventricular reverse remodeling after restrictive annuloplasty. J Am Soc Echocardiogr. 2011;24:1365–75.
32. Menicanti L, Di Donato M, Frigiola A, Buckberg G, Santambrogio C, Ranucci M, et al.; RESTORE Group. Ischemic mitral regurgitation: intraventricular papillary muscle imbrication without mitral ring during left ventricular restoration. J Thorac Cardiovasc Surg. 2002;123:1041–50.
33. Castelvecchio S, Parolari A, Garatti A, Gagliardotto P, Mossuto E, Canziani A, et al. Surgical ventricular restoration plus mitral valve repair in patients with ischemic heart failure. Risk factors for early and mid-term outcome. Oral presentation at 29th EACTS annual meeting, Amsterdam, 3–7 Oct 2015.
34. Schurr P, Boeken U, Limathe J, Akhyari P, Feindt P, Lichtenberg A. Impact of mitral valve repair in patients with mitral regurgitation undergoing coronary artery bypass grafting. Acta Cardiol. 2010;65:441–7.
35. Kang DH, Kim MJ, Kang SJ, Song JM, Song H, Hong MK, et al. Mitral valve repair versus revascularization alone in the treatment of ischemic mitral regurgitation. Circulation. 2006;114(1 Suppl):I499–503.
36. Deja MA, Grayburn PA, Sun B, Rao V, She L, Krejca M, et al. Influence of mitral regurgitation repair on survival in the surgical treatment for ischemic heart failure trial. Circulation. 2012;125:2639–48.
37. Kron IL, Hung J, Overbey JR, Bouchard D, Gelijns AC, Moskowitz AJ, et al. Predicting recurrent mitral regurgitation after mitral valve repair for severe ischemic mitral regurgitation. J Thorac Cardiovasc Surg. 2015;149:752–61.
38. Kron IL, Green GR, Cope JT. Surgical relocation of the posterior papillary muscle in chronic ischemic mitral regurgitation. Ann Thorac Surg. 2002;74:600–1.
39. Choi JO, Daly RC, Lin G, Lahr BD, Wiste HJ, Beaver TM, et al. Impact of surgical ventricular reconstruction on sphericity index in patients with ischemic cardiomyopathy: follow-up from the STICH trial. Eur J Heart Fail. 2015;17:453–63.

Percutaneous Approaches to Functional Mitral Regurgitation

14

Michele De Bonis and Elisabetta Lapenna

Abstract

Many patients with functional (or secondary) mitral regurgitation (MR) are not eligible for surgery due to advanced age, comorbidities and severe left ventricular dysfunction. For these reasons, over the past few years, several transcatheter techniques have been developed to treat secondary MR with less invasive approaches. Currently, the procedure with the widest clinical application is the percutaneous edge-to-edge repair performed with the MitraClip System, which mimics the surgical edge-to-edge repair by implanting a clip via a transatrial transfemoral access under fluoroscopic and transesophageal echocardiographic guidance. This technique has provided good results in terms of safety and symptoms improvement and is now considered a viable option to treat high-risk and inoperable symptomatic patients. A careful selection of the patients from an anatomical and clinical point of view is essential to achieve efficacy and avoid futility. Residual or recurrent MR remains an issue which needs to be addressed. In addition, randomized studies are necessary to clarify whether percutaneous correction of secondary MR in high-risk patients provides clinical and prognostic benefit in comparison with optimal medical therapy.

Beyond the MitraClip system, other percutaneous approaches to secondary MR include indirect and direct annuloplasty procedures. However, their clinical application is currently not comparable to the MitraClip therapy and for this reason most of this chapter will be focused on the percutaneous edge-to-edge mitral valve repair.

Keywords

Secondary mitral regurgitation • Percutaneous edge-to-edge repair • Trans-catheter annuloplasty • MitraClip

M. De Bonis, MD (✉) • E. Lapenna, MD
Department of Cardiac Surgery, San Raffaele "Vita e Salute" University Medical School, IRCCS San Raffaele Hospital, Via Olgettina 60, Milan 20132, Italy
e-mail: debonis.michele@hsr.it

K.M.J. Chan (ed.), *Functional Mitral and Tricuspid Regurgitation*,
DOI 10.1007/978-3-319-43510-7_14

Principles of Treatment

Functional (or secondary) mitral regurgitation (MR) is a consequence of annular dilatation and geometrical distortion of the sub-valvular apparatus secondary to left ventricular (LV) remodelling and dyssynchrony, most usually associated with cardiomyopathy or coronary artery disease.

The best surgical treatment for secondary MR remains controversial because the prognosis of the patients is more related to the cardiomyopathic process than to MR itself. Mitral repair performed with an undersized rigid complete ring is the reference standard and can be performed with acceptable peri-operative risk and significant symptomatic improvement in carefully selected patients [1, 2]. Recurrent MR is the main disadvantage [3], which may underlie the lack of observed survival benefit compared to medical therapy [4]. Several predictors of repair failure have been identified [5] and their presence should prompt the use of concomitant techniques besides annuloplasty to improve durability or lead to replacement rather than repair of the mitral valve [6–8].

The Euro Heart Survey conducted by the European Society of Cardiology (ESC) showed that a large number of patients with severe MR are denied surgical treatment because they are considered to be at too high risk for surgery owing to advanced age or comorbidities [9].

For these reasons, over the past few years, several transcatheter techniques have been developed to treat secondary MR with less invasive approaches. Currently, the procedure with the widest clinical experience is the percutaneous edge-to-edge repair performed with the MitraClip System (Abbott Laboratories, Abbott Park, Illinois) (Fig. 14.1). The technology has received CE mark in 2008 and is available for clinical use in Europe. It has been included in the ESC/EACTS Valvular Heart Disease Guidelines as a treatment option for high-risk and inoperable patients as decided by a dedicated Heart Team [5]. In the US, FDA approval was achieved only for degenerative MR (DMR) and the device still remains investigational for the treatment of functional MR (FMR). The first case was performed in 2003 and nowadays more than 20,000 patients have been treated with this approach worldwide.

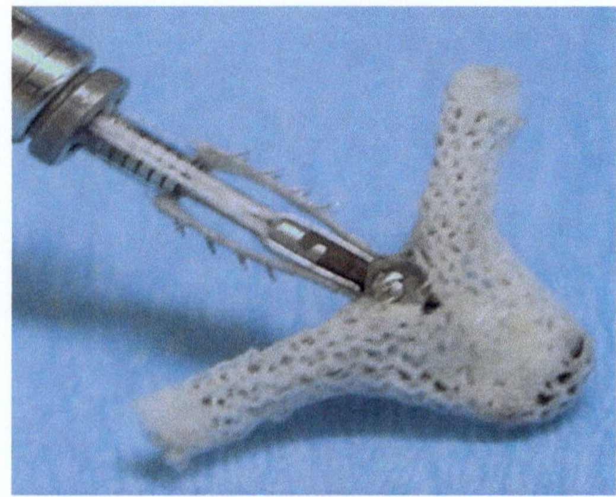

Fig. 14.1 Close up of the MitraClip device

Beyond the MitraClip system, other percutaneous approaches to FMR include indirect and direct annuloplasty procedures. The indirect annuloplasty systems are in various stages of development, have no surgical equivalent and their efficacy needs to be proven. Conversely, percutaneous direct annuloplasty reproduces surgical techniques and can be achieved with annular plication or commissure-to-commissure implant.

Their clinical application is currently not comparable to the MitraClip therapy and for this reason most of this chapter will be focused on the percutaneous edge-to-edge mitral valve repair.

Technique

Percutaneous Edge-to-Edge Repair

The MitraClip delivery system is made up of a sophisticated tri-axial catheter system (steerable guide catheter and clip delivery system catheter) and an implantable clip, available in one single size. The clip delivery system, which can be steered in four directions, has the MitraClip device attached to its distal end. The guide catheter is 24 Fr at the level of the groin and 22 Fr at the atrial septum. The device is a cobalt-chromium implant with two arms and two "grippers" adjacent to each arm to independently secure the leaf-

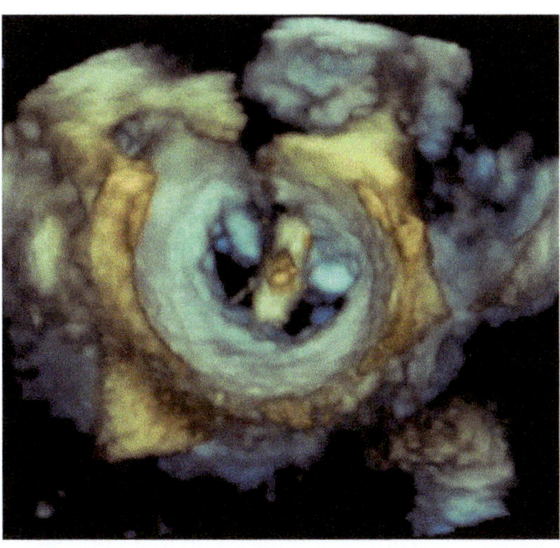

Fig. 14.2 3D Transesophageal view of the MitraClip correctly oriented with the arms perpendicular to the line of coaptation

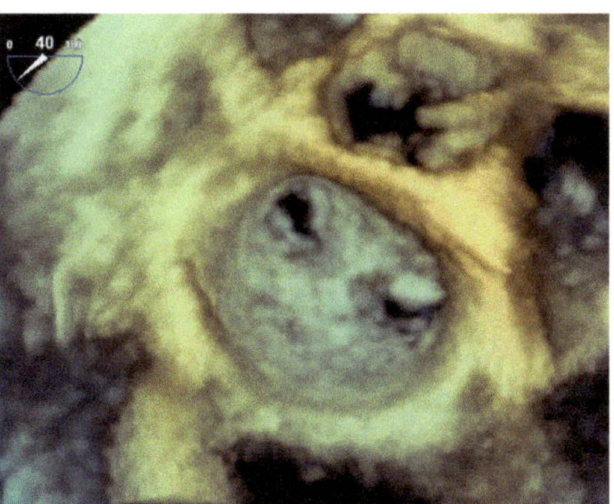

Fig. 14.3 3D Transesophageal view of a double-orifice mitral valve after MitraClip implantation

lets following grasping. The clip arms and grippers are covered with polyester to enhance healing (Fig. 14.1). The MitraClip is implanted under general anesthesia, guided by transesophageal echocardiography (TEE) and fluoroscopy. Currently, many procedures are performed under real-time 3D echocardiography with fusion imaging techniques, which makes them easier and more intuitive. After peripheral venous access at the groin, the atrial septum is crossed using diathermy in the mid-superior and posterior aspect of the fossa ovalis, to achieve proper alignment of the system. The location of the transseptal puncture is critical to reach the mitral valve leaflets with coaxial alignment to the long axis of the heart. Following trans-septal puncture, a steerable guide catheter is advanced into the left atrium. Afterwards, the clip delivery system is inserted and the MitraClip device is steered towards the mitral valve, at the origin of the regurgitant jet. The clip arms are opened and positioned perpendicularly to the line of coaptation; symmetric implantation is fundamental for an effective and durable repair (Fig. 14.2). The clip is advanced into the left ventricle and then retracted and partially closed to a "V" shape to engage the leaflets. Leaflets are grasped by gentle retraction of the clip toward the left atrium. To secure the leaflets into the device, the grippers are dropped and the clip is closed at approximately 60° to allow assessment of leaflet insertion. This step is still reversible and is used to assess symmetry and efficacy of the position. When the clip is closed, the final effect on MR reduction is evaluated using full-volume 3D color Doppler and, if the result of the implant is satisfactory, the clip is deployed (Fig. 14.3). However, if necessary, at this stage the clip can still be reopened, inverted to release the leaflets and repositioned. Alternatively, a second clip can be used, but it is rare for more than two clips to be used in order to avoid mitral valve stenosis. Once the procedure is completed, percutaneous vascular closure is performed, and the patient is weaned from general anesthesia.

Percutaneous Annuloplasty

Undersized ring annuloplasty has been extensively used for the surgical treatment of FMR. On the basis of this surgical background, several trans-catheter percutaneous technologies have been developed to perform a percutaneous annuloplasty procedure. They can be essentially divided into direct and indirect annuloplasty systems.

Direct Annuloplasty

Percutaneous direct annuloplasty tries to reproduce surgical annuloplasty techniques:

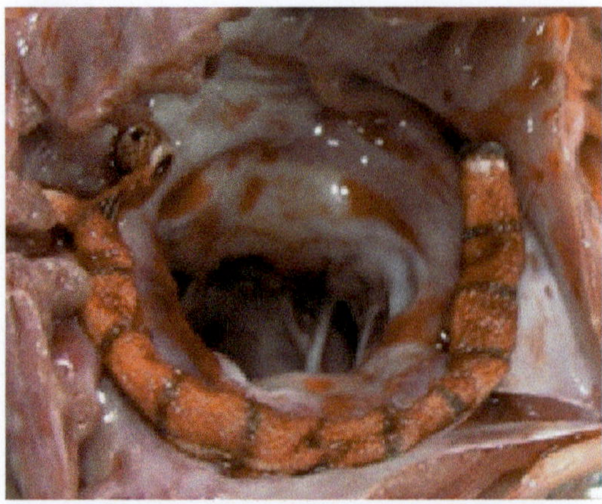

Fig. 14.4 Implanted Cardioband in an animal model

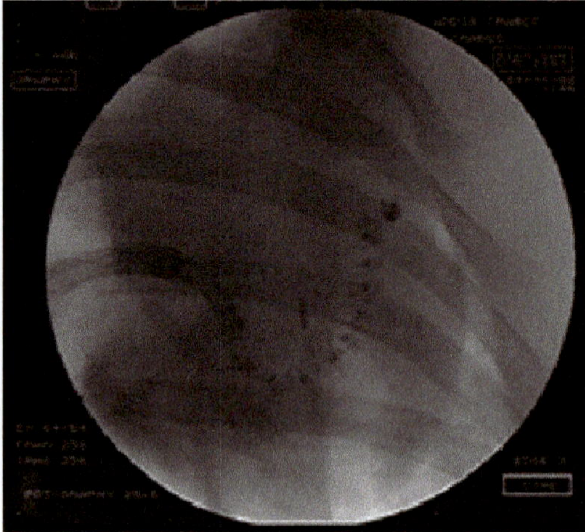

Fig. 14.5 Angiographic image of Cardioband after implantation

Cardioband (Valtech Cardio Inc., Or Yehuda, Israel) is an adjustable, catheter-deliverable, sutureless Dacron band that is inserted percutaneously [10]. The insertion requires a steerable guide and device delivery system that is similar to the MitraClip system. Through a transseptal approach the band is anchored to the atrial side of the mitral annulus via multiple helical anchors, from trigone to trigone (Figs. 14.4 and 14.5). After delivery, the implant is tensioned to create posterior annuloplasty with septal-lateral dimension reductions of approximately 30% and to achieve adequate leaflet coaptation and MR reduction. The first-in-human procedure was performed in 2013 in Milan, Italy, and a European multi-center CE Mark trial is underway.

The **Mitralign** Percutaneous Annuloplasty System (Mitralign Inc., Tewksbury, MA USA) is a suturing plicating system, originally designed to plicate the mitral annulus at P1 and P3 level from a retrograde ventricular approach with a guide catheter inserted across the aortic valve [11]. Two pledgeted anchors are inserted with the aid of a radiofrequency wire puncture of the annulus and then pulled together to shorten or plicate the annulus and fixed with a stainless steel lock. Two sets of paired anchors are placed at both commissures. In a phase 1 report, septal-lateral dimension was reduced up to 8 mm. Since the Mitralign is a true suturing system, multiple plicating pledgets can be implanted along the annulus and different applications may be speculated. A multicenter CE Mark trial in Germany, Poland, Brazil, and Colombia has completed enrollment.

The **Accucinch** device (Guided Delivery System Inc., Santa Clara, CA, USA) also uses a retrograde ventricular approach to implant a series of anchors beneath the mitral annulus in the basal ventricular myocardium and connect them with a nitinol wire that is then used to cinch the mitral annulus and the basal ventricular wall. The Accucinch is currently under clinical evaluation.

Other devices in this category remain preclinical including the BOA RF catheter (QuantumCor Inc, Bothell, WA) which uses radiofrequency energy delivered via a transseptal catheter to heat shrink the collagen within the mitral annulus to mimic surgical ring annuloplasty. In animals, a 20–25% reduction in anterior-posterior dimension was achieved with 6-month durability. A first-in-human validation study during open heart surgery is planned.

Indirect Annuloplasty

The basic principle of indirect annuloplasty is to apply tension on the coronary sinus in order to indirectly reduce the mitral annulus dimension and improve leaflet coaptation. Unfortunately this approach has shown to have serious limitations. Early attempts led to a modest reduction in MR severity and a high incidence of adverse

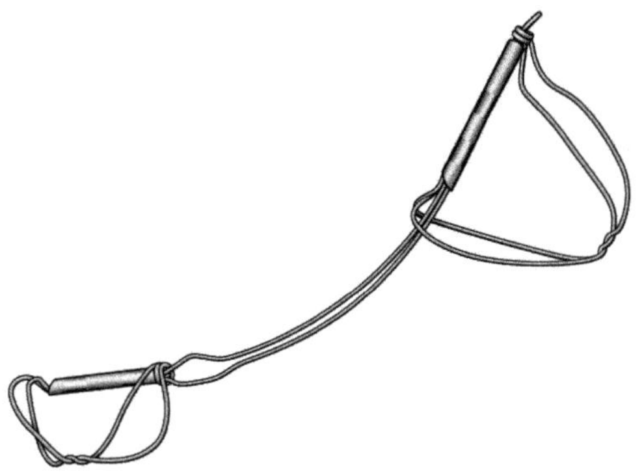

Fig. 14.6 Carillon indirect annuloplasty device

cardiovascular events, including early and late myocardial infarction as well as coronary sinus rupture [12, 13]. The limited efficacy is likely related to the variable distance between the coronary sinus and the mitral annulus and due to the high risk of coronary artery compression. For these reasons coronary sinus devices have gradually lost appeal in favour of direct annuloplasties. Nonetheless, it is possible that some superresponders may be identifiable on the basis of careful preprocedure imaging and could gain benefit from this technique.

Among the indirect annuloplasty devices which have been developed, only the **Carillon** (Cardiac Dimensions Inc., Kirkland, WA, USA) remains currently available for clinical use after having obtained CE mark (Fig. 14.6). This device has anchors placed permanently in the coronary sinus, which are then pulled toward each other with a cinching device to reduce the mitral annular circumference by traction. In the Amadeus feasibility study, the device was successfully implanted in 30 of 48 (62.5 %) patients with modest improvement of MR, a 15 % rate of coronary compromise and death in 1 patient [14]. A newer version of the device was evaluated in the Transcatheter Implantation of Carillon Mitral Annuloplasty Device (TITAN) trial [15]. Among 53 enrolled subjects with secondary (61 % ischemic) MR, the device was successfully implanted in 36 patients (68 %). At 6 and 12 months a significant improvement in the degree of MR, LV dimension, functional status, and quality of life was documented. Comparison was made with baseline and with the 17 patients who were enrolled in the trial but did not receive implants.

Results of Treatment

Although very promising, not enough data are available at the moment to judge the clinical value of the percutaneous annuloplasty devices. On the other hand, many studies have been published on the early and mid-term outcomes of the percutaneous edge-to-edge repair. When assessing the results of the MitraClip therapy, however, it is important to consider that this is also a relatively new technique with limited follow-up. In addition, most studies about the MitraClip have included mixed populations of patients with both degenerative and functional MR, making assessment of specific outcomes in different subgroups more complex.

For instance, in the randomized EVEREST II (Endovascular Valve Edge-to-Edge Repair of Mitral Regurgitation Study) trial, 184 patients were designated (2:1) to receive MitraClip therapy and 95 patients to undergo surgical repair or replacement [16]. However, most of the patients were low-risk patients with primary MR (FMR being present in only 27 % of the cases).

Major adverse events at 30 days were significantly less frequent with MitraClip therapy (9.6 % versus 57 % with surgery, P<0.0001), although much of this difference was attributable to the greater need for blood transfusion with surgery. The primary end point of freedom from death, mitral valve surgery, and MR severity >2+ at 12 months in patients with initial clinical success was similar, but by intent to treat analysis was lower with MitraClip (55 %) as compared with surgery (73 %, P=0.0007). At 4 years, overall mortality was similar in the 2 groups, mitral valve surgery was used more often after MitraClip (25 % versus 5 % after surgery), and moderate or severe MR was more common after transcatheter therapy. The primary combined end point of freedom from death, surgery, or 3+ or 4+ MR in the intention-to-treat population was lower (40 %) with percutaneous repair and 53 % with surgery (P=0.070). However, patients with a good result after MitraClip had sustained improvement for 4 years [17]. For the reasons mentioned above, the EVEREST II trial does not provide the best evidence for high risk patients with mitral regurgitation secondary to LV remodelling and dysfunction. Nevertheless secondary MR represents currently the most common indication for percutaneous EE repair (65–75 % of patients) [18].

One of the studies suggesting a potential prognostic benefit in high-risk patients treated with the MitraClip in both the degenerative and functional MR has been the High-Risk Registry of the EVEREST II study. Patients treated with the MitraClip had a better survival rate at 1 year compared to a matched group managed with optimal medical treatment alone. In addition, the registry demonstrated a significant reduction in heart failure hospitalization by a factor of approximately 50 % as compared to the year before implantation, improvement in clinical symptoms, and significant LV reverse remodeling over 12 months in patients submitted to MitraClip therapy [19].

Another very important study for the assessment of the results of the MitraClip therapy in the setting of secondary MR is the ACCESS-EU registry [18]. In this series 393 patients with secondary MR, severe LV dysfunction and congestive heart failure were enrolled. Mortality was 3 % at 30-days which is notably low, especially if we consider that the majority of patients were at high surgical risk (Logistic EuroSCORE I 23 ± 18 %) and affected by FMR secondary to chronic heart failure. One-year mortality was 17 % with significant complications (stroke, resuscitation and tamponade) in 1–2 % of cases. Efficacy was similar to previous findings in degenerative MR with residual MR grade 3–4 in 8 % and 22 % at discharge and 12 month follow up, respectively. The majority (69 %) were in NYHA class I/II at 12 months with demonstrable reverse LV and left atrial remodeling but residual MR grade 2+ in almost 50 %.

Satisfactory clinical results have also been reported by the German TRAnscatheter MItral valve interventions (TRAMI) registry [20] that enrolled 1,064 patients (525 patients ≥76 years and 539 patients <76 years; more than 70 % with FMR). Age was the most frequent reason for non-surgical treatment in the elderly. The in-hospital MACCE (death, myocardial infarction, stroke) was low in both groups (3.5 % vs. 3.4 %) and the proportion of non-severe mitral regurgitation at discharge was similar (95.8 % vs. 96.4 %, p = 0.73). A logistic regression model did not reveal any significant impact of age on acute efficacy and safety of MitraClip therapy, showing that elderly and younger patients have similar clinical benefits.

The Transcatheter Valve Treatment Sentinel Pilot Registry [21], a prospective, independent, consecutive collection of individual patient data, enrolled a total of 628 patients (mean age 74.2 ± 9.7 years) who underwent transcatheter edge-to-edge between January 2011 and December 2012 in 25 centers in 8 European countries. The prevalent pathogenesis was functional mitral regurgitation (FMR) (72.0 %). The majority of patients (85.5 %) were highly symptomatic (New York Heart Association functional class III or higher), with a high logistic EuroSCORE I (20.4 ± 16.7 %). In-hospital mortality was low (2.9 %) and the estimated 1-year mortality was 15.3 %, which was similar for FMR and degenerative mitral regurgitation. The estimated 1-year rate of re-hospitalization because of heart failure was 22.8 %. Paired echocardiographic data from the 1-year follow-up, available for 368 consecutive patients, showed a persistent reduction in the degree of mitral regurgitation at 1 year, with 6.0 % of patients with severe mitral regurgitation.

Of course direct comparisons between percutaneous edge-to-edge repair and surgery in secondary MR are difficult since patients treated with either strategy are significantly different. Two small non-randomized series reported higher efficacy of surgery compared to percutaneous intervention [22, 23]. In contrast, post-hoc analysis of the EVEREST II trial demonstrated equivalence of the two strategies in this setting [16, 17]. However, in the absence of a medical therapy control group, it is not possible to establish whether either treatment has positive impact on survival – ongoing randomized studies will address this question.

Which Patients Should Have This Procedure?

In secondary MR, percutaneous edge-to-edge repair is a low risk option to reduce symptoms and induce reverse LV remodeling but commonly associated with residual and recurrent MR. Thus, according to the 2012 ESC/EACTS guidelines on Valvular heart disease [5], it may be considered only in patients with symptomatic severe secondary MR (despite optimal medical therapy – including CRT if indicated), with anatomical suitability, who are judged inoperable or at high surgical risk by a team of cardiologists and cardiac surgeons, and with a life expectancy greater than 1 year (recommendation class IIb, level of evidence C). On the other hand, in the United States, MitraClip received Food and Drug Administration approval in October 2013 only for patients with primary (degenerative) MR who are deemed prohibitive risk for surgery by a multidisciplinary heart team. Recent ACC/AHA guidelines recommend (class IIb, level of evidence B) consideration of transcatheter repair for severely symptomatic patients with chronic severe primary MR, reasonable life expectancy, and prohibitive surgical risk attributable to severe comorbidities [24].

A multidisciplinary Heart Team (interventional cardiologists, cardiac surgeons, anaesthetists, imaging and heart failure specialists) should evaluate the pros and cons of surgical, percutaneous and conservative approaches in all high-risk patients with MR, assessing the risk/benefit ratio of each option whilst incorporating relevant comorbidities and individualized life expectancy. The possible futility of intervention in very high-risk subjects must also be considered – some will not benefit from surgical or percutaneous intervention and conservative management (and possible palliative care) is more appropriate.

Risk assessment is fundamental to decision-making. However, definitions of 'high surgical risk' and the "inoperable patient" remain elusive and significantly influenced by surgeon and centre experience. In addition, while most procedural risk scores discriminate between high and low-risk, they were not developed in large cohorts with valvular heart disease and are poorly calibrated in high-risk subjects [25]. With those limitations in mind, the best established risk scores (e.g. STS, Euroscore) should be utilised in conjunction with other factors (e.g., frailty, porcelain aorta) as recommended by the VARC-2 consensus document [26] and a tailored approach for individual patients remains appropriate.

Table 14.1 EVEREST II main anatomic eligibility criteria for percutaneous edge-to-edge repair in secondary MR

Moderate to severe mitral regurgitation (grade 3/4 or more)
Pathology in A2-P2 zone
Coaptation length >2 mm
Coaptation depth <11 mm
Mitral valve orifice area >4 cm^2
Mobile leaflet length >1 cm

Table 14.2 Most common unfavorable anatomical conditions for percutaneous edge-to-edge repair

Commissural lesions
Short posterior leaflet
Severe asymmetric tethering
Calcification in the grasping area
Severe annular calcification
Cleft
Severe annular dilatation
Severe left ventricular remodeling
Large (>50 %) intercommissural extension of regurgitant jet

Transesophageal echocardiography is essential to confirm whether a high-risk or inoperable patient with secondary MR is anatomically eligible for percutaneous EE repair. No specific guidelines are currently available and the EVEREST II trial anatomical inclusion criteria are the principal reference (Table 14.1). Although still useful as a guideline, these criteria are not considered strictly mandatory anymore: as a matter of fact, they do not seem to be clearly associated with acute or long-term results and are currently not respected in a vast proportion of patients. Indeed, percutaneous treatment outside these criteria (including commissural MR, advanced LV remodelling, anatomic cleft, asymmetric tethering) is now common, although certain anatomical conditions predict failure or suboptimal outcome and need to be carefully assessed before intervention (Table 14.2).

Conclusions

Transcatheter edge-to-edge mitral repair with the MitraClip System is the most widely used percutaneous approach to treat secondary MR. It has provided good results in terms of safety and symptoms improvement and is now considered a viable option to treat high-risk and inoperable symptomatic patients. Residual or recurrent MR remains an issue which needs to be addressed. In future, the combination of the edge-to-edge repair with percutaneous annuloplasty, might improve efficacy and durability. However randomized studies are needed to clarify whether percutaneous correction of FMR in high-risk patients provides clinical and prognostic benefit in comparison with optimal medical therapy. To answer this question, a randomized trial (Clinical Outcomes Assessment of the MitraClip Percutaneous Therapy for High Surgical Risk Patients [COAPT]) is underway.

References

1. Bolling SF, Deeb GM, Brunsting LA, Bach DS. Early outcome of mitral valve reconstruction in patients with end-stage cardiomyopathy. J Thorac Cardiovasc Surg. 1995;4:676–83.
2. Spoor MT, Geltz A, Bolling SF. Flexible versus nonflexible mitral valve rings for congestive heart failure. Circulation. 2006;114(Suppl I):I67–71.
3. McGee EC, Gillinov AM, Blackstone EH, Rajeswaran J, Cohen G, Najam F, Shiota T, Sabik JF, Lytle BW, McCarthy PM, Cosgrove DM. Recurrent mitral regurgitation after annuloplasty for functional ischemic mitral regurgitation. J Thorac Cardiovasc Surg. 2004;128:916–24.
4. Wu AH, Aaronson KD, Bolling SF, Pagani FD, Welch K, Koelling TM. Impact of mitral valve annuloplasty on mortality risk in patients with mitral regurgitation and left ventricular systolic dysfunction. J Am Coll Cardiol. 2005;45:381–7.
5. Joint Task Force on the Management of Valvular Heart Disease of the European Society of Cardiology (ESC); European Association for Cardio-Thoracic Surgery (EACTS), Vahanian A, Alfieri O, Andreotti F, Antunes MJ, Barón-Esquivias G, Baumgartner H, Borger MA, Carrel TP, De Bonis M, Evangelista A, Falk V, Iung B, Lancellotti P, Pierard L, Price S, Schäfers HJ, Schuler G, Stepinska J, Swedberg K, Takkenberg J, Von Oppell UO, Windecker S, Zamorano JL, Zembala M. Guidelines on the management of valvular heart disease (version 2012). Eur Heart J. 2012;33:2451–96.
6. Borger MA, Murphy PM, Alam A, Armstrong S, Maganti M, David TE. Initial results of the chordal-cutting operation for ischemic mitral regurgitation. J Thorac Cardiovasc Surg. 2007;133:1483–92.
7. Langer F, Kunihara T, Hell K, Schramm R, Schmidt KI, Aicher D, Kindermann M, Schäfers HJ. RING+STRING: successful repair technique for ischemic mitral regurgitation with severe leaflet tethering. Circulation. 2009;120:S85–91.
8. Acker MA, Parides MK, Perrault LP, Moskowitz AJ, Gelijns AC, Voisine P, Smith PK, Hung JW, Blackstone EH, Puskas JD, Argenziano M, Gammie JS, Mack M, Ascheim DD, Bagiella E, Moquete EG, Ferguson TB, Horvath KA, Geller NL, Miller MA, Woo YJ, D'Alessandro DA, Ailawadi G, Dagenais F, Gardner TJ, O'Gara PT, Michler RE, Kron IL. Mitral-valve repair versus replacement for severe ischemic mitral regurgitation. N Engl J Med. 2014;370:23–32.
9. Mirabel M, Iung B, Baron G, Messika-Zeitoun D, Détaint D, Vanoverschelde JL, Butchart EG, Ravaud P, Vahanian A. What are the characteristics of patients with severe, symptomatic, mitral regurgitation who are denied surgery? Eur Heart J. 2007;28:1358–65.
10. Maisano F, La Canna G, Latib A, Denti P, Taramasso M, Kuck KH, et al. First-in-Man trans-septal implantation of a "surgical-like" mitral valve annuloplasty device for functional mitral regurgitation. JACC Cardiovasc Interv. 2014;7(11):1326–8.
11. Siminiak T, Dankowski R, Baszko A, Lee C, Firek L, Kałmucki P, Szyszka A, Groothuis A. Percutaneous direct mitral annuloplasty using the Mitralign Bident system: description of the method and a case report. Kardiol Pol. 2013;71:1287–92.
12. Harnek J, Webb JG, Kuck KH, Tschope C, Vahanian A, Buller CE, James SK, Tiefenbachere CP, Stone GW. Transcatheter implantation of the MONARC coronary sinus device for mitral regurgitation. J Am Coll Cardiol Interv. 2011;4:115–22.
13. Sack S, Kahlert P, Bilodeau L, Pièrard LA, Lancellotti P, Legrand V, Bartunek J, Vanderheyden M, Hoffmann R, Schauerte P, Shiota T, Marks DS, Erbel R, Ellis SG. Percutaneous transvenous mitral annuloplasty: initial human experience with a novel coronary sinus implant device. Circ Cardiovasc Interv. 2009;2: 277–84.
14. Schofer J, Siminiak T, Haude M, Herrman JP, Vainer J, Wu JC, Levy WC, Mauri L, Feldman T, Kwong RY, Kaye DM, Duffy SJ, Tübler T, Degen H, Brandt MC, Van Bibber R, Goldberg S, Reuter DG, Hoppe UC. Percutaneous mitral annuloplasty for functional mitral regurgitation: results of the CARILLON Mitral Annuloplasty Device European Union Study. Circulation. 2009;120:326–33.
15. Siminiak T, Wu JC, Haude M, Hoppe UC, Sadowski J, Lipieci J, Fajadet J, Shah AM, Feldman T, Kaye DM, Goldberg SL, Levy WC, Soloman SD, Reuter DG. Treatment of functional mitral regurgitation by percutaneous annuloplasty: results of the TITAN trial. Eur J Heart Fail. 2012;14:1090–6.
16. Feldman T, Foster E, Glower DD, Kar S, Rinaldi MJ, Fail PS, Smalling RW, Siegel R, Rose GA, Engeron E, Loghin C, Trento A, Skipper ER, Fudge T, Letsou GV, Massaro JM, Mauri L. Percutaneous repair or surgery for mitral regurgitation. N Engl J Med. 2011;364: 1395–406.
17. Mauri L, Foster E, Glower DD, Apruzzese P, Massaro JM, Herrmann HC, Hermiller J, Gray W, Wang A,

Pedersen WR, Bajwa T, Lasala J, Low R, Grayburn P, Feldman T. 4-year results of a randomized controlled trial of percutaneous repair versus surgery for mitral regurgitation. J Am Coll Cardiol. 2013;62:317–28.
18. Maisano F, Franzen O, Baldus S, Schafer U, Hausleiter J, Butter C, Ussia GP, Sievert H, Richardt G, Widder JD, Moccetti T, Schillinger W. Percutaneous mitral valve interventions in the real world: early and 1-year results from the ACCESS-EU, a prospective, multicenter, nonrandomized post-approval study of the MitraClip therapy in Europe. J Am Coll Cardiol. 2013;62:1052–61.
19. Glower DD, Kar S, Trento A, Lim DS, Bajwa T, Quesada R, Whitlow PL, Rinaldi MJ, Grayburn P, Mack MJ, Mauri L, McCarthy PM, Feldman T. Percutaneous mitral valve repair for mitral regurgitation in high-risk patients: results of the EVEREST II study. J Am Coll Cardiol. 2014;64:172–81.
20. Schillinger W, Hunlich M, Baldus S, Ouarrak T, Boekstegers P, Hink U, Butter C, Bekeredjian R, Plicht B, Sievert H, Schofer J, Senges J, Meinertz T, Hasenfuss G. Acute outcomes after MitraClip therapy in highly aged patients: results from the German TRAnscatheter Mitral valve Interventions (TRAMI) Registry. EuroIntervention. 2013;9:84–90.
21. Nickenig G, Estevez-Loureiro R, Franzen O, Tamburino C, Vanderheyden M, Lüscher TF, Moat N, Price S, Dall'Ara G, Winter R, Corti R, Grasso C, Snow TM, Jeger R, Blankenberg S, Settergren M, Tiroch K, Balzer J, Petronio AS, Büttner HJ, Ettori F, Sievert H, Fiorino MG, Claeys M, Ussia GP, Baumgartner H, Scandura S, Alamgir F, Keshavarzi F, Colombo A, Maisano F, Ebelt H, Aruta P, Lubos E, Plicht B, Schueler R, Pighi M, Di Mario C; Transcatheter Valve Treatment Sentinel Registry Investigators of the EURObservational Research Programme of the European Society of Cardiology. Percutaneous mitral valve edge-to-edge repair: in-hospital results and 1-year follow-up of 628 patients of the 2011–2012 Pilot European Sentinel Registry. J Am Coll Cardiol. 2014;64:875–84.
22. Taramasso M, Denti P, Buzzati N, De Bonis M, La Canna G, Colombo A, Alfieri O, Maisano F. Mitraclip therapy and surgical mitral repair in patients with moderate to severe left ventricular failure causing functional mitral regurgitation: a single-center experience. Eur J Cardiothorac Surg. 2012;42(6):920–6.
23. De Bonis M, Taramasso M, Lapenna E, Denti P, La Canna G, Buzzatti N, Pappalardo F, Di Giannuario G, Cioni M, Giacomini A, Alfieri O. MitraClip therapy and surgical edge-to-edge repair in patients with severe left ventricular dysfunction and secondary mitral regurgitation: mid-term results of a single-centre experience†. Eur J Cardiothorac Surg. 2016;49(1):255–62.
24. Nishimura RA, Otto CM, Bonow RO, Carabello BA, Erwin III JP, Guyton RA, O'Gara PT, Ruiz CE, Skubas NJ, Sorajja P, Sundt III TM, Thomas JD. 2014 AHA/ACC guideline for the management of patients with valvular heart disease: a report of the American College of Cardiology/American Heart Association Task Force on Practice Guidelines. J Am Coll Cardiol. 2014;63:e57–185.
25. Rosenhek R, Iung B, Tornos P, Antunes MJ, Prendergast BD, Otto CM, Kappetein AP, Stepinska J, Kaden JJ, Naber CK, Acartürk E, Gohlke-Bärwolf C. ESC Working Group on Valvular Heart Disease Position Paper: assessing the risk of interventions in patients with valvular heart disease. Eur Heart J. 2012;33:822–8.
26. Kappetein AP, Head SJ, Genereux P, Piazza N, van Mieghem NM, Blackstone EH, Brott TG, Cohen DJ, Cutlip DE, van Es GA, Hahn RT, Kirtane AJ, Krucoff MW, Kodali S, Mack MJ, Mehran R, Rodes-Cabau J, Vranckx P, Webb JG, Windecker S, Serruys PW, Leon MB. Updated standardized endpoint definitions for transcatheter aortic valve implantation: the Valve Academic Research Consortium-2 consensus document. Eur Heart J. 2012;33:2403–18.

What Determines Outcome of Functional Ischemic Mitral Regurgitation?

15

K.M. John Chan

Abstract

The outcome of functional ischemic mitral regurgitation and its surgical treatment is influenced by many factors including the severity of the mitral regurgitation, the degree of leaflet tethering, and left ventricular size, function and viability, amongst others. Papillary muscle geometry, function and viability may also affect outcomes in functional ischemic mitral regurgitation.

Keywords

Functional ischemic mitral regurgitation • Leaflet tethering • Papillary muscle geometry • Left ventricular viability • Mitral annuloplasty

The outcome of functional ischemic mitral regurgitation is dependent on several factors including the severity of the mitral regurgitation; the size, function, geometry and viability of the left ventricle; the geometry, function and viability of the papillary muscles; and the geometry of the mitral valve leaflets. These factors influence the natural history of functional ischemic mitral regurgitation, the type of intervention which would best treat the condition, and the outcome of the treatment chosen.

K.M.J. Chan, BM BS, MSc, PhD, FRCS CTh
Department of Cardiothoracic Surgery, Gleneagles Hospital, Jalan Ampang, Kuala Lumpur 50450, Malaysia
e-mail: kmjohnchan@yahoo.com

Mitral Regurgitation Severity

The severity of the mitral regurgitation has an important influence on the outcome of functional ischemic mitral regurgitation. The greater the severity of the mitral regurgitation, the higher the probability of death and of hospital admissions for heart failure, with medical treatment alone [1–4]. However, it is unclear whether eliminating the mitral regurgitation by mitral valve repair or replacement improves survival, although there is evidence that symptoms and functional capacity is improved, and there is also left ventricular reverse remodeling [5–7]. Eliminating mitral regurgitation appears to be important to allow left ventricular reverse remodeling to occur [8]. The severity of the mitral regurgitation also determines the need for, and the durability of mitral valve annuloplasty.

K.M.J. Chan (ed.), *Functional Mitral and Tricuspid Regurgitation*,
DOI 10.1007/978-3-319-43510-7_15

In mild-to-moderate functional ischemic mitral regurgitation, mitral valve annuloplasty in addition to CABG may not be necessary; these patients appear to do just as well with isolated coronary artery revascularization alone, although their survival is still worse compared to those without mitral regurgitation [9–13]. In more severe functional ischemic mitral regurgitation, intervention on the mitral valve is necessary. Mitral valve annuloplasty is an effective and durable repair technique in those with an effective regurgitant orifice area (ERO) of up to 40 mm^2 and results in improved symptoms and functional capacity with reversal of left ventricular remodeling [5, 14]. However, in the more severe mitral regurgitation group, those with an ERO of more than 40 mm^2, a high recurrence rate of moderate or more mitral regurgitation has been reported with mitral annuloplasty alone. In this group, additional repair techniques on the subvalvular apparatus may be necessary, or alternatively, a mitral valve replacement may be the preferred treatment [15].

Left Ventricular Size, Function, Geometry and Viability

The influence of left ventricular viability on left ventricular reverse remodelling and improvement in left ventricular function in patients with ischaemic heart disease is well established, although less work on this has been done in patients with functional ischaemic mitral regurgitation. However, the underlying pathologies are similar in patients with functional ischaemic mitral regurgitation and those with left ventricular dysfunction secondary to ischaemic heart disease. Patients with functional ischaemic mitral regurgitation can be thought of as being in the more advanced end of the spectrum of severity of ischemic heart disease. In these patients, the amount of non-viable scarred myocardial segments has a strong determinant on the outcome of the patient. One study using positron emission tomography (PET) to assess left ventricular viability reported that patients with five or more viable left ventricular segments had a significantly lower 6-month mortality rate compared to patients with less than five viable left ventricular segments following CABG and mitral valve annuloplasty for functional ischaemic mitral regurgitation (4 % versus 43 %, $p<0.01$). Ejection fraction decreased significantly in those with less than five viable left ventricular segments following surgery but remained unchanged in the others [16]. A meta-analysis of patients with left ventricular dysfunction undergoing coronary artery revascularisation reported a lower annual mortality of 3 % in those with significant amounts of viable myocardium compared to 8 % ($p<0.001$) in those without significant viable myocardium as detected by thallium, PET or dobutamine stress echocardiography [17].

Cardiovascular magnetic resonance is an established tool used in patients with ischaemic heart failure to identify viable myocardium and predict functional recovery following coronary artery revascularisation. The degree of functional recovery is related to the amount of scar tissue present as evidenced by the extent of late gadolinium enhancement (LGE) in each of the left ventricular segments. A recovery of 77.8 % of dysfunctional left ventricular segments can be expected following coronary artery revascularisation if no LGE is present compared to 56.6 % if 1–25 % LGE is present, 41.8 % if 26–50 % LGE is present, 10.5 % if 51–75 % LGE is present, and 1.7 % if 76–100 % LGE is present [18]. The presence of LGE has also been independently associated with increased major adverse cardiac events and mortality. In one study, the presence of even small amounts of LGE affecting just 1.4 % of left ventricular mass was associated with a seven fold increased risk of major adverse cardiac events ($p<0.001$) [19]. As the majority of patients with functional ischaemic mitral regurgitation have LGE, a worse outcome can be expected for these patients compared to the majority of patients with coronary artery disease but no LGE. Indeed, several observational studies have reported an increased incidence of heart failure admissions and decreased survival in patients with even mild functional ischaemic mitral regurgitation despite successful coronary artery revascularisation [1, 3, 9, 11]. Assessment of left ventricular viability is therefore of major importance in functional ischaemic mitral regurgitation and has a strong influence on the outcome of the patient. Based on other studies on ischaemic left ventricular dysfunction, assessing left ventricular viability by cardiovascular magnetic resonance LGE may also be useful in predicting future cardiac events and estimating prognosis in functional ischaemic mitral regurgitation.

The size and geometry of the left ventricle also has an impact on the outcome of surgical treatment for functional ischemic mitral regurgitation. An excessively dilated left ventricle (left ventricular end diastolic diameter greater than 65 mm) is a predictor of reduced survival and poorer left ventricular reverse remodelling following restrictive mitral annuloplasty [7, 8, 20, 21]. Increased volumes and sphericity of the left ventricle have also been associated with recurrence of mitral regurgitation following mitral annuloplasty [21–23]. More recently, the presence of dyskinesia or aneurysm at the base of the left ventricle was predictive of recurrent mitral regurgitation following mitral annuloplasty [24]. In these patients, some additional procedures on the left ventricle may be necessary for optimal outcomes, such as a left ventricular restoration surgery [25, 26].

Papillary Muscle Geometry, Function and Viability

The geometry, function and viability of the papillary muscles are likely to have a significant influence on the outcome of functional ischemic mitral regurgitation, although there have been few studies on this to date. However, changes in papillary muscle geometry, such as papillary muscle displacement, will manifest in the more commonly assessed mitral leaflet tethering indices and left ventricular volumes. Displacement of the papillary muscles laterally or posteriorly, for example, is likely to result in increased mitral leaflet tethering with increase in tenting areas and volumes. Similarly, increased separation of the papillary muscles is likely the result of increased left ventricular volumes and sphericity. This has been reported to be a predictor of recurrent mitral regurgitation following mitral annuloplasty [27]. The direction of displacement of the papillary muscles may help provide guidance on the need for, and choice of, subvalvular repair techniques, for example papillary muscle sling or papillary muscle relocation techniques [28, 29].

Mitral Valve Geometry

The severity of mitral leaflet tethering has a significant influence on the outcome of functional ischemic mitral regurgitation. Patients with limited tethering of the mitral valve, as indicated by a small tethering distance or tethering area, are unlikely to show an increase in the mitral regurgitation severity with coronary artery revascularisation alone; concomitant mitral valve repair may not result in much additional benefit in these patients [10]. On the other hand, patients with greater tethering of the mitral valve, as indicated by a large tethering distance or tethering area, are likely to show an increase in the mitral regurgitation severity with coronary artery revascularisation alone, and are likely to benefit from concomitant mitral valve repair or replacement [5, 23]. However, it should be noted that patients with a large tethering area or tethering distance also have a higher risk of developing recurrent mitral regurgitation following mitral valve annuloplasty [23, 30, 31]. Kongsaerepong et al. reported that a tethering area greater than 1.6 cm^2 was an independent risk factor for significant recurrent mitral regurgitation following concomitant CABG and mitral valve annuloplasty for functional ischemic mitral regurgitation, while Gelsomino et al. reported that a tethering distance of 1.1 cm or more was a significant risk factor [30, 31]. Ciarka, et al., reported that increased leaflet angles were a predictor of recurrent mitral regurgitation [23]. In all of these patients who are at a higher risk of developing recurrent mitral regurgitation with mitral annuloplasty, additional subvalvular repair techniques may be necessary to ensure long term durability, or alternatively, a mitral valve replacement may be a better option.

References

1. Aronson D, Goldsher N, Zukermann R, Kapeliovich M. Ischemic mitral regurgitation and risk of heart failure after myocardial infarction. Arch Intern Med. 2006;166:2362–8.
2. Grigioni F, Detaint D, Avierinos J-F, Scott C, Tajik J, Enriquez-Sarano M. Contribution of ischemic mitral regurgitation to congestive heart failure after myocardial infarction. J Am Coll Cardiol. 2005;45:260–7.
3. Lamas GA, Mitchell GF, Flaker GC, Smith SC, Gersh BJ. Clinical significance of mitral regurgitation after acute myocardial infarction. Circulation. 1997;96(3):827–33.
4. Perez de Isla L. Prognostic significance of functional mitral regurgitation after a first non-ST-segment elevation acute coronary syndrome. Eur Heart J. 2006; 27(22):2655.
5. Chan KMJ, Punjabi PP, Flather M, et al. Coronary artery bypass surgery with or without mitral valve annuloplasty in moderate functional ischemic mitral regurgitation: final results of the randomized ischemic mitral evaluation (RIME) trial. Circulation. 2012;126: 2502–10.
6. Fattouch K, Guccione F, Sampognaro R, et al. Efficacy of adding mitral valve annuloplasty to coronary artery bypass grafting in patients with moderate ischemic mitral valve regurgitation: a randomized trial. J Thorac Cardiovasc Surg. 2009;138:278–85.
7. Braun J, van de Veire NR, Klautz RJM, et al. Restrictive mitral annuloplasty cures ischemic mitral regurgitation and heart failure. Ann Thorac Surg. 2008;85:430–7.
8. Mikuckaite L, Vaskelyte J, Radauskaite G, Zaliunas R, Benetis R. Left ventricular remodelling following ischemic mitral valve repair: predictive factors. Scand Cardiovasc J. 2009;43:57–62.
9. Schroder JN, Williams ML, Hata JA, Muhlbaier LH, Swaminathan M. Impact of mitral valve regurgitation evaluated by intraoperative transoesophageal echocardiography on long term outcomes after coronary artery bypass grafting. Circulation. 2005;112(Suppl I):I-293–8.
10. Smith PK, Puskas JD, Ascheim DD, et al. Surgical treatment of moderate ischemic mitral regurgitation. N Engl J Med. 2014;371:2178–88.
11. Grossi EA, Crooke GA, Di Giorgi PL, Schwartz CA. Impact of moderate functional mitral insufficiency in patients undergoing surgical revascularization. Circulation. 2006;114(1):I573.
12. Di Mauro M, Di Giammarco G, Vitolla G, Contini M. Impact of no-to-moderate mitral regurgitation on late results after isolated coronary artery bypass grafting in patients with ischemic cardiomyopathy. Ann Thorac Surg. 2006;81(6):2128.
13. Ryden T, Bech-Hanssen O, Brandrup-Wognsen G, Nilsson F, Svensson S, Jeppsson A. The importance of grade 2 ischemic mitral regurgitation in coronary artery bypass grafting. Eur J Cardiothorac Surg. 2001;20:276–81.
14. Beeri R, Yosefy C, Guerrero L, et al. Early repair of moderate ischemic mitral regurgitation reverses left ventricular remodelling. A functional and molecular study. Circulation. 2007;116(Suppl I):I-288–93.
15. Goldstein D, Moskowitz AJ, Gelijns AC, et al. Two year outcomes of surgical treatment of severe ischemic mitral regurgitation. N Engl J Med. 2016;374(4): 344–53.
16. Pu M, Thomas JD, Gillinov AM, Griffin BP, Brunken RC. Importance of ischemic and viable myocardium for patients with chronic ischemic mitral regurgitation and left ventricular dysfunction. Am J Cardiol. 2003;92:862–4.
17. Allman KC, Shaw LJ, Hachamovitch R, Udelson JE. Myocardial viability testing and impact of revascularisation on prognosis in patients with coronary artery disease and left ventricular dysfunction: a meta-analysis. J Am Coll Cardiol. 2002;39:1151–8.
18. Kim RJ, Wu E, Rafael A, Chen E-L. The use of contrast-enhanced magnetic resonance imaging to identify reversible myocardial dysfunction. N Engl J Med. 2000;343:1445–53.
19. Kwong RY, Chan AK, Brown KA, et al. Impact of unrecognised myocardial scar detected by cardiac magnetic resonance imaging on event free survival in patients presenting with signs or symptoms of coronary artery disease. Circulation. 2006;113:2733–43.
20. Braun J, Bax JJ, Versteegh MIM, Voigt PG. Preoperative left ventricular dimensions predict reverse remodelling following restrictive mitral annuloplasty in ischemic mitral regurgitation. Eur J Cardiothorac Surg. 2005;27:847–53.
21. Ueno T, Sakata R, Iguro Y, et al. Preoperative advanced left ventricular remodelling predisposes to recurrence of ischemic mitral regurgitation with less reverse remodelling. J Heart Valve Dis. 2008;17:36–41.
22. Hung J, Papakostas L, Tahta SA, Hardy BG. Mechanism of recurrent ischemic mitral regurgitation after annuloplasty. Continued LV remodelling as a moving target. Circulation. 2004;110(Suppl II): II-85–90.
23. Ciarka A, Braun J, Delgado V, et al. Predictors of mitral regurgitation recurrence in patients with heart failure undergoing mitral annuloplasty. Am J Cardiol. 2010;106:395–401.
24. Kron IL, Hung J, Overbey JR, et al. Predicitng recurrent mitral regurgitation after mitral valve repair for severe ischemic mitral regurgitation. J Thorac Cardiovasc Surg. 2015;149:752–61.
25. Menicanti L, Donato MD, Castelvecchio S, Santambrogio C. Functional ischemic mitral regurgitation in anterior ventricular remodelling: results of surgical ventricular restoration with and without mitral repair. Heart Fail Rev. 2005;9(4):317–27.
26. Shudo Y, Taniguchi K, Takeda K, et al. Restrictive mitral annuloplasty with or without surgical ventricular restoration in ischemic dilated cardiomyopathy with severe mitral regurgitation. Circulation. 2011;124 Suppl 1:S107–14.

27. Roshanali F, Mandegar H, Yousefnia MA, Rayatzadeh H, Alaeddini F. A prospective study of predicting factors in ischemic mitral regurgitation recurrence after ring annuloplasty. Ann Thorac Surg. 2007;84:745–9.
28. Fattouch K, Murana G, Castrovinci S, et al. Mitral valve annuloplasty and papillary muscle relocation oriented by 3-dimensional tranesophagel echocardiography for severe functional mitral regurgitation. J Thorac Cardiovasc Surg. 2012;143:S38–42.
29. Hvass U, Tapia M, Baron F, Pouzet B. Papillary muscle sling: a new functional approach to mitral repair in patients with ischemic left ventricular dysfunction and functional mitral regurgitation. Ann Thorac Surg. 2003;75:809–11.
30. Gelsomino S, Lorusso R, Caciolli S, et al. Insights on left ventricular and valvular mechanisms of recurrent ischemic mitral regurgitation after restrictive annuloplasty and coronary artery bypass grafting. J Thorac Cardiovasc Surg. 2008;136(2):507–18.
31. Kongsaerepong V. Echocardiographic predictors of successful versus unsuccessful mitral valve repair in ischemic mitral regurgitation. Am J Cardiol. 2006; 98(4):504.

Which Treatment is Best for Functional Ischemic Mitral Regurgitation?

16

K.M. John Chan

Abstract

Functional ischemic mitral regurgitation is primarily caused by myocardial ischaemia or infarction with secondary effects on the mitral valve apparatus and the left ventricle leading to mitral regurgitation and left ventricular dilatation and dysfunction. A range of treatment options are available to treat this condition and these must be tailored to each individual patient. It must be appreciated that functional ischaemic mitral regurgitation is a heterogeneous condition with a range of severity of the different pathologies.

Keywords

Functional ischemic mitral regurgitation

Functional ischemic mitral regurgitation has an adverse outcome with an increased probability of death and of heart failure, which is related to the severity of the mitral regurgitation [1–3]. The greater the severity of the mitral regurgitation, the higher the probability of death and of heart failure. The aim of any intervention in this condition is therefore twofold: to improve survival, and to improve symptoms and functional status. To achieve this, it is necessary to correct any myocardial ischemia which was responsible for causing this condition, and to correct the mitral regurgitation if it is significant. Addressing these two pathologies successfully would lead to left ventricular reverse remodeling, which should translate to an improvement in symptoms, functional status and survival. Several treatment options are available and successful treatment of this condition would necessitate a combination of these interventions so that each of the underlying pathologies is adequately addressed: (1) optimal medical treatment for coronary artery disease and heart failure, (2) coronary artery revascularization, (3) mitral valve repair or replacement, and (4) left ventricular restoration surgery.

Functional ischemic mitral regurgitation is a heterogeneous condition (Table 16.1). Patients present with varying severity of the mitral

K.M.J. Chan, BM BS, MSc, PhD, FRCS CTh
Department of Cardiothoracic Surgery,
Gleneagles Hospital, Jalan Ampang,
Kuala Lumpur 50450, Malaysia
e-mail: kmjohnchan@yahoo.com

K.M.J. Chan (ed.), *Functional Mitral and Tricuspid Regurgitation*,
DOI 10.1007/978-3-319-43510-7_16

Table 16.1 The heterogeneity of functional ischemic mitral regurgitation

Parameter	Range of values
1. Mitral regurgitation severity	Mild Moderate (ERO < 20 mm^2) Severe (ERO 20–40 mm^2) Very severe (ERO > 40 mm^2)
2. Mitral leaflet tethering	None Mild (tethering distance < 10 mm) Severe (tethering distance ≥ 10 mm)
3. Left ventricle viability	Fully viable Mostly viable (>5 LV segments viable) Mostly non-viable (≤5 LV segments viable)
4. Left ventricle size	Mildly dilated Moderately dilated Severely dilated (LVEDD > 65 mm)
5. Left ventricle function	Mildly impaired Moderately impaired Severely impaired (LVEF < 30 %)

ERO effective regurgitation orifice area, *LV* left ventricle, *LVEDD* left ventricular end diastolic diameter, *LVEF* left ventricular ejection fraction

regurgitation: from mild, to moderate, to severe, to the very severe mitral regurgitation. There are varying degrees of mitral leaflet tethering, and of left ventricle viability, size and function. Each of these factors has a significant impact on the natural history of the condition, and on the response to coronary artery revascularization alone, concomitant mitral valve repair or replacement, and the need for additional interventions on the left ventricle. Treatment therefore needs to be tailored to each individual patient taking into consideration all of these factors. Furthermore, the American Heart Association (AHA) and the American College of Cardiology (ACC) has recently revised its grading of the severity of functional ischemic mitral regurgitation (Table 16.2) [4]. In addition to mitral valve hemodynamics, valve and left ventricular anatomy and geometry, as well as associated cardiac findings and symptoms are now taken into consideration in the grading of functional ischemic mitral regurgitation severity. These are all considerations which need to be taken into account when deciding on the best treatment for the patient with functional ischemic mitral regurgitation (Table 16.3).

Grade A Ischemic Mitral Regurgitation

Using the recent AHA/ACC guidelines classification, these patients are at risk of mitral regurgitation; they do not have significant mitral regurgitation and have only a small mitral regurgitant jet at most. The mitral valve leaflet geometry is relatively normal and the left ventricle is normal in size or only mildly dilated [4]. These patients do not require any intervention on the mitral valve. They need to be optimized on medical treatment for ischemic heart disease and coronary artery revascularization performed if appropriate. In observational studies, only 12 % of these patients had progression of their mitral regurgitation severity [5]. However, the long term survival of these patients remains worse compared to patients who do not have mitral regurgitation, although the mitral regurgitation in these cases may not be the cause of the worse prognosis, but may just be a marker of a more dilated left ventricle with poorer function [6].

Grade B Ischemic Mitral Regurgitation

These patients are referred to as having progressive mitral regurgitation in the AHA/ACC guidelines. The mitral regurgitation is mild-to-moderate in severity with an effective regurgitant orifice area (ERO) of less than 20 mm^2, the mitral leaflet tethering is mild and the left ventricle is only mildly dilated with some systolic dysfunction [4]. In these patients, if the left ventricle myocardium is fully viable, left ventricular function is likely to recover with complete coronary artery revascularization in addition to optimal medical therapy, and the mitral regurgitation will likely reduce as a result, with reverse remodeling of the left ventricle. This was demonstrated in the

Table 16.2 AHA/ACC grading of functional ischemic mitral regugitation severity

Grade	Definition	Valve anatomy	Valve hemodynamics	Associated cardiac findings	Symptoms
A.	At risk of MR	Normal valve leaflets, chords, and annulus in a patient with coronary disease or cardiomyopathy	No MR jet or small central jet area <20 % LA on Doppler, Small vena contracta <0.30 cm	Normal or mildly dilated LV size with fixed (infarction) or inducible (ischemia) regional wall motion abnormalities Primary myocardial disease with LV dilation and systolic dysfunction	Symptoms due to coronary ischemia or HF may be present that respond to revascularization and appropriate medical therapy
B.	Progressive MR	Regional wall motion abnormalities with mild tethering of mitral leaflet. Annular dilation with mild loss of central coaptation of the mitral leaflets	ERO < 0.20 cm^2 Regurgitant volume <30 mL Regurgitant fraction <50 %	Regional wall motion abnormalities with reduced LV systolic function. LV dilation and systolic dysfunction due to primary myocardial disease	Symptoms due to coronary ischemia or HF may be present that respond to revascularization and appropriate medical therapy
C.	Asymptomatic severe MR	Regional wall motion abnormalities and/or LV dilation with severe tethering of mitral leaflet. Annular dilation with severe loss of central coaptation of the mitral leaflets	ERO >0.20 cm^2 Regurgitant volume >30 mL Regurgitant fraction >50 %	Regional wall motion abnormalities with reduced LV systolic function LV dilation and systolic dysfunction due to primary myocardial disease	Symptoms due to coronary ischemia or HF may be present that respond to revascularization and appropriate medical therapy
D.	Symptomatic severe MR	Regional wall motion abnormalities and/or LV dilation with severe tethering of mitral leaflet. Annular dilation with severe loss of central coaptation of the mitral leaflets	ERO >0.20 cm^2 Regurgitant volume >30 mL Regurgitant fraction >50 %	Regional wall motion abnormalities with reduced LV systolic function. LV dilation and systolic dysfunction due to primary myocardial disease	HF symptoms due to MR persist even after revascular-ization and optimization of medical therapy. Decreased exercise tolerance. Exertional dyspnea

From Nishimura et al. [4]. With permission from Elsevier

Table 16.3 Recommended interventions according to the severity of ischemic mitral regurgitation and other parameters (when there is an indication for coronary artery revascularisation)

MR severity grade	Other parameters	Interventions
A. At risk of MR		Coronary revascularisation
B. Progressive MR	LV all viable	Coronary revascularisation
	Significant non-viable LV	Consider mitral annuloplasty in addition to CABG
C. & D. Severe MR	Tethering distance < 10 mm	Mitral annuloplasty + CABG
	Tethering distance ≥ 10 mm	Mitral annuloplasty + subvalvular repair + CABG or mitral valve replacement + CABG
	LVEDD ≥ 65 mm	Consider left ventricular restoration surgery
Very severe MR	ERO > 40 mm^2	Mitral annuloplasty + subvalvular repair + CABG or mitral valve replacement + CABG

MR mitral regurgitation, *LV* left ventricle, *LVEDD* left ventricle end diastolic diameter, *CABG* coronary artery bypass graft surgery

Cardiothoracic Surgical Network (CTSN) Moderate Mitral Regurgitation randomized trial where 70 % of patients receiving isolated coronary artery bypass graft surgery (CABG) showed an improvement in their mitral regurgitation severity at 1 year, and there was similar reductions in left ventricular volumes regardless of whether the patients received isolated CABG or concomitant CABG plus mitral valve annuloplasty [7]. However, if significant non-viable myocardium is present, recovery of left ventricular function is less likely to occur, leaving the patient with persistent mitral regurgitation and absence of left ventricular reverse remodeling; in these patients, concomitant mitral annuloplasty should be considered at the time of CABG.

Grades C and D Ischemic Mitral Regurgitation

The AHA/ACC guidelines refer to this group of patients as having severe ischemic mitral regurgitation. They may be asymptomatic (Grade C) or symptomatic (Grade D) [4]. These patients have significant mitral regurgitation with an ERO greater than 20 mm^2 and require an intervention on the mitral valve, as demonstrated in the Randomised Ischemic Mitral Evaluation (RIME) Trial, where patients randomized to concomitant CABG plus mitral annuloplasty had significantly better functional capacity, symptoms, and left ventricular reverse remodeling at 1 year compared to patients who received isolated CABG [8]. Provided the correct surgical principles are followed and there is no severe mitral leaflet tethering (tethering distance less than 10 mm), and the left ventricle is not overly dilated (left ventricular end diastolic diameter less than 65 mm), mitral annuloplasty in this group of patients is very successful and durable; the freedom from moderate or more mitral regurgitation at 1 year in the RIME Trial was 96 % [8, 9]. However, if significant mitral leaflet tethering is present (tethering distance greater than 10 mm), some additional subvalvular repair techniques may be necessary in addition to mitral annuloplasty to ensure a durable repair [10]. Alternatively, a mitral valve replacement may be the preferred operation. If the left ventricle is severely dilated (LVEDD greater than 65 mm), additional left ventricular restoration surgery may be necessary to improve the survival of the patient [9].

Very Severe Mitral Regurgitation

This refers to the group of patients with an ERO greater than 40 mm^2. This group of patients are not distinguished from those with lesser severity of mitral regurgitation (ERO 20–40 mm^2) in the recent AHA/ACC guidelines; both groups are considered as having severe ischemic mitral regurgitation [4]. However, the two groups behave very differently and so should be considered separately when deciding on the choice of surgical interventions. The CTSN Severe Ischemic Mitral

Regurgitation Trial demonstrated that mitral annuloplasty in patients with an ERO greater than 40 mm [2] did not have a very good durability; the freedom from moderate or more mitral regurgitation at 2 years was only 64 %, and patients receiving a mitral annuloplasty had significantly more heart failure episodes compared to patients who received a mitral valve replacement [11]. Mitral valve replacement is therefore the preferred intervention in this group of patients, or alternatively, additional subvalvular repair procedures in addition to an annuloplasty are necessary if mitral valve repair is to be performed. On the other hand, patients with lesser severity of mitral regurgitation (ERO 20–40 mm^2), but who are still considered as having severe ischemic mitral regurgitation according to current guidelines, do very well with a mitral annuloplasty at the time of CABG [4]. The RIME Trial demonstrated a 96 % freedom from moderate or more recurrent mitral regurgitation at 1 year following concomitant mitral annuloplasty plus CABG in this group of patients, with corresponding improvements in functional capacity, symptoms and left ventricular reverse remodeling compared to those receiving isolated CABG [8].

References

1. Aronson D, Goldsher N, Zukermann R, Kapeliovich M. Ischemic mitral regurgitation and risk of heart failure after myocardial infarction. Arch Intern Med. 2006;166:2362–8.
2. Lamas GA, Mitchell GF, Flaker GC, Smith SC, Gersh BJ. Clinical significance of mitral regurgitation after acute myocardial infarction. Circulation. 1997;96(3):827–33.
3. Grigioni F, Detaint D, Avierinos J-F, Scott C, Tajik J, Enriquez-Sarano M. Contribution of ischemic mitral regurgitation to congestive heart failure after myocardial infarction. J Am Coll Cardiol. 2005;45:260–7.
4. Nishimura RA, Otto CM, Bonow RO, et al. 2014 AHA/ACC guideline for the management of patients with valvular heart disease: a report of the American College of Cardiology/American Heart Association Task Force on Practice Guidelines. J Am Coll Cardiol. 2014;63(22):e57–185.
5. Campwala SZ, Bansal RC, Wang N, Razzouk A, Pai RG. Mitral regurgitation progression following isolated coronary artery bypass surgery: frequency, risk factors, and potential prevention strategies. Eur J Cardiothorac Surg. 2006;29(3):348.
6. Grossi EA, Crooke GA, Di Giorgi PL, Schwartz CA. Impact of moderate functional mitral insufficiency in patients undergoing surgical revascularization. Circulation. 2006;114(1):I573.
7. Smith PK, Puskas JD, Ascheim DD, et al. Surgical treatment of moderate ischemic mitral regurgitation. N Engl J Med. 2014;371:2178–88.
8. Chan KMJ, Punjabi PP, Flather M, et al. Coronary artery bypass surgery with or without mitral valve annuloplasty in moderate functional ischemic mitral regurgitation: final results of the randomized ischemic mitral evaluation (RIME) trial. Circulation. 2012;126:2502–10.
9. Braun J, van de Veire NR, Klautz RJM, et al. Restrictive mitral annuloplasty cures ischemic mitral regurgitation and heart failure. Ann Thorac Surg. 2008;85:430–7.
10. Fattouch K, Murana G, Castrovinci S, et al. Mitral valve annuloplasty and papillary muscle relocation oriented by 3-dimensional tranesophagel echocardiography for severe functional mitral regurgitation. J Thorac Cardiovasc Surg. 2012;143:S38–42.
11. Goldstein D, Moskowitz AJ, Gelijns AC, et al. Two year outcomes of surgical treatment of severe ischemic mitral regurgitation. N Engl J Med. 2016;374(4):344–53.

Future Directions in Functional Mitral Regurgitation

17

K.M. John Chan

Abstract

Newer mitral valve repair techniques have emerged in recent years and long term results of these are needed. The indications for these repair techniques in addition to mitral valve annuloplasty also need to be better defined. The role of myocardial viability in guiding management of this condition also needs further investigation. Longer term follow up is also needed in studies comparing mitral valve repair versus replacement in functional ischaemic mitral regurgitation. Further studies are also needed on the role of ventricular restoration surgery in those with very dilated left ventricles as well as the longer term results of percutaneous treatment of mitral regurgitation.

Keywords

Functional ischemic mitral regurgitation • Mitral annuloplasty • Mitral valve replacement • Myocardial viability • Percutaneous mitral valve repair

Functional ischemic mitral regurgitation is one of the most challenging conditions to manage. Unlike organic mitral regurgitation where there is purely a mechanical problem, and correcting the mitral regurgitation either by mitral valve repair or replacement, results in a cure for most patients, functional ischemic mitral regurgitation has many pathologies, each of which must be adequately addressed to achieve the best outcome for the patient. These include the coronary artery disease, myocardial ischemia and myocardial infarction, left ventricular dilatation, dysfunction and scarring, and the tethering of the mitral valve apparatus, in addition to the mitral regurgitation. The problem is that not all of the pathologies can be effectively treated in every patient, and unlike in degenerative mitral regurgitation where excellent and durable valve repair techniques are in existence, in functional ischemic mitral regurgitation, a consistent, durable valve repair for every

K.M.J. Chan, BM BS, MSc, PhD, FRCS CTh
Department of Cardiothoracic Surgery,
Gleneagles Hospital, Jalan Ampang,
Kuala Lumpur 50450, Malaysia
e-mail: kmjohnchan@yahoo.com

K.M.J. Chan (ed.), *Functional Mitral and Tricuspid Regurgitation*,
DOI 10.1007/978-3-319-43510-7_17

patient remains elusive. Although the technique of mitral valve repair by mitral annuloplasty is well established, and is efficacious in many cases of ischaemic mitral regurgitation, particularly if the mitral regurgitation is not too severe and the leaflets not too severely restricted, several studies have reported limited durability of this valve repair technique in cases of very severe mitral regurgitation, those with severe tethering of the mitral valve leaflets, and those with severely dilated left ventricles [1, 2]. Newer repair techniques on the subvalvular apparatus are in use to address the severely tethered leaflets, e.g., papillary muscle repositioning, but long term results of this is still awaited and studies comparing it to conventional mitral annuloplasty are needed [3].

Functional ischaemic mitral regurgitation is a disease of the left ventricle (LV). However, adequate assessment of the LV is usually not performed in many studies on ischaemic mitral regurgitation and in clinical practice. A recent randomised controlled trial reported similar outcomes in patients with moderate functional ischemic mitral regurgitation receiving coronary artery bypass grafting alone and in those receiving combined coronary artery bypass grafting and mitral annuloplasty [4]. However, there was no assessment of LV viability in this study and it is likely that most patients in this study had non-infarcted viable left ventricles which recovered its function with successful coronary artery revascularisation. On the contrary, another randomised trial reported better outcomes in those who received combined coronary artery bypass graft surgery and mitral annuloplasty [1]. In this study, LV viability assessment was done on all patients and most had non-viable scarred myocardium in the inferior LV wall. Further studies are needed to determine if the assessment of myocardial viability or presence of scar tissue may help distinguish those who would improve with successful coronary artery revascularisation alone, and those in whom a concomitant valve repair is needed.

Recent studies have suggested that mitral valve replacement may be superior to mitral valve repair in those with very severe mitral regurgitation and dilated left ventricles in terms of valve durability [2]. However, many of these patients received a bioprosthetic valve which is known to have a limited durability, and longer term results beyond 10 years are needed to truly determine if mitral valve replacement or repair is better, or if the two surgical treatments are equivalent. Comparisons with other repair techniques besides mitral annuloplasty are also needed particularly in those with severely restricted leaflets where papillary muscle procedures may be beneficial.

Further studies are also needed on the use of left ventricular restoration surgery in patients with severe functional ischaemic mitral regurgitation and very dilated left ventricles. It has been reported that long term survival is not as good in this group of patients compared to those with less dilated left ventricles when CABG and mitral annuloplasty alone are used [5]. It has been suggested that this group of patients would benefit from adding LV restoration surgery but further more objective studies are needed including randomised trials comparing the two procedures directly.

Percutaneous techniques have been developed and are showing promise in functional ischemic mitral regurgitation. However, there is a continuing problem with residual or recurrent mitral regurgitation. Randomised trials are also needed to determine if it is beneficial compared to optimal medical therapy and conventional valve repair or replacement operations.

References

1. Chan KMJ, Punjabi PP, Flather MF, Wage R, Symmonds K, Roussin I, Rahman-Haley S, Pennell DJ, Kilner PJ, Dreyfus GD, Pepper JR. Coronary artery bypass surgery with or without mitral valve annuloplasty in moderate functional ischemic mitral regurgitation: final results of the Randomized Ischemic Mitral Evaluation (RIME) Trial. Circulation. 2012;126:2502–10.
2. Acker MA, Parides MK, Perrault LP, Moskowitz AJ, Gelijns AC, Voisine P, Smith PK, Hung JW, Blackstone EH, Puskas JD, Argenziano M, Gammie JS, Mack M, Ascheim DD, Bagiella E, Moquete EG, Ferguson TB, Horvath KA, Geller NL, Miller MA, Woo YJ, D'Alessandro DA, Ailawadi G, Dagenais F, Gardner TJ, O'Gara PT, Michler RE, Kron IL, CTSN. Mitral

valve repair versus replacement for severe ischemic mitral regurgitation. N Engl J Med. 2014;370:23–32.
3. Kron IL, Green GR, Cope JT. Surgical relocation of the posterior papillary muscle in chronic ischemic mitral regurgitation. Ann Thorac Surg. 2002;74: 600–1.
4. Smith PK, Puskas JD, Ascheim DD, Voisine P, Gelijns AC, Moskowitz AJ, Hung J, Parides MK, Ailawadi G, Perrault LP, Acker MA, Argenziano M, Thourani V, Gammie JS, Miller MA, Page P, Overbey JR, Bagiella E, Dagenais F, Blackstone EH, Kron IL, Goldstein DJ, Rose EA, Moquete EG, Jeffries N, Gardner TJ, O'Gara PT, Alexander JH, Michler RE. Surgical treatment of moderate ischemic mitral regurgitation. N Engl J Med. 2014;371:2178–88.
5. Braun J, van de Veire NR, Klautz RJM, Versteegh MIM, Holman ER, Westenberg JM, Boersma E, van der Wall EE, Bax JJ, Dion RAE. Restrictive mitral annuloplasty cures ischemic mitral regurgitation and heart failure. Ann Thorac Surg. 2008;85:430–7.

Part II

Functional Tricuspid Regurgitation

Anatomy of the Tricuspid Valve and Pathophysiology of Functional Tricuspid Regurgitation

18

K.M. John Chan

Abstract

Understanding the anatomy of the tricuspid valve is fundamental to an understanding of the pathophysiology of functional tricuspid regurgitation and the surgical treatment for it. The tricuspid valve apparatus consists of the tricuspid valve leaflets, annulus, chordae, and papillary muscles. Functional tricuspid regurgitation occurs secondary to left sided heart valve disease which leads to raised pulmonary artery pressures, tricuspid annular dilatation and tethering of the leaflets due to remodeling of the right ventricle. Leaflet adaptation also occurs. Three stages of functional tricuspid regurgitation can be recognized.

Keywords

Tricuspid valve • Functional tricuspid regurgitation • Tricuspid annular dilatation • Tricuspid leaflet tethering • Right ventricular remodelling

An understanding of the anatomy of the tricuspid valve is necessary to understand the pathophysiology of functional tricuspid regurgitation (FTR). This is crucial to the understanding of how best to manage FTR, allowing us to tailor the appropriate treatment according to the pathology and stage of the disease.

K.M.J. Chan, BM BS, MSc, PhD, FRCS CTh
Department of Cardiothoracic Surgery,
Gleneagles Hospital, Jalan Ampang,
Kuala Lumpur 50450, Malaysia
e-mail: kmjohnchan@yahoo.com

Anatomy of the Tricuspid Valve

The tricuspid valve is located in the right atrioventricular junction. It comprises of three leaflets, the annulus, chordae and papillary muscles. The anterior leaflet is the largest of the leaflets, followed by the posterior leaflet; the septal leaflet is the smallest (Fig. 18.1). The leaflets are separated by clefts or commissures. Smaller commissural leaflets are found in between the three leaflets [1]. The leaflets attach at their base to the annulus, and at their free edge and body to chordae, which in turn attach to papillary muscles. Chordae from the septal leaflet as well as the septal half of the anterior leaflet attach directly to the septum [2]. The large anterior

K.M.J. Chan (ed.), *Functional Mitral and Tricuspid Regurgitation*,
DOI 10.1007/978-3-319-43510-7_18

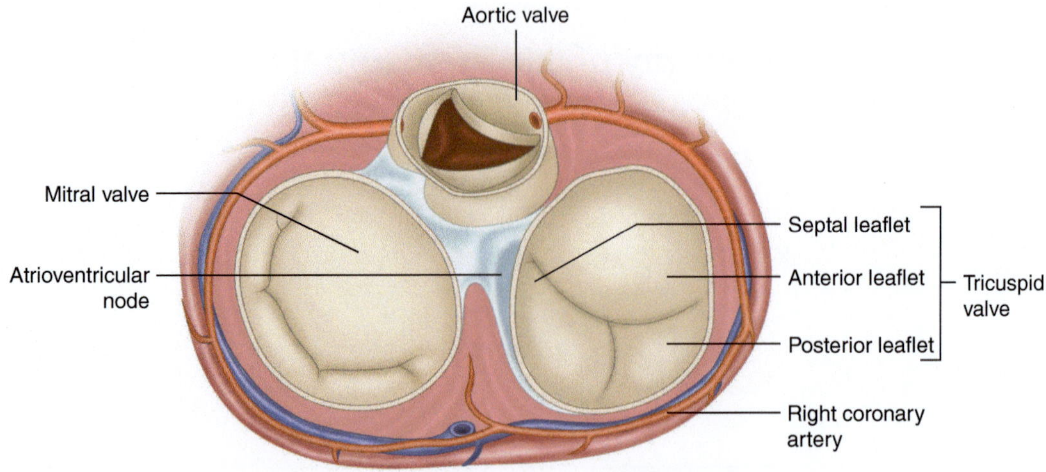

Fig. 18.1 Anatomy of the tricuspid valve and surrounding structures (Adapted from Carpentier et al. [28])

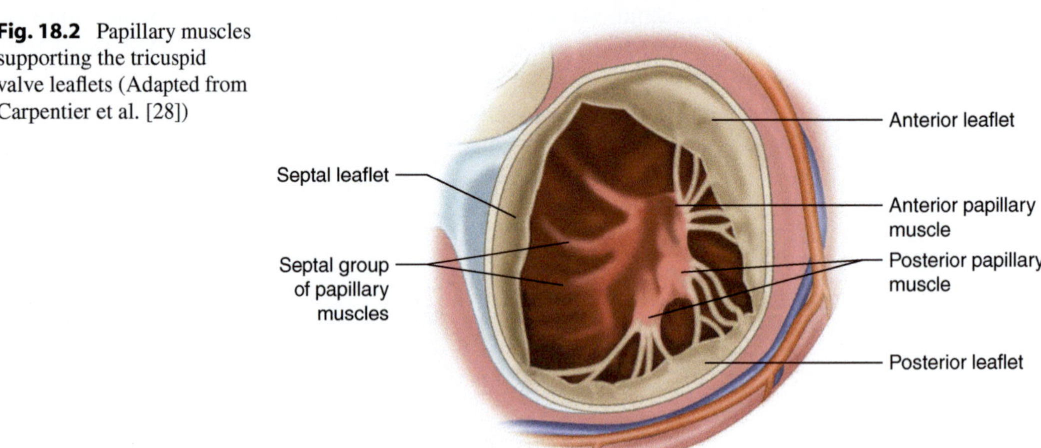

Fig. 18.2 Papillary muscles supporting the tricuspid valve leaflets (Adapted from Carpentier et al. [28])

papillary muscle arises from the anterior wall of the right ventricle, gives rise to chordae which support the commissure between the anterior and posterior leaflets (Fig. 18.2). In about half of normal individuals, the anterior papillary muscle only supports the anterior leaflet, with a smaller papillary muscle providing chords to the commissure between the anterior and posterior leaflets [3]. The small medial papillary muscle, also known as the papillary muscle of conus, or the muscle of Lancisi, supports the coaptation zone between the septal and anterior leaflets [3]. This papillary muscle marks the entrance of the right bundle branch into the subendocardial layer of the right ventricle [3]. The atrial-ventricular conduction axis is located at the apex of the triangle of Koch, formed by the coronary sinus as its base, the tendon of Todaro deep to the Eustachian valve forming one arm of the triangle, and the hinge point of the septal leaflet forming the other arm. Care must be taken during suture placement for tricuspid valve replacement surgery in this area to avoid conduction problems. A smaller posterior or inferior papillary muscle, or more commonly multiple muscles, supports the commissure between the posterior and septal leaflets [3]. The papillary muscles are attached to the free wall of the right ventricle and septum [1]. Changes in the size and geometry of the right ventricle, particularly with increased eccentricity, can therefore cause leaflet tethering with reduced coaptation resulting in functional TR [4, 5]. Most of the tricuspid annulus lies on the muscular atrioventricular junction. The tricuspid annulus lies in close proximity to the right coronary artery in the region of the antero-posterior commissure; care must be taken to avoid too deep suture placement in this region to avoid injury to the right coronary artery.

Pathophysiology of Functional Tricuspid Regurgitation

Functional tricuspid regurgitation (FTR) occurs due to loss of leaflet coaptation as a result of two pathologies: dilatation of the tricuspid annulus and/or leaflet tethering, both of which occur due to right ventricular remodeling and dilatation as a result of raised pulmonary artery pressures from left sided heart valve disease [6, 7]. These two pathologies may co-exist, with one pathology leading to the other, or they may be distinct. Tricuspid annular dilatation can also be caused by long standing atrial fibrillation [8]. It is referred to as functional as the leaflets are normal in morphology but their function is impaired due to dilatation of the tricuspid annulus which pulls them apart, or right ventricular dilatation, elongation and altered geometry which displaces the papillary muscles laterally and apically, tethering the leaflets and preventing adequate leaflet coaptation [9]. Raised pulmonary artery pressures due to left sided heart valve disease contribute to these pathologies and exacerbates the severity of FTR [9, 10]. The severity of TR is greatest when both tricuspid annular dilatation and leaflet tethering are present.

Due to the high compliance of the right ventricular chamber, changes in preload, afterload and right ventricular contractility can affect the severity of TR and tricuspid annular dimensions significantly. Assessment of these parameters should therefore be done preoperatively in the awake patient and not during general anesthesia as this can induce vasodilatation and venodilatation with reductions in afterload and preload and hence TR severity.

Tricuspid Annular Dilatation

Early morphological changes in the heart secondary to left sided heart valve disease and atrial fibrillation which eventually leads to TR include an enlargement of the left and right atrium, the right ventricle and the tricuspid annulus [6, 11]. As the tricuspid annulus starts to dilate, it also assumes a more circular configuration, losing its 3-dimensional geometry [6, 11, 12]. In addition, the normal tricuspid annulus decreases in size during systole; this dynamic motion of the tricuspid annulus is lost in functional TR and may be another mechanism contributing to it [12].

In the early stages, right ventricular and annular remodeling occur without significant TR [6]. The anterior tricuspid annulus can dilate up to 40 % while the posterior annulus can dilate up to 80 %; the septal annulus is relatively fixed due to its anatomical relationship to the fibrous skeleton of the heart. [13] Right ventricular dilatation also occurs and can be significant [14, 15]. Dilatation of the tricuspid annulus is the most common cause of FTR [10]. The severity of TR increases with increasing tricuspid annular diameter size [4, 16]. Pulmonary hypertension secondary to left sided valvular heart disease is an important contributing factor [9, 11, 17].

Tricuspid annular dilatation pulls the tricuspid valve leaflets apart, particularly the anterior and posterior leaflets, decreasing leaflet coaptation (Fig. 18.3). Functional TR ensues once the annulus is dilated by more than 40 % its normal size [4, 5]. Increasing annular size results in increasing TR [11]. The degree of annular dilatation and hence the severity of TR can vary depending on the preload and afterload conditions, and also right ventricular (RV) contractility. Once the tricuspid annulus is dilated, it is unlikely to be reversible.

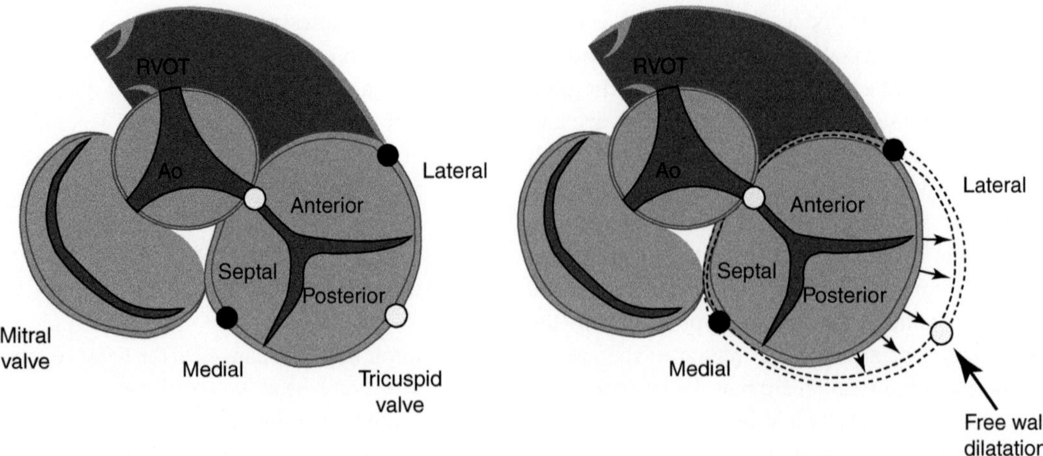

Fig. 18.3 Tricuspid valve seen from the right atrium showing the direction of tricuspid annular dilatation which mainly involves the anterior and posterior annulus (From Ton-Nu et al. [27])

Tricuspid Leaflet Tethering

Tethering of the tricuspid leaflet is another cause of FTR [10]. As the right ventricle dilates due to raised pulmonary artery pressures, it can assume a more elongated or eccentric geometry, thereby pulling the anterior papillary muscle apically and laterally, and tethering the tricuspid valve leaflets as a result, preventing adequate leaflet coaptation [9, 18]. Right ventricular eccentricity has been shown to be independently associated with TR severity [4]. This pathology is distinct from tricuspid annular dilatation although the two can co-exist, with tricuspid annular dilatation progressing to leaflet tethering with progressive RV dilatation and eccentricity [6]. The reverse is also true and leaflet tethering can progress to annular dilatation. Increased right ventricular sphericity can also result; here the septal papillary muscles are also displaced laterally, i.e., towards the left ventricle [9].

Tricuspid Leaflet Adaptation

It has recently been demonstrated that right ventricular pressure overload and remodeling was associated with an increase in tricuspid valve leaflet size by as much as 49 % compared to controls, and when this increase in size was inadequate to cover the tricuspid valve closure area, a graded increase in TR severity was observed [19]. Inadequate leaflet enlargement in response to annular dilatation may be another mechanism of functional tricuspid regurgitation, although further studies are needed to confirm this hypothesis. Similar observations were previously made in functional mitral regurgitation [20]. The biological mechanism for increased leaflet area was previously demonstrated in a sheep model in which mechanical leaflet tethering or stress caused by papillary muscle retraction reactivated embryonic pathways for leaflet growth [19, 21].

Stages of Functional Tricuspid Regurgitation

Three stages of FTR can be recognized depending on the degree of tricuspid annular dilatation and the presence or absence of leaflet tethering: [22, 23]

Stage 1: *The tricuspid annulus is not dilated, the leaflets coapt normally from body to body, there is no leaflet tethering.*

There is usually no TR or the TR is usually mild.

Stage 2: *The tricuspid annulus is dilated to more than 40 mm, the leaflets coapt abnormally from edge to edge only, there is no leaflet tethering or leaflet tethering is mild (less than 8 mm)*

TR is usually mild or moderate but may increase in severity depending on right ventricular preload, afterload and contractility.

Stage 3: *The tricuspid annulus is dilated to more than 40 mm, there is no leaflet coaptation, leaflet tethering is significant (greater than 8 mm)*

TR is usually severe under all physiological conditions.

TR can also occur due to leaflet thickening and commissural fusion as may occur in rheumatic heart disease and carcinoid infiltration. There may be accompanying tricuspid stenosis.

Hemodynamic Effects of Tricuspid Regurgitation

A recent study demonstrated that patients with TR have impaired exercise and functional capacity and this was related to an inability to adequately increase cardiac output with stress in proportion to metabolic needs [24]. This would be consistent with studies showing a poorer NYHA functional class in patients in whom TR was not addressed at the time of left sided heart valve surgery and in those who develop progressive TR [25]. At rest, TR subjects had lower pulmonary blood flow, increased right atrial pressure and higher pulmonary capillary wedge pressure compared to controls. With exercise, TR subjects displayed lower peak oxygen consumption, an objective measure of functional capacity, and also lower pulmonary blood flow, and less increase in pulmonary blood flow relative to peak oxygen consumption. There was also higher pulmonary capillary wedge pressures [24]. In addition, there was also inadequate left ventricular diastolic filling with exercise. A previous study also reported that subjects with TR have reduced cardiac output, and cardiac output became lower as TR progressed from mild to severe [26].

References

1. Joudinaud TM, Flecher EM, Duran CMG. Functional terminology for tricuspid valve. J Heart Valve Dis. 2006;15:382–8.
2. Seccombe JF, Cahill DR, Edwards WD. Quantitative morphology of the normal human tricuspid valve: autopsy study of 24 cases. Clin Anat. 1993;6:203–12.
3. Tretter JT, Sarwark AE, Anderson RH, Spicer DE. Assessment of the anatomical variation to be found in the normal tricsupid valve. Clin Anat. 2016;29:399–407.
4. Kim HK, Kim YJ, Park JS, Kim KH, Kim KB, Ahn H, Sohn DW, Oh BH, Park YB, Choi YS. Determinants of the severity of functional tricuspid regurgitation. Am J Cardiol. 2006;98:236–42.
5. Spinner EM, Shannon P, Buice D, Jimenez JH, Veledar E, del Nido PJ, Adams DH, Yoganathan AP. In vitro characterization of the mechanisms responsible for functional tricuspid regurgitation. Circulation. 2011;124:920–9.
6. Said SM, Burkhart HM, Schaff HV, Johnson JN, Connolly HM, Dearani JA. When should a mechanical tricuspid valve replacement be considered? J Thorac Cardiovasc Surg. 2014;148:603–8.
7. Fukuda S, Saracino G, Matsumura Y, Daimon M, Tran H. Three-dimensional geometry of the tricuspid annulus in healthy subjects and in patients with functional tricuspid regurgitation: a real-time, 3-dimensional echocardiographic study. Circulation. 2006;114:I492.
8. Najib MQ, Vinales KL, Vittala SS, Challa S, Lee HR, Chaliki HP. Predictors for the development of severe tricuspid regurgitation with anatomically normal valve in patients with atrial fibrillation. Echocardiography. 2011;29:140–6.
9. Spinner EM, Lerakis S, Higginson J, Pernetz M, Howell S, Veledar E, Yoganathan AP. Correlates of tricuspid regurgitation as determined by 3D echocardiography: pulmonary arterial pressure, ventricle geometry, annular dilatation, and papillary muscle displacement. Circ Cardiovasc Imaging. 2012;5:43–50.
10. Park YH, Song JM, Lee EY, Kim YJ, Kang DH, Song JK. Geometric and haemodynamic determinant of functional tricuspid regurgitation: a real time three dimensional echocardiographic study. Int J Cardiol. 2008;124:160–5.
11. Nemoto N, Lesser JR, Pedersen WR, Sorajja P, Spinner E, Garberich RF, Vock DM, Schwartz RS. Pathogenic structural heart changes in early tricuspid regurgitation. J Thorac Cardiovasc Surg. 2015;150:323–30.
12. Ring L, Rana BS, Kydd A, Boyd J, Parker K and Rusk RA. Dynamics of the tricuspid valve annulus in normal and dilated right hearts: a three-dimensional transoesophageal echocardiography study. Eur Heart J Cardiovasc Imaging. 2012;13(9):756–62.
13. Deloche A, Guerinon J, Fabiani JN, Morillo F, Caramanian M, Carpentier A. Anatomical study of rheumatic tricuspid valves: application to the study of various valvulopathies. Ann Chir Thorac Cardiovasc. 1973;12:343–9.
14. Nath J, Forster E, Heidenreich PA. Impact of tricuspid regurgitation on long term survival. J Am Coll Cardiol. 2004;43:405–9.

15. Topilsky Y, Nkomo VT, Vatury O, Michelena HI, Letourneau T, Suri R, Pislaru S, Park S, Mahoney DW, Biner S, Enriquez-Sarano M. Clinical outcome of isolated tricuspid regurgitation. JACC Cardiovasc Imaging. 2014;7:1186–94.
16. Goldstone AB, Howard JL, Cohen JE, MacArthur JW, Atluri P, Kirkpatrick JN, Woo YJ. Natural history of coexistent tricuspid regurgitation in patients with degenerative mitral valve disease: implications for future guidelines. J Thorac Cardiovasc Surg. 2014;148:2802–10.
17. Mutlak D, Aronson D, Lessick J, Reisner SA, Dabbah S, Agmon Y. Functional tricuspid regurgitation in patients with pulmonary hypertension. Is pulmonary hypertension the only determinant of regurgitant severity? Chest. 2009;135:115–21.
18. Topilsky Y, Khanna A, Le Tourneau T, Park S, Michelena H, Suri R, Mahoney DW, Enriquez-Sarano M. Clinical context and mechanism of functional tricuspid regurgitation in patients with and without pulmonary hypertension. Circ Cardiovasc Imaging. 2012;5:314–23.
19. Afilalo J, Grapsa J, Nihoyannopoulos P, Beaudoin J, Gibbs JSR, Channick RN, Langleben D, Rudski LG, Hua L, Handschumacher MD, Picard MH, Levine RA. Leaflet area as a determinant of tricuspid regurgitation severity in patients with pulmonary hypertension. Circ Cardiovasc Imaging. 2015;8, e002714.
20. Chaput M, Handschumacher MD, Tournoux F, Hua L, Guerrero JL, Vlahakes GJ, Levine RA. Mitral leaflet adaptation to ventricular remodelling. Occurence and adequacy in patients with functional mitral regurgitation. Circulation. 2008;118:845–52.
21. Dal-Bianco JP, Aikawa E, Bischoff J, Guerrero JL, Handschumacher MD, Sullivan S, Johnson B, Titus J, Iwamoto Y, Wylie-Sears J, Levine RA, Carpentier A. Active adaptation of the tethered mitral valve: insights into a compensatory mechanism for functional mitral regurgitation. Circulation. 2009;120: 334–42.
22. Dreyfus GD, Chan KMJ. Functional tricuspid regurgitation: a more complex entity than it appears. Heart. 2009;95:868–9.
23. Dreyfus GD, Martin RP, Chan KMJ, Dulguerov F. Functional tricuspid regurgitation: a need to revise our understanding. J Am Coll Cardiol. 2015;65: 2331–6.
24. Andersen MJ, Nishimura RA, Borlaug BA. The hemodynamic basis of exercise intolerance in tricuspid regurgitation. Circ Heart Fail. 2014;7:911–7.
25. Dreyfus GD, Corbi PJ, Chan KMJ, Bahrami TB. Secondary tricuspid regurgitation or dilatation: which should be the criteria for surgical repair? Ann Thorac Surg. 2005;79:127–32.
26. Hansing CE, Rowe GG. Tricuspid insufficiency. A study of hemodynamics and pathogenesis. Circulation. 1972;45:793–9.
27. Ton-Nu TT, Levine RA, Handschumacher MD. Geometric determinants of functional tricuspid regurgitation: insights from 3-dimensional echocardiography. Circulation. 2006;114:143–9.
28. Carpentier A, Adams D, Filsoufi F. Carpentier's reconstructive valve surgery. 1st ed. Maryland Heights: Elsevier; 2010.

Natural History of Functional Tricuspid Regurgitation

19

K.M. John Chan

Abstract

Functional tricuspid regurgitation is a common condition. It is benign in most people when only mild in severity, but when moderate or more in severity, tricuspid regurgitation is associated with reduced survival. If left untreated, moderate tricuspid regurgitation will progress, with impact on symptoms, functional capacity and survival.

Keywords

Functional tricuspid regurgitation, right ventricular function • natural history • survival • tricuspid annular dilatation

Tricuspid regurgitation (TR) is a common finding present in 80–90 % of healthy individuals according to the Framingham study [1]. The most common cause of greater than mild TR, accounting for about 80–90 % of cases, is secondary or functional TR, which occurs as a consequence of left sided heart valve disease, cardiomyopathy and atrial fibrillation [2]. Primary or organic TR is less common and is due to rheumatic heart valve disease, infective endocarditis, endocardial device leads, tricuspid leaflet prolapse, Ebstein's anomaly, carcinoid heart disease, and trauma, amongst others [2].

K.M.J. Chan, BM BS, MSc, PhD, FRCS CTh
Department of Cardiothoracic Surgery,
Gleneagles Hospital, Jalan Ampang,
Kuala Lumpur 50450, Malaysia
e-mail: kmjohnchan@yahoo.com

The presence of greater than mild TR carries an adverse prognosis. This was shown in a study by Nath, et al., who reported 1-year survival of 91.7 % in those with no TR, 90.3 % in mild TR, 78.9 % in moderate TR, and 63.9 % in severe TR (Fig. 19.1) [3]. Moderate or greater TR was associated with increased mortality independent of pulmonary artery systolic pressures and left ventricular ejection fraction. When adjusted for age, left ventricular ejection fraction, inferior vena cava size, and right ventricular size and function, survival was worse for patients with moderate and severe TR compared to those with no TR [3]. Similar findings were made by Topilsky, et al., who reported that the survival of patients with isolated severe TR was significantly worse compared to those with milder TR severity. The 10 year survival and freedom from cardiac events of those with severe TR was significantly worse compared to those with milder TR

K.M.J. Chan (ed.), *Functional Mitral and Tricuspid Regurgitation*,
DOI 10.1007/978-3-319-43510-7_19

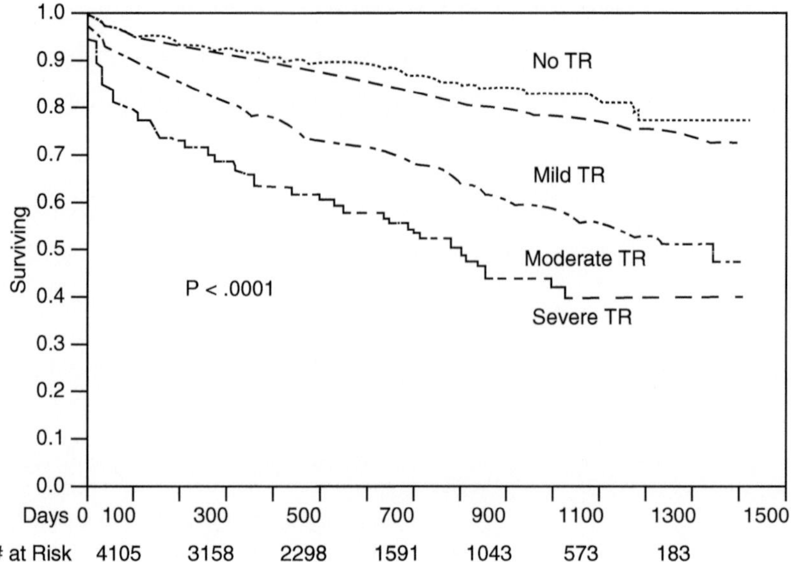

Fig. 19.1 Survival curves according to severity of tricuspid regurgitation (From Nath et al. [3], with permission from Elsevier)

severity, and was independent of right ventricular size and function, pulmonary artery pressures, co-morbidities, and lower than expected for the general population [4]. A strength of this study compared to others was that patients with left sided heart valve disease such as mitral regurgitation were excluded thus suggesting that the TR itself was an important cause of reduced survival and cardiac events independent of associated left sided heart valve disease and pathology [4]. Tricuspid regurgitation is therefore not a benign condition and has to be adequately managed and addressed.

Functional TR is a progressive disease and if left untreated, will progress with worse survival [5]. In a recent study by Song et al., involving 638 patients who underwent left sided heart valve surgery without tricuspid valve surgery, moderate or severe TR was present at 5 years in 7.3% of those who had none or trace TR at their initial surgery, and in 20% of those who had mild TR [6]. Survival was significantly worse in those who developed late TR. Similarly, Dreyfus et al. reported that significant late TR developed in 34% of patients who underwent mitral valve repair without tricuspid valve surgery and this was associated with worse NYHA functional class [7]. Matsunaga and Duran meanwhile reported an incidence of moderate or severe TR in 75% of patients 3 years after mitral valve repair for functional ischaemic mitral regurgitation [8]. Calafiore et al. reported that TR progressed in 40% of patients following mitral valve surgery without tricuspid valve surgery and this was associated with worse survival and functional class [9]. Yilmaz et al. meanwhile reported that mean TR grade increased significantly from a mean of 1.84–2.11 (p=0.03) 5 years after isolated mitral valve surgery without concomitant tricuspid valve surgery, and 29.4% of patients had moderate or more TR at 5 years compared to 16.5% pre-operatively [10].

Important factors which may influence the progression of TR include the presence of annular dilatation, leaflet tethering and atrial fibrillation [11, 12]. TR is likely to progress if tricuspid annular dilatation or leaflet tethering are present and not addressed at the time of left sided heart valve surgery [11]. Conversely, TR is unlikely to progress in patients with mild TR and no significant annular dilatation, leaflet tethering or atrial fibrillation [11].

References

1. Singh JP, Evans JC, Levy D. Prevalence and clinical determination of mitral, tricuspid, and aortic regurgitation (the Framingham Heart Study). Am J Cardiol. 1999;83:897–902.
2. Ong K, Yu G, Jue J. Prevalence and spectrum of conditions associated with severe tricuspid regurgitation. Echocardiography. 2013;31:558–62.

3. Nath J, Forster E, Heidenreich PA. Impact of tricuspid regurgitation on long term survival. J Am Coll Cardiol. 2004;43:405–9.
4. Topilsky Y, Nkomo VT, Vatury O, Michelena HI, Letourneau T, Suri R, Pislaru S, Park S, Mahoney DW, Biner S, Enriquez-Sarano M. Clinical outcome of isolated tricuspid regurgitation. JACC Cardiovasc Imaging. 2014;7:1186–94.
5. Calafiore AM, Gallina S, Iaco AL, Contini M, Bivona A, Gagliardi M, Bosco P, Di Mauro M. Mitral valve surgery for functional mitral regurgitation: should moderate or more tricuspid regurgitation be treated? A propensity score analysis. Ann Thorac Surg. 2009;87:698–703.
6. Song H, Kim M-J, Chung CH, Choo SJ. Factors associated with development of late significant tricuspid regurgitation after successful left sided valve surgery. Heart. 2009;95:931–6.
7. Dreyfus GD, Corbi PJ, Chan KMJ, Bahrami TB. Secondary tricuspid regurgitation or dilatation: which should be the criteria for surgical repair? Ann Thorac Surg. 2005;79:127–32.
8. Matsunaga A, Duran CMG. Progression of tricuspid regurgitation after repaired functional ischemic mitral regurgitation. Circulation. 2005;112:I453–7.
9. Calafiore AM, Gallina S, Iaco AL, Contini M, Bivona A, Gagliardi M, Bosco P, Di Mauro M. Mitral valve surgery for functional mitral regurgitation: should moderate or more tricuspid regurgitation be treated? A propensity score analysis. Ann Thorac Surg. 2009;87:698–703.
10. Yilmaz OG, Suri RMS, Dearani JA, Sundt TM, Daly RC, Burkhart HM, Enriquez-Sarano M, Schaff HV. Functional tricuspid regurgitation at the time of mitral valve repair for degenerative leaflet prolapse: the case for a selective approach. J Thorac Cardiovasc Surg. 2011;142:608–13.
11. Van de Veire NR, Braun J, Delgado V, Versteegh MIM, Dion RA, Klautz RJM, Bax JJ. Tricuspid annuloplasty prevents right ventricular dilatation and progression of tricuspid regurgitation in patients with tricuspid annular dilatation undergoing mitral valve repair. J Thorac Cardiovasc Surg. 2011;141:1431–9.
12. Kwak J-J, Kim Y-J, Kim M-K, Kim H-K, Park JS, Kim HK, Kim K-B, Ahn H, Sohn D-W, Oh BH, Park Y-B. Development of tricuspid regurgitation late after left-sided valve surgery: a single center experience with long-term echocardiographic examinations. Am Heart J. 2008;155:732–7.

Imaging Assessment of Functional Tricuspid Regurgitation

20

Amin Yehya, Venkateshwar Polsani, and Randolph P. Martin

Abstract

Functional tricuspid regurgitation (TR) is mainly due to disruption in the geometry of the tricuspid annulus secondary to tricuspid annular dilatation and right ventricular enlargement with or without pulmonary hypertension. Multiple imaging modalities have been used to evaluate the severity of functional TR. Echocardiography remains the most widely utilized modality for TR assessment but there is a growing role for cardiac magnetic resonance imaging which has better spatial and temporal resolution. Multi-modality imaging techniques are sometimes needed for adequately assessing the severity of functional TR.

Keywords

Tricuspid regurgitation • Heart Failure • Functional tricuspid regurgitation • Echocardiography • Cardiac MRI

A. Yehya, MD, MS, FACC (✉)
Piedmont Heart Institute, Samsky Advanced Heart Failure Center, 95 Collier Rd, Suite 3000, Atlanta, GA, USA
e-mail: amin.yehya@yahoo.com

V. Polsani, MD, FACC, FASE
Piedmont Heart Institute, Piedmont Atlanta Hospital, 275 Collier Road,
Atlanta, GA 30309, USA
e-mail: Venkateshwar.polsani@piedmont.org

R.P. Martin, MD, FACC, FASE, FESC
Piedmont Heart Institute, Marcus Valve Center, 95 Collier Raod, Suite 2065,
Atlanta, GA 30309, USA
e-mail: randy.martin@piedmont.org

Tricuspid Valve Anatomy

Tricuspid valve (TV) apparatus consists of the TV leaflets (anterior, posterior and septal), TV fibrous annulus, chordae tendinae, and the right ventricular (RV) papillary muscles [1]. For a proper functioning TV, all the units have to be intact and work harmoniously. The anterior TV leaflet is the largest and is quadrangular in shape while the posterior leaflet is triangular with multiple scallops. The anterior and the posterior leaflets are anchored to the anterior papillary muscle. On the other hand, the septal leaflet is semicircular and is relatively fixed. The TV leaflets have various chordae attached to the interventricular

K.M.J. Chan (ed.), *Functional Mitral and Tricuspid Regurgitation*,
DOI 10.1007/978-3-319-43510-7_20

septum and the RV free wall. When the TV annulus or RV dilates, it results in disruption of normal TV leaflets coaptation producing marked malalignment, especially of the anterior and posterior leaflets leading to tricuspid regurgitation (TR) [2, 3].

Fukuda et al. noted on 3D transthoracic studies that the TV annulus in healthy subjects was nonplanar and elliptical with a depressed center (postero-septal being the lowest-closest to the RV apex, and antero-septal being the highest) [4]. On the other hand, patients with functional TR had more of a planar and dilated annulus in the septal-lateral direction creating more of a circular shape [3].

TR is either primary or secondary [5]. Primary can be isolated or attributed to an intrinsic abnormality involving the valves, leaflet perforation, flail leaflet, congenital malformation (Ebstein's anomaly) etc. [6]. The etiology of isolated TR is not well understood. The diagnosis can be established quickly when it's noted that the regurgitant jet is holosystolic, there is no associated pulmonary hypertension (PH), no identifiable primary causes of TR, and the patient has had no prior interventions or trauma to the tricuspid valve [7]. Functional TR, while it can be due to intrinsic RV pathology or secondary to left heart disease with or without PH, it also can occur in long-standing atrial fibrillation [8]. The severity of the TR is affected by the RV preload, afterload and the underlying RV function [9].

Imaging Anatomy of the Tricuspid Valve Apparatus

The anatomic evaluation of the TV should not only include imaging the tricuspid leaflets themselves, but also all of the supporting structures associated with the tricuspid leaflets, including the dimensions and anatomic structure of the tricuspid annulus, RA size and function, RV size and function, and important information should be gathered on the inferior vena cave (IVC) and the coronary sinus [5].

In addition to the anatomic evaluation of the TV and tricuspid apparatus, it is equally important to assess flow and flow profiles across the TV and the RV outflow tract. These are primarily accomplished by the use of state-of-the-art cardiac ultrasound Doppler echocardiography, as well as magnetic resonance imaging capabilities for determining flow.

Imaging modalities used in the assessment of the tricuspid apparatus and functional TR include:

1. Echocardiogram,
   A. Transthoracic Echocardiogram (TTE);
   B. Transesophageal Echo (TEE);
2. Cardiac Magnetic Resonance (CMR) Imaging; and
3. Cardiac Computed Tomography (CT).

Transthoracic and Transesophageal Echocardiogram

Transthoracic echo (2D-TTE) is noninvasive, readily available, and is the most widely used imaging modality to initially assess tricuspid valve anatomy and function, as well as right-sided pressures and right-sided chamber anatomy and function. It is well recognized that 2D-TTE is operator-dependent and having access to appropriate acoustic windows can pose challenges [10]. Also, there is inter-observer variability in both the performance and interpretation of the echocardiographic findings. Saying that, it is still the procedure of choice for the initial evaluation of the TV apparatus and the associated cardiac anatomic structures. The cornerstone of 2D-TTE is not only anatomic evaluation of the tricuspid apparatus, RA, and RV, but also Doppler interrogation of tricuspid regurgitant flow, right-sided pressures, as well as evaluation of flow and flow-dependent parameters in the right ventricular outflow tract [11]. Three-dimensional TTE (3D-TTE) was intended not only to give a more anatomically correct view of the tricuspid apparatus, but also to improve spatial resolution.

TEE can be a superior modality to assess TV anatomy through a better field of view, yet it is not widely applicable as the initial echocardiographic test of choice. However, it is known that

3D-TEE has become the standard for assessing functional anatomy of the mitral apparatus. Its utilization to assess TV anatomy is limited, due to the unfamiliarity of the echocardiographic world with tricuspid patho-physiology. There clearly, though, appears to be a role that 3D-TEE will have in better evaluating the tricuspid apparatus across the spectrum of patients who present with combined left and right-sided valvular abnormalities, as well as isolated TV abnormalities. It is also important to note that both TTE and TEE have temporal resolution in the order of 3–20 ms, enabling visualization of very small, fine structures on the TV leaflets [12].

Cardiac Magnetic Resonance Imaging (MRI)

Cardiac MRI has high spatial (1–2 mm) and temporal resolution (20–30 ms) with a wide field of view that can adequately evaluate the TV anatomy in multiple planes and its relation to other cardiac structures (RA, IVC, pulmonary artery (PA)). It is a radiation free technology, with significant test-to-test reproducibility, accurate RV volume assessment and a distinct soft tissue resolution improving visualization of the myocardium, valves, and the blood pool [13].

The main limitation is that it is time consuming, expensive, not readily available, and cannot be used in patients with intra cardiac defibrillators or pacemakers unless they have MRI compatible devices.

Contrast Enhanced Computer Tomography (CT)

CT has the best spatial resolution (<5 mm) but has limited temporal resolution (70–150 ms). New generation (dual source) CT scanners have better temporal resolution. Iodinated contrast is necessary to improve the soft tissue resolution to assess the tricuspid valve, RV and RA anatomy. To assess the motion of the RV, RA and valve leaflets retrospective cardiac gated scan needs to be done. Retrospective gating increases the amount of radiation exposure to the patient. Currently, CT is not done to assess the anatomy of the native TV. It has better utility in valvular assessment in patients with prosthetic valves [14].

Characteristics of Functional Tricuspid Insufficiency

It must be emphasized that functional TR is the result of abnormalities of either the RV or the tricuspid annulus, which thereby affect the functional anatomy of the tricuspid apparatus itself (Table 20.1).

When specifically looking at functional TR, it is very important to assess annular dilatation (>40 mm is abnormal), the height of coaptation of the tricuspid leaflets from the valve annular plane (>8 mm is abnormal), the tenting area (>6 cm^2 is abnormal), the presence or absence of edge-to-edge coaptation of the valve leaflets, and the regurgitant jet area. To evaluate the functional TR with 2D-TTE, in at least 2 orthogonal planes. For example; the RV inflow view, apical or subcostal views are the preferred planes to assess TR jet [3].

Table 20.1 2D- TTE parameters for TR assessment

Parameter	Mild TR	Severe TR
Regurgitant jet	Thin and central	Large and dense central or wall hugging eccentric jet
Coaptation mode	Normal (body-to-body) No tethering	No coaptation with or without tethering
Jet density	Soft and parabolic	Dense, triangular with early peaking
Vena contracta width (mm)	Not defined	>6.5
Annular diameter (mm)	<40	>40
PISA radius (mm) At Niquist limit 28 m/s	≤5	>9
Hepatic vein flow	Systolic dominance	Systolic flow reversal
ERO area mm^2	Not defined	≥40

Modified from Lancellotti et al. [15]

Color and Spectral Doppler are the main echocardiographic modalities to qualitatively and quantitatively assess the severity and impact of TR, while color Doppler evaluation of the presence and size of the TR jet in the RA is primarily utilized to qualitatively assess its severity [15]. The functional TR jet is usually central and is classified as either mild, if the area occupying of the TR jet in the RA is <5 cm^2, or severe, if the regurgitant area is >10 cm^2 [5]. There are major limitations, in that the color jet is only a mean velocity map and is influenced by many factors, the foremost of which is the ability to accurately image the TR jet, as well as hemodynamic state of the patient. In an attempt to improve the quantification of the TR color jet as a marker of severity, the recent ACC/AHA guidelines in 2014 have emphasized utilizing the vena contracta (VC) – a measurement of the width of the high velocity regurgitant jet on the atrial side of the tricuspid apparatus – as a marker of severity. VC is usually imaged in apical four-chamber view at an adapted Nyquist limit, with narrow sector scan with zoom in mode for better temporal resolution [16]. Average measurement of VC>6.5 mm is usually associated with severe TR (Fig. 20.1).

It is easy to understand how there are limitations with this method, especially if there are multiple TR jets present or if the orifice is elliptical, not circular. In an attempt to further semi-quantitate the assessment of the severity of TR by echocardiographic Doppler, the PISA, or Proximal Isovelocity Surface Area radius, has also been utilized. While this has been widely applied to assessing the severity of mitral regurgitation, it has not been proven to be useful or reproducible in the evaluation of TR. The apical four-chamber view and the parasternal long- and short-axis views are recommended. Eccentric TR jets may limit the ability of an accurate radius of PISA to be measured. But, currently, most believe that a PISA radius of >9 mm at Nyquist limit is indicative of significant TR. Recently, many have emphasized trying to accurately quantitate TR by measuring an effective regurgitant orifice (ERO), but again, the variability and reproducibility of these measurements is difficult. An ERO area >40 mm^2 is suggestive of severe TR (Fig. 20.2). A simple way of evaluating severity of TR is to evaluate the presence of systolic flow reversal in the hepatic vein – also an indication of severe TR [17].

Spectral Doppler has been utilized to evaluate the flow velocity of the TR jet. From this, one can calculate RV and PA systolic pressures. The key measurement, though, is to get an accurate TR jet velocity profile, as this may vary, not only from acoustic window utilized (parasternal position versus apical position), but also from the direction of interrogation of the TR jet by the continuous wave Doppler. Saying that, it is widely utilized as a calculation of RV and, hence, PA systolic pressure, even though it does have limitations. For accurate calculation of right RV or PA systolic pressures it is important to appropriately estimate RA pressure. Various methods are utilized to estimate RA pressure based upon the size of the IVC, as well as the ability to show inspiratory collapse. Mutlak et al. noted that elevated PA systolic pressures are associated with more severe TR [18].

RV function can be assessed in four-chamber view by measuring end-diastolic area and the end-systolic area to calculate the RV fractional area change [3]. RV function is also analyzed by tricuspid annular plane systolic excursion (TAPSE), as well as tissue evaluation of the tricuspid annulus (S'). All of these measurements are utilized in clinical practice, but have important limitations in both proper acquisition of images, as well as proper measurements. TTE with strain analysis of RV function has shown promise at being able to accurately evaluate global RV function, but has not been widely clinically utilized [19, 20]. Measurements of RA size and dimension give some insight into the chronicity of the functional TR [20].

Doppler parameters have also been utilized to evaluate pulmonary vascular resistance (PVR), which is especially important when trying to evaluate patients who have adult congenital heart disease or congestive heart failure. PVR is directly related to the trans pulmonary pressure gradient and inversely related to trans pulmonary flow and can be measured noninvasively by Doppler when there is suspected elevation of the right-sided pressures, known or suspected increase inflow across the pulmonary valve, or

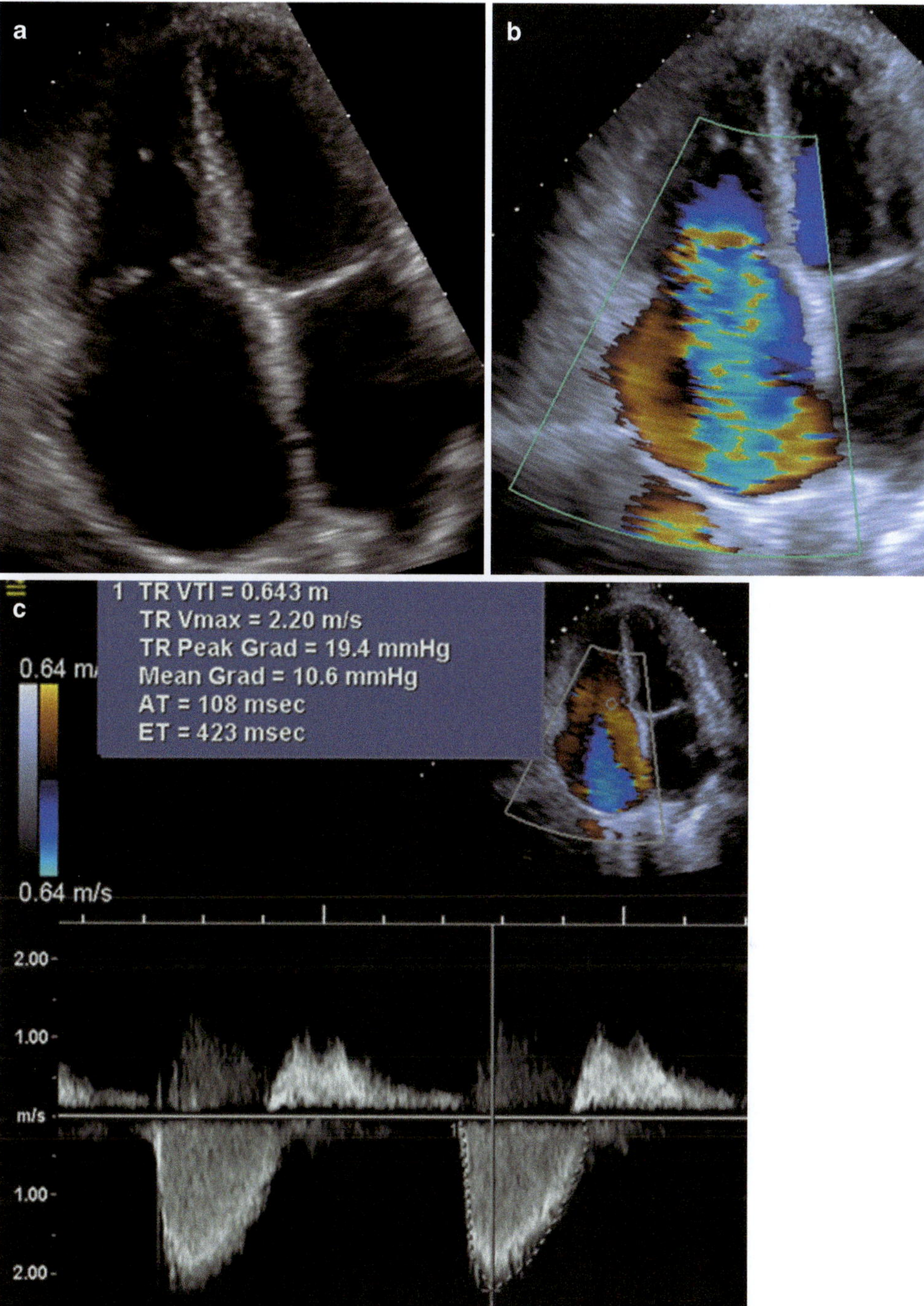

Fig. 20.1 Image **a** shows the apical four chamber view in systole showing poor co-aptation of septal and anterior leaflets of the tricuspid valve and also shows enlargement of right atrium (RA). Image **b** shows the color Doppler of the tricuspid valve insufficiency. The TR jet occupies most of the RA and extends to the roof of the RA. Image **c** shows the continuous wave Doppler with the "triangular spectral envelope" which is consistent with severe TR and had low peak velocity due to rapid equalization of pressures in RV and RA. Image **d** shows the sub-costal view of the dilated IVC with hepatic vein flow reversal by color Doppler. Image **e** shows the spectral Doppler with systolic reversal in hepatic vein flow. Images **f** and **g** are mid esophageal short-axis TEE images showing the non-coaptation of leaflets and severe TR

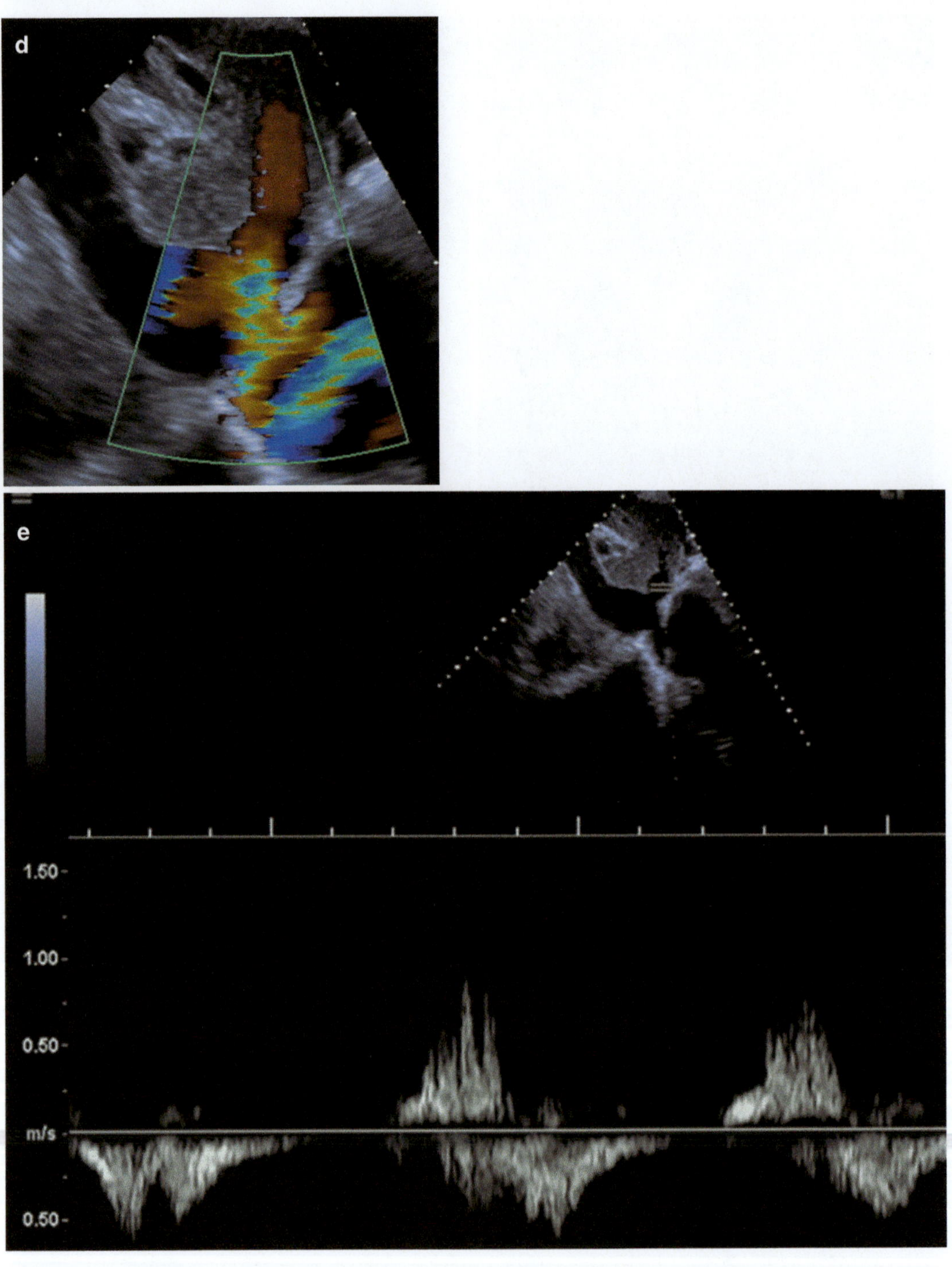

Fig. 20.1 (continued)

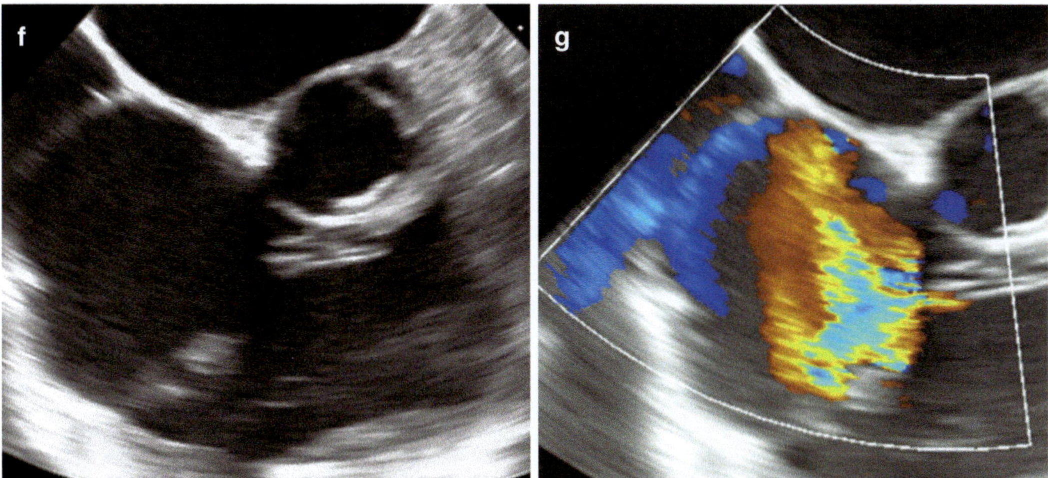

Fig. 20.1 (continued)

any high output situation. The easiest way to measure that is by using an algorithm, whereby the ratio of tricuspid regurgitant velocity divided by the Velocity Time Integral (VTI) in the RV outflow tract is assessed and if that ratio exceeds 0.2, then it is suspected that one might have increased PVR. Spectral Doppler can also be utilized to evaluate flow parameters in the RV outflow tract. Being able to calculate a RV VTI does allow for the assessment of mean PA pressures. Importantly, the shape of the RV outflow tract pulse wave Doppler tracing gives a qualitative assessment of the presence or absence of PH, but being able to calculate RV outflow tract VTI may be very important to assess the functional reserve of the RV [21].

Assessment of Right Ventricular Volume

Adequate imaging of the RV is crucial in evaluating the severity of the TR [5]. Pulmonary hypertension causes RV remodeling through tethering of the TV leaflets. On the other hand, RV failure leads to annular dilatation affecting the tricuspid annulus [22, 23].

Historically, 2D- TTE has been used to qualitatively assess RV volume and pressure overload. This is done primarily by looking at the interventricular septal motion in diastole and systole, where a persistent flattening of the interventricular septum has been shown to be indicative of both RV volume and pressure overload, whereas, intermittent flattening of the septum has been associated more with volume than with pressure overload [5]. While 3D- TEE has been utilized by some to try to better evaluate global RV function and volumes, and while this technique has shown some success when compared to the gold standard of CMR in assessment of RV volume and function, it has not been widely utilized in clinical practice.

Cardiac MRI is the current gold standard for accurate and reproducible volumetric evaluation of the cardiac chambers due to its high spatial resolution and the ability to scan in multiple planes (Fig. 20.3). MRI has the advantages of directly assessing flow across the pulmonary valve and pulmonary artery, using phase contrast technique [24]. Flow in the PA can be utilized to indirectly quantitate the regurgitant volume of TR and hence the severity of TR by subtracting the volume of flow through PA from RV stroke volume. Another modality for direct assessment of TV inflow is through calculation of the area of anatomic non-coaptation of the tips of the valve leaflets. In addition, cardiac MRI is important in determining the hemodynamic and anatomic consequences of TR. This information will be crucial when a surgical intervention is opted (Fig. 20.4).

Retrospective contrast enhanced gated CT can be used for assessment of RV volumes and dimensions. One situation where it may have a role is in patients with left ventricular assist devices (LVAD). Patients with LVAD tend to have poor acoustic windows by TTE and cannot be scanned by cardiac MRI. So gated CTA can be used to assess function in this subgroup of patients.

Multi-modality imaging approach with various imaging techniques as described above should be used to accurately assess the anatomy of TV apparatus (annulus dimensions, tenting area and height, RV and RA volumes), severity of functional TR (regurgitant volume and fraction), hemodynamic consequences (PA pressures and PVR) and help with planning future intervention.

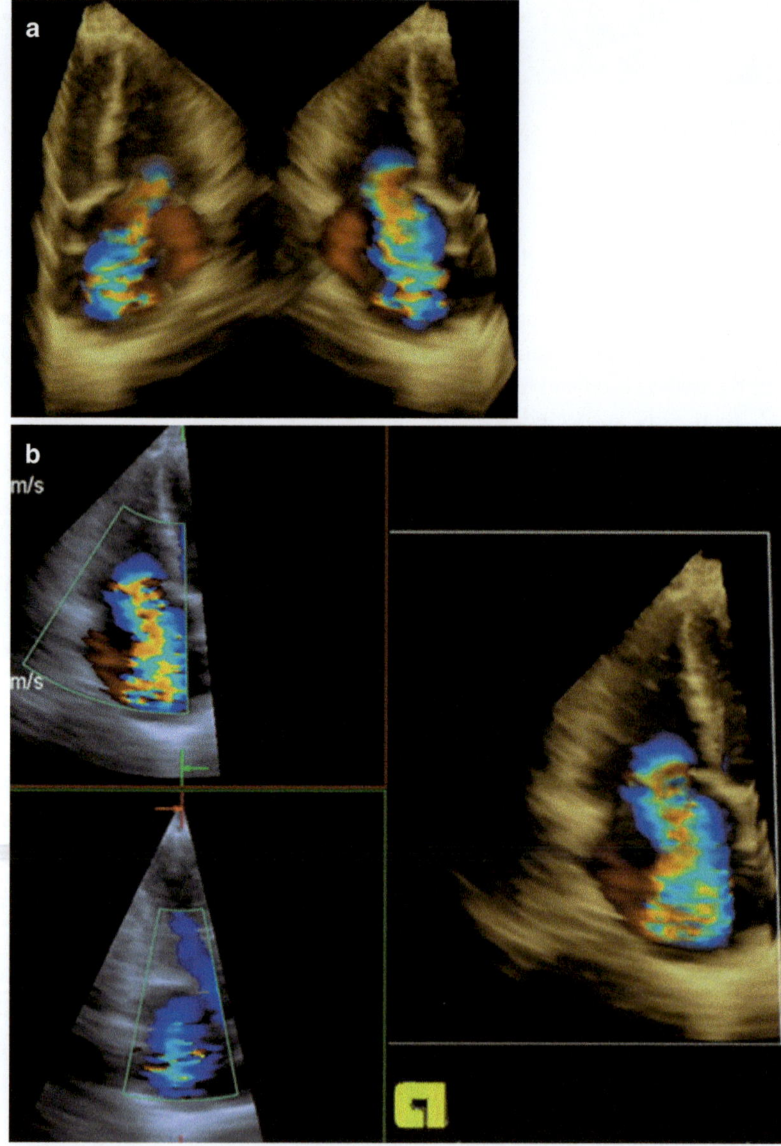

Fig. 20.2 Image **a** shows the three dimensional orthogonal views of the RV and RA showing the TR jet. Images **b** and **c** show the process of assessment of 3D effective regurgitant orifice area (EROA) by proximal iso-velocity surface (PISA) area method. In this patient 3D-EROA is 1.1 sq. cm

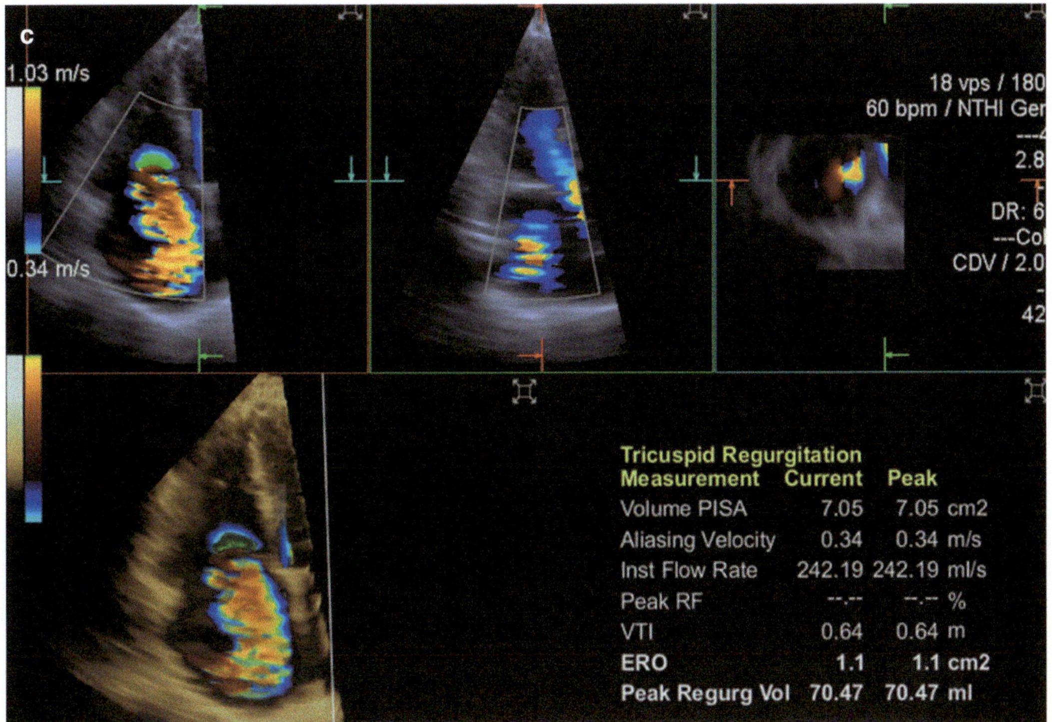

Fig. 20.2 (continued)

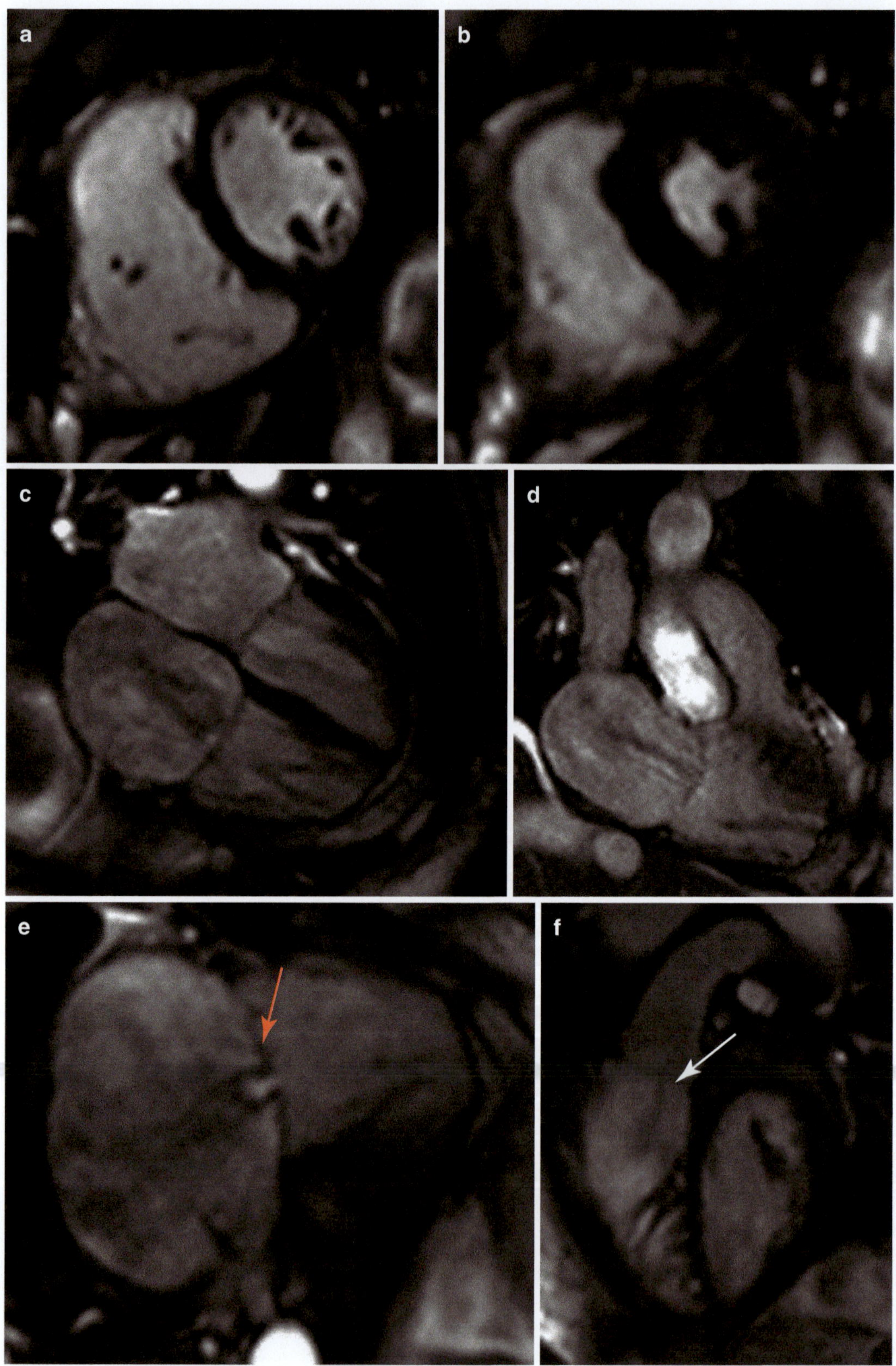
a
b
c
d
e
f

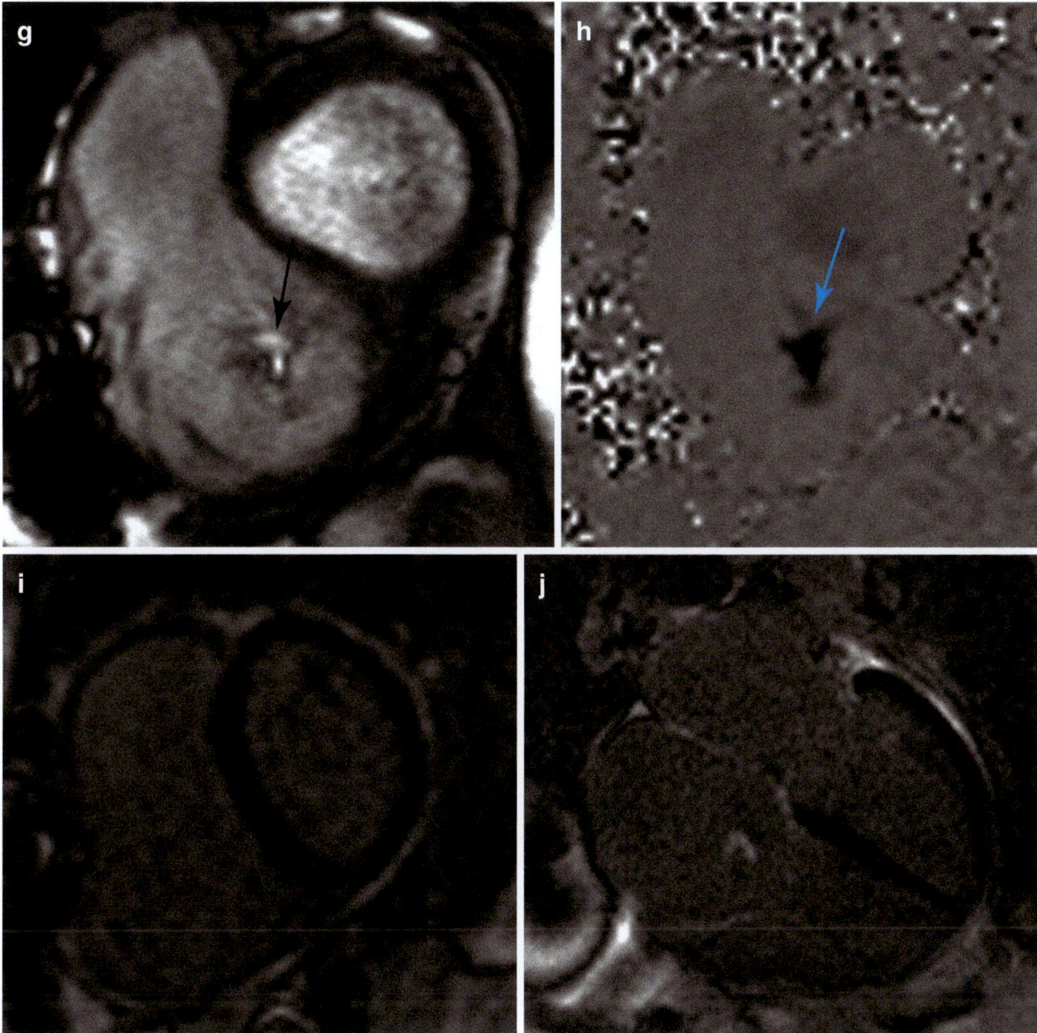

Fig. 20.3 (continued)

Fig. 20.3 Images **a** and **b** are steady state free precision (SSFP) frames in diastole and systole of the mid-short axis of the heart showing the enlarged RV. The RV endiastolic volume is 248 ml. Image **c** (SSFP four chamber), image **d** (SSFP RV inflow view) and image **e** (SSFP RV two chamber view) showing the TR jet (*red arrow*) due to dephasing of protons. Image **f** is the RV outflow showing the pulmonic valve and the pulmonic insufficiency jet (*white arrow*). Image **g** shows the short axis view of the RV with anatomic area of coaptation defect (*black arrow*). Image **h** shows the systolic frame of thru-plane phase contrast imaging showing the TR jet (*blue arrow*). Images **i** and **j** show the delayed hyper-enhancement images with no evidence of macroscopic scar in RV and LV

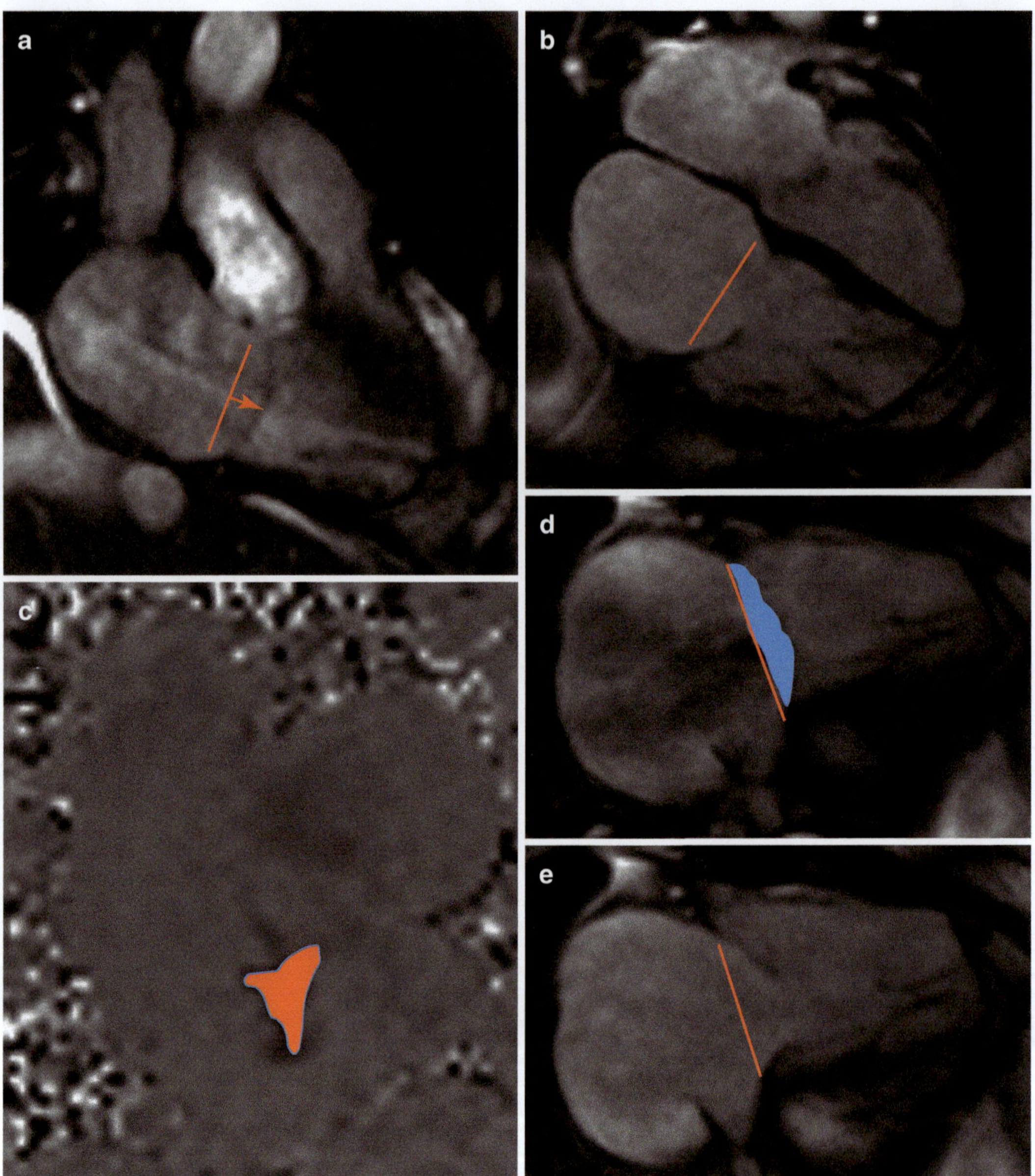

Fig. 20.4 Images **a** and **d** are systolic frames of RV inflow and two chamber views showing the methods to measure the tenting area (*blue area*) and coaptation distance (*red arrow*) from the tricuspid annulus plane. Images **b** and **e** show the methods to measure the septal to infero-lateral wall and the intercommisural dimensions of the tricuspid annulus. Image **c** is the phase image of the thru plane phase contrast image done at the tips of the tricuspid valve showing the anatomic regurgitant orifice area (*red area*)

References

1. Silver MD, Lam JH, Ranganathan N, Wigle ED. Morphology of the human tricuspid valve. Circulation. 1971;43:333–48.
2. Dreyfus GD, Martin RP, Dulguerov F, Chan KM, Alexandrescu C. Functional tricuspid regurgitation: a need to revise our understanding. J Am Coll Cardiol. 2015;65(21):2331–6.
3. Rogers JH, Bolling SF. The tricuspid valve: current perspective and evolving management of tricuspid regurgitation. Circulation. 2009;119:2718–25.
4. Fukuda S, Saracino G, Matsumara Y, Daimon M, Tran H, Greenberg NL, Hozumi T, Yoshikawa J, Thomas JD, Shiota T. Three-dimensional geometry of the

tricuspid annulus in healthy subjects and in patients with functional tricuspid regurgitation: a real-time, 3-dimensional echocardiographic study. Circulation. 2006;114:I-492–8.

5. Badano LP, Muraru D, Enriquez-Sarano M. Assessment of functional tricuspid regurgitation. Eur Heart J. 2013;34:1875–85.
6. Mutlak D, Lessick J, Reisner SA, Aronson D, Dabbah S, Agmon Y. Echocardiography-based spectrum of severe tricuspid regurgitation: the frequency of apparently idiopathic tricuspid regurgitation. J Am Soc Echocardiogr. 2007;20:405–8.
7. Galie N, Hoeper MM, Humbert M, et al. Guidelines for the diagnosis and treatment of pulmonary hypertension: the Task Force for the Diagnosis and Treatment of Pulmonary Hypertension of the European Society of Cardiology (ESC) and the European Respiratory Society (ERS), endorsed by the International Society of Heart and Lung Transplantation (ISHLT). Eur Heart J. 2009;30: 2493–537.
8. Topilsky Y, Nkomo V, Vatury O, Michelena H, Letourneau T, Suri R, Pislaru S, Park S, Mahoney D, Biner S, Enriquez-Sarano M. Clinical outcome of isolated tricuspid regurgitation. J Am Coll Cardiol Img. 2014;7:1185–94.
9. Waller BF. Etiology of pure tricuspid regurgitation. Cardiovasc Clin. 1987;17:53–95.
10. Hung J. The pathogenesis of functional tricuspid regurgitation. Semin Thorac Cardiovasc Surg. 2010; 22:76–8.
11. Klein A, Burstow D, Tajik A, Zachariah P, Taliercio C, Taylor C, Bailey K, Seward J. Age-related prevalence of valvular regurgitation in normal subjects: a comprehensive color-flow examination in 118 volunteers. J Am Soc Echocardiogr. 1990;3:54–63.
12. Shiota T, Jones M, Chikada M, Fleishman CE, Castellucci JB, Cotter B, et al. Real-time three-dimensional echocardiography for determining right ventricular stroke volume in an animal model of chronic right ventricular volume overload. Circulation. 1998;97:1897–900.
13. Morello A, Gelfand EV. Cardiovascular magnetic resonance imaging for valvular heart disease. Curr Heart Fail Rep. 2009;6(3):160–6.
14. Jenkins WS, Chin C, Rudd JH, Newby DE, Dweck MR. What can we learn about valvular heart disease from PET/CT? Future Cardiol. 2013;9(5):657–67.
15. Lancellotti P, Moura L, Pierard LA, Agricola E, Popescu BA, Tribuilloy C, Hagendorff A, Monin JL, Badano LP, Zamorano JL. European Association of Echocardiography recommendations for the Assessment of valvular regurgitation. Part 2: mitral and tricuspid regurgitation (native valve diseases). Eur J Echocardiogr. 2010;11:307–32.
16. Tribouilloy CM, Enriquez-Sarano M, Bailey KR, Tajik AJ, Seward JB. Quantification of tricuspid regurgitation by measuring the width of the vena contracta with Doppler color flow imaging: a clinical study. J Am Coll Cardiol. 2000;36:472–8.
17. Mascherbauer J, Maurer G. The forgotten valve: lessons to be learned in tricuspid regurgitation. Eur Heart J. 2010;31:2841–3.
18. Mutlak D, Aronson D, Lessick J, Reisner SA, Dabbah S, Agmon Y. Functional tricuspid regurgitation in patients with pulmonary hypetension: is pulmonary artery pressure the only determinant of regurgitation severity? Chest. 2009;135:115–21.
19. Gondi S, Dokainish H. Right ventricular tissue Doppler and strain imaging: ready for clinical use? Echocardiography. 2007;24:522–32.
20. Haddad F, Hunt SA, Rosenthal DN, Murphy DJ. Right ventricular function in cardiovascular disease, part I: anatomy, physiology, aging, and functional assessment of the right ventricle. Circulation. 2008;117:1436–48.
21. Zoghbi WA, Enriquez-Sarano M, Foster E, Grayburn PA, Kraft CD, Levine RA, Nihoyannopoulos P, Otto CM, Quinones MA, Rakowski H, Stewart WJ, Waggoner A, Weissman NJ. Recommendations for evaluation of the severity of native valvular regurgitation with two dimensional and Doppler echocardiography. J Am Soc Echocardiogr. 2003;16(7):777–802.
22. Fukuda S, Song JM, Gillinov AM, et al. Tricuspid valve tethering predicts residual tricuspid regurgitation after tricuspid annuloplasty. Circulation. 2005;111:975–9.
23. Kim HK, Kim YJ, Park JS, et al. Determinants of the severity of functional tricuspid regurgitation. Am J Cardiol. 2006;98:236–42.
24. Lopez-Mattei JC, Shah DJ. The role of cardiac magnetic resonance in valvular heart disease. Methodist Debakey Cardiovasc J. 2013;9(3):142–8.

21 Tricuspid Ring Annuloplasty for Functional Tricuspid Regurgitation

K.M. John Chan

Abstract

Tricuspid ring annuloplasty is the most common technique of tricuspid valve repair with consistent reproducible results. It is indicated at the time of left sided heart valve surgery when tricuspid regurgitation is severe or when it is associated with tricuspid annular dilatation or raised pulmonary artery pressures. It can be performed safely with a very low risk of complications. If left untreated, functional tricuspid regurgitation will progress with adverse effects on symptoms, functional capacity, right ventricular remodeling and survival. Results are best when the operation is performed at an early stage.

Keywords

Tricuspid annuloplasty • Tricuspid valve repair • Tricuspid regurgitation • Tricuspid annular dilatation • Ring annuloplasty

Tricuspid annuloplasty is the most common technique of tricuspid valve repair in functional tricuspid regurgitation (TR). An increasing number of concomitant tricuspid annuloplasty procedures are being performed in recent years due to a more aggressive approach to the treatment of functional tricuspid regurgitation as recommended in the guidelines [1]. However, as functional TR is a sequelae of long standing mitral valve disease, the need for concomitant tricuspid valve surgery may decrease with time as more mitral valve repairs are being performed earlier in asymptomatic patients.

Indications for Concomitant Tricuspid Valve Repair

Tricuspid valve repair is indicated during left sided heart valve surgery in patients with severe TR, or in those with greater than mild TR and a dilated tricuspid annulus, or pulmonary hypertension, particularly if the leaflet coaptation mode is abnormal i.e., occurring only between the leaflet edges and not between the body of the leaflets [2–4].

K.M.J. Chan, BM BS, MSc, PhD, FRCS CTh
Department of Cardiothoracic Surgery,
Gleneagles Hospital, Jalan Ampang,
Kuala Lumpur 50450, Malaysia
e-mail: KMJohnChan@yahoo.com

K.M.J. Chan (ed.), *Functional Mitral and Tricuspid Regurgitation*,
DOI 10.1007/978-3-319-43510-7_21

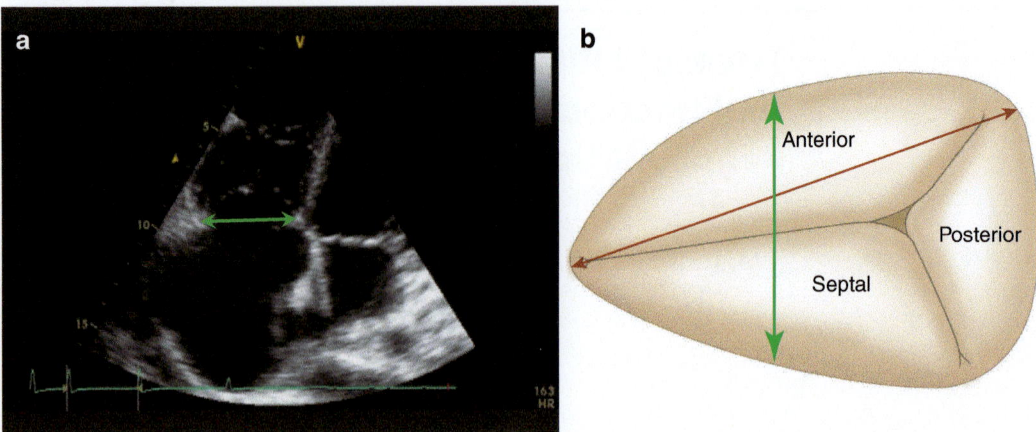

Fig. 21.1 (**a**) Measurement of the tricuspid annular diameter by transthoracic echocardiography from an apical four chamber view in mid-diastole. This measures the tricuspid annulus from approximately the middle of the septal annulus to the middle of the anterior annulus (*green arrow*). The corresponding positions on the tricuspid annulus are shown in (**b**). (**b**) Measurement of the tricuspid annulus surgically during the operation. This measures the tricuspid annulus from the antero-septal commissure to the antero-posterior commissure with the heart fully stretched out (*red arrows*)

Determining the Size of the Tricuspid Annulus

Measurement of the tricuspid annulus by transthoracic echocardiography is typically done from an apical four chamber view in diastole. This measures the distance between the middle of the septal annulus and the middle of the anterior annulus (Fig. 21.1a). This is in contrast with the surgical measurement of the tricuspid annular diameter which measures the tricuspid annulus from the antero-septal commissure to the antero-posterior commissure, two fixed points which can be easily identified (Fig. 21.1b). As a guide, an annular diameter of 40 mm measured by transthoracic echocardiography from an apical four chamber view roughly corresponds to an annular diameter of 70 mm measured by surgical assessment intraoperatively. An annular diameter of 40 mm measured by transthoracic echocardiography or 70 mm measured by surgical assessment has been taken as the threshold beyond which the tricuspid annulus is considered to be dilated and surgical intervention on the tricuspid valve is indicated in patients undergoing left sided valve surgery [3]. It has also been suggested that an indexed tricuspid annular diameter corrected for body surface area can be used to guide the need for concomitant tricuspid annuloplasty at the time of mitral valve surgery with various authors recommending a threshold size for concomitant tricuspid valve repair surgery of 21–27 mm/m^2 [5–8]. The guidelines recommend a threshold size of 21 mm/m^2 [9]. In one study, almost all patients with an indexed tricuspid annular diameter greater than 21 mm/m^2 had at least moderate tricuspid regurgitation [10]. The use of an indexed tricuspid annular diameter corrected for body surface area may be more suitable in patients of small body size. Measurements of the tricuspid annular diameter and severity of TR should be done pre-operatively in the awake patient as general anesthesia can lead to a reduction in TR severity as a result of reduction in the afterload and preload from vasodilatation and venodilatation [10].

What Do the Guidelines Recommend?

The American Heart Association/American College of Cardiology 2014 guidelines on valvular heart disease recommend tricuspid valve surgery in the following situations [3]:

1. Patients with severe TR undergoing left sided valve surgery (Class 1 recommendation, Level of Evidence C),
2. Patients with mild, moderate or greater functional TR at the time of left sided valve surgery when either tricuspid annular dilatation or prior evidence of right heart failure is present (Class IIa recommendation, Level of Evidence B),
3. Patients with symptoms due to severe primary TR that are unresponsive to medical therapy (Class IIa recommendation, Level of Evidence C),
4. Patients with moderate functional TR and pulmonary hypertension at the time of left-sided valve surgery (Class IIb recommendation, Level of Evidence C),
5. Asymptomatic or minimally symptomatic patients with severe primary TR and progressive degrees of moderate or greater right ventricular dilatation and/or systolic dysfunction (Class IIb recommendation, Level of Evidence C),
6. Patients with persistent symptoms due to severe TR who have undergone previous left sided valve surgery and who do not have severe pulmonary hypertension or significant right ventricular systolic dysfunction (Class IIb recommendation, Level of Evidence C).

The classes of recommendation are as follows:

Class I: Benefits outweigh the risk. Procedure should be performed.
Class IIa: Benefits outweigh the risk but additional studies with focused objectives are needed. It is reasonable to perform the procedure.
Class IIb: Benefits may outweigh the risk or may be equivalent. Additional studies with broad objective are needed; additional registry data would be helpful. Procedure may be considered.

The levels of evidence are as follows:

Level A: Multiple populations evaluated. Data derived from multiple randomized controlled trials or meta analyses.
Level B: Limited populations evaluated. Data derived from a single randomized controlled trial or non-randomized studies.
Level C: Very limited populations evaluated. Only consensus opinion of experts, case studies, or standards of care available.

Progression of Untreated Tricuspid Regurgitation

The recommendation to intervene on the tricuspid valve when the tricuspid annulus is dilated in the absence of significant tricuspid regurgitation (TR) was first made by Dreyfus, et al., in 2005 [11]. In an observational study on 311 patients undergoing mitral valve repair in whom tricuspid annuloplasty was also performed if the tricuspid annulus was dilated to more than 70 mm measured intra-operatively (from the antero-septal commissure to the antero-posterior commissure), it was observed that NYHA functional class was significantly better at 5 years in those in whom a concomitant tricuspid annuloplasty was performed. In addition, TR progressed in those who did not have a concomitant tricuspid annuloplasty but not in those who did [11]. The observation that mild or moderate FTR progresses in 15–40 % of patients if left untreated has been reported in numerous other studies including a meta-analysis [7, 10, 12–25]. Goldstone, et al., reported that the proportion of patients with moderate or more TR increased from 7.9 % at baseline to 36 % 9 years after isolated mitral valve surgery, and this was associated with right ventricular dysfunction [10]. Of note, the mean tricuspid annular diameter is this study was 40.1 mm, which is the current threshold size at which concomitant tricuspid valve repair is recommended. The study also reported that FTR progressed in those with only mild TR if the baseline indexed tricuspid annular diameter was greater than 21 mm/m^2 [10]. Tricuspid annular dilation, TR severity, right ventricular dysfunction, pulmonary hypertension, atrial fibrillation, enlarged left and right atria and rheumatic etiology are amongst the common risk factors for TR progression which have been identified [7, 10, 22, 23, 26, 27]. In a randomized trial of patients with mild tricuspid regurgitation and tricuspid annular dilatation undergoing mitral valve surgery, patients randomized to receive a tricuspid annuloplasty had less TR progression, improved right ventricular reverse remodeling, and better functional outcomes compared to patients who did not receive a tricuspid annuloplasty [15]. Similar observations have been made in a few other studies [18, 28]. Importantly, several studies have reported an association with reduced survival in those with significant late TR or those in whom there is progression of TR [13, 14, 16, 21, 27, 29]. Re-operations on the tricuspid valve in those who subsequently develop symptomatic severe TR also carries a high hospital mortality of between 14 and 35 % [30–32].

Benefits of Tricuspid Annuloplasty

Correction of significant TR has been shown to improve right ventricular geometry and function, and pulmonary artery pressures [28, 33, 34]. Studies have also shown an improvement in functional capacity and survival following tricuspid annuloplasty [11, 13]. Prophylactic tricuspid annuloplasty performed when the tricuspid annulus is dilated but before the onset of severe TR also prevents the progression of TR and right ventricular dilatation, improves the functional capacity and survival of the patient, and avoids the need for future re-operative tricuspid valve surgery which carries a high operative risk [11, 13, 18].

Surgical Technique

Tricuspid annuloplasty can be performed using either a tricuspid annuloplasty ring or band, or by various suture annuloplasty techniques. Several studies have reported a lower recurrence rate of TR when an annuloplasty ring is used as compared to suture annuloplasty, and some have reported improved survival when an annuloplasty ring is used for tricuspid valve repair [35, 36]. Tricuspid ring annuloplasty will be described in this chapter. Tricuspid suture annuloplasty is covered in a separate chapter.

The tricuspid annulus can be sized by measuring its leaflet area by pulling on the anterior papillary muscle which supports both the anterior and posterior leaflets and using an obturator to determine this size (Fig. 21.2a). It can also be sized by measuring the orifice area by matching the corresponding notches of the obturator to the antero-septal and postero-septal commissures i.e., the length of the septal annulus (Fig. 21.2b). If there is a discrepancy in size between the two measurements, then the size obtained by using the orifice area i.e., the septal annulus length, should be used as this is relatively fixed in size and does not dilate. A discrepancy in size with the leaflet area being smaller than the orifice area is also an indication for tricuspid valve repair as this suggests that the leaflets are of insufficient size to achieve valvular competence [9].

In the presence of severe FTR, the annuloplasty ring can be undersized to increase leaflet coaptation [37]. For example, if the annulus is sized at 34 mm, a 32 mm ring could be used instead. However, caution must be exercised particularly in elderly patients with weak tissue as the excess tension can cause annular dehiscence particularly at the septal annulus [38]. A series of 2/0 ethibond sutures or equivalent are placed around the tricuspid annulus except at the region of the conduction tissues at the septal annulus (Fig. 21.3). The sutures are then in turn passed through the tricuspid annuloplasty ring. Care is needed around the posterior annulus to avoid the right coronary artery, and in the region of the anterior annulus where too deep a suture may cause injury to the aortic wall and aortic valve leaflets. As a precaution, traction can be exerted on the sutures placed in the posterior leaflet annulus after placement to ensure that there is no visible distortion of the right coronary artery. If any suggestion of distortion or occlusion of the right coronary artery is suggested by this maneuver, the sutures should be removed and placed again carefully.

Several commercially available tricuspid annuloplasty rings are available with the newer rings shaped geometrically into a 3-dimensional configuration to match the normal geometry of the tricuspid annulus. Care must be taken during

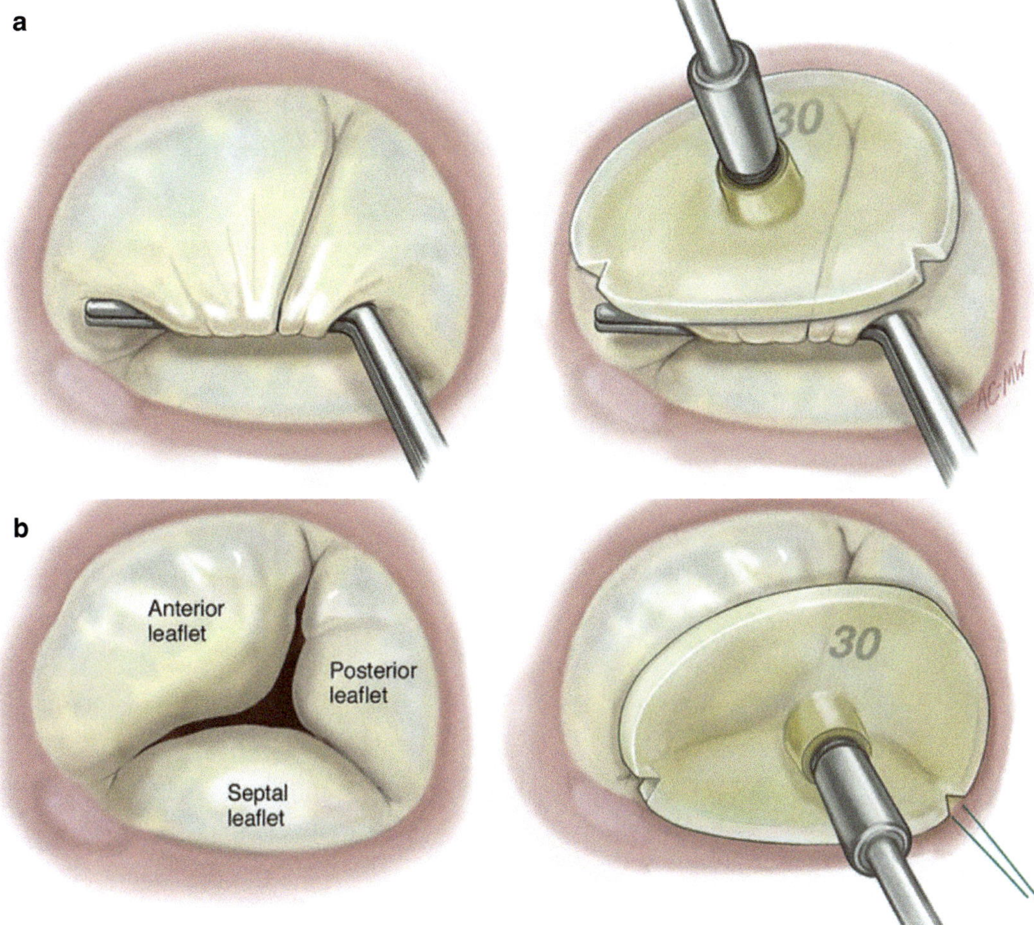

Fig. 21.2 (**a**) Measuring the tricuspid annular size by pulling on the anterior papillary muscle; this usually supports the anterior leaflet and half of the posterior leaflet, although sometimes, it may only support the anterior leaflet. An obturator of the same size is used to determine the size of the annuloplasty ring to use. (**b**) Measuring the tricuspid annular size by determining the length of the septal annulus. A suture placed in the postero-septal commissure is useful to facilitate this. An obturator is then used to match the corresponding positions on it to the anteroseptal commissure and the posteroseptal commissure to determine the size of the annuloplasty ring to use (From Carpentier et al. [51], with permission from Elsevier)

suture placement to ensure that the sutures are passed through the annuloplasty ring at their corresponding positions on the tricuspid annulus so as not to distort the tricuspid valve. Two important landmarks are the anteroposterior commissure and the posteroseptal commissures which should pass through the corresponding positions in the tricuspid annuloplasty ring. The annuloplasty ring is then lowered and the sutures tied. A water test is performed while occluding the pulmonary artery to confirm valve competency. To minimize myocardial ischaemia times, the tricuspid valve annuloplasty can be done after the release of the aortic cross clamp and during the period of rewarming and reperfusion.

Early Results

In less than severe TR, where the indication for intervention on the tricuspid valve is tricuspid annular dilatation, adding tricuspid annuloplasty to left sided heart valve surgery does not increase operative risk and can be performed safely with

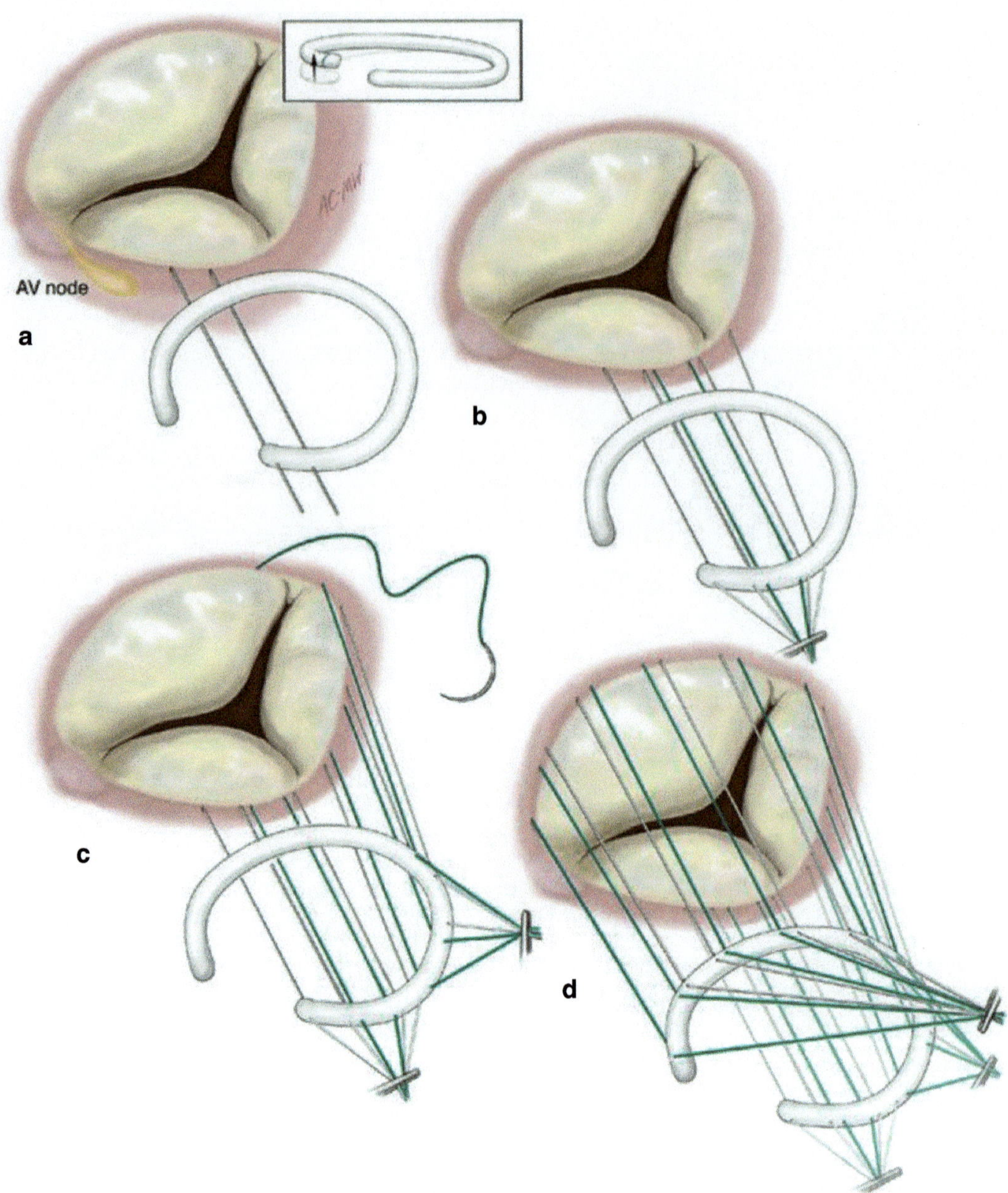

Fig. 21.3 (**a**) 2/0 ethibond sutures or equivalent are placed around the tricuspid annulus. The tricuspid annuloplasty ring is designed such that no sutures are placed in the region of the conduction tissues. (**b–d**) Care is taken to ensure that sutures placed in the annulus are passed through the corresponding positions in the annuloplasty ring; the fixed landmarks to guide this are the commissural sutures which should be placed at the corresponding positions on the annuloplasty ring. This ensures that the tricuspid valve is not distorted as a result of performing the annuloplasty (From Carpentier et al. [51], with permission from Elsevier)

an operative mortality of less than 1 % [11, 25, 28, 32]. This is despite patients undergoing concomitant tricuspid valve annuloplasty plus mitral valve surgery being older, having worse right and left ventricular function and higher pulmonary artery pressures, and being more likely to be in atrial fibrillation compared to patients having isolated mitral valve surgery [28].

In more severe TR, where the indication for intervention on the tricuspid valve is severe TR, the operative mortality and complication rates are higher but still similar for those undergoing concomitant tricuspid and mitral valve surgery and isolated mitral valve surgery according to the Society of Thoracic Surgeons database [39]. One study did report higher operative mortality in those having concomitant tricuspid and mitral valve surgery compared to isolated mitral valve surgery [40]. However, this was a non-randomized study and it is likely that the higher mortality and complication rates in those undergoing combined mitral and tricuspid valve surgery was due to the fact that these were a sicker and higher risk group of patients compared to those who underwent isolated mitral valve surgery.

Several risk factors for increased operative mortality for tricuspid valve surgery have been identified namely NYHA functional class IV and the presence of liver cirrhosis, and also renal failure, cerebrovascular disease, chronic lung disease, congestive heart failure, non-elective presentation, and reoperation [39, 41]. In one study, the presence of liver disease increased operative mortality from 9.4 to 22.9 % [1]. Yiu, et al., reported that indices of leaflet tethering and right ventricular geometry also had an impact on outcomes with increasing right ventricular size and leaflet tethering being independently associated with adverse outcomes (including heart failure and death) at 1 year, after correcting for age and NYHA functional class III/IV [42].

Complications

Complications relating directly to the tricuspid valve annuloplasty is not common but do occur and include injury to the right coronary artery from too deep placement of the annuloplasty sutures in the region of the posterior annulus, injury to the aortic wall from too deep annuloplasty sutures in the aortic area of the anterior annulus, annular and ring dehiscence in the septal annulus due to friable tissue, and need for a permanent pacemaker, amongst others [38, 43]. Ring dehiscence was reported to be more common following rigid ring annuloplasty compared to flexible band annuloplasty (8.7 % versus 0.9 %) and always occurred in the septal annulus possibly due to the increased shearing forces in this area. [38] Adequate depth and number of sutures should therefore be ensured in this area. The risk of requiring a permanent pacemaker following tricuspid valve repair is between 2.4 and 9.5 % and is similar to that of isolated mitral valve surgery [1, 28, 39].

Injury to the right coronary artery should be suspected if the patient becomes unstable and there are signs of inferior myocardial ischaemia after tricuspid valve annuloplasty. It can occur due to distortion of the right coronary artery due to plication of the annulus by sutures placed at the annulus, away from the right coronary artery itself. It can also be caused by direct injury to the right coronary artery by sutures placed through it or going around it and occluding it. Patients with a very dilated tricuspid annulus are most at risk of this complication due to distortion of the course of the right coronary artery, and also those with very calcified coronary arteries which may make them more susceptible to kinking [44]. Caution should be exercised to avoid too deep sutures in the region of the anteroposterior commissure and avoiding placing sutures in the atrial wall. Options for management in these cases include coronary artery bypass graft surgery, or removal of the annuloplasty ring and sutures if the patient is still in the operating theatre, or if the patient is in the intensive care unit already, coronary angiography to confirm the diagnosis, and percutaneous coronary intervention (PCI). Distortion of the right coronary artery can occur from annular plication away from the right coronary artery itself, in which case, PCI may be successful in restoring coronary flow. However, if the right coronary artery has been occluded or narrowed due to an annuloplasty suture passing around or through it, PCI is unlikely to be successful and coronary artery bypass graft surgery or removal of the annuloplasty ring and sutures would be necessary [43].

Long Term Results

The long term results of tricuspid ring annuloplasty are excellent when performed for tricuspid annular dilatation when the TR is not severe [21, 28]. Dreyfus, et al. report that TR progresses in only 2 % of these patients after ring annuloplasty and the mean TR grade at 5 years was 0.4 [11]. Similarly, Chikwe, et al., report freedom from moderate or more TR of 97 % at 7 years [28]. Kim et al. also reported freedom from moderate-to-severe TR at 5 years of 93 % [21].

However, when performed for severe FTR, about 10 % of patients leave hospital with moderate or more residual TR, and a 15–20 % recurrence rate of significant TR is reported [45]. Risk factors for residual TR and TR recurrence include a higher pre-operative TR grade, poor left ventricular function, permanent pacemaker and severe leaflet tethering [35, 36, 45–47]. Re-operations in these patients carry a very high risk with a hospital mortality of up to 18–35 % [30, 31]. It is now recommended that additional repair techniques in addition to ring annuloplasty are needed in patients with significant leaflet tethering to ensure long term durability [2]. This is described in the next chapter. However, it must be recognized that this is a higher risk group of patients; increased heart failure and mortality have been reported in patients with significant leaflet tethering or a dilated right ventricle mid cavity following tricuspid annuloplasty [42].

Results of tricuspid annuloplasty using a rigid ring appear better compared to annuloplasty using a flexible band or suture annuloplasty. Matsunaga and Duran reported a high recurrence rate of TR of 45 % with the use of flexible band or suture annuloplasty for greater than moderate functional TR [20]. Another study showed increased right atrial and right ventricular reverse remodeling, and decreased tricuspid annular diameter and tethering indices following rigid ring annuloplasty compared to flexible band annuloplasty [48]. In a systematic review, Khorsandi, et al., reported that of all relevant papers reviewed, 7 studies showed better results with rigid ring annuloplasty over De Vega's suture annuloplasty in terms of rate of recurrence leading to re-operation and long term mortality in patients with severe TR, 5 studies showed similar results between the two techniques, and 2 studies showed better results with De Vega's suture annuloplasty. The authors concluded that there was good evidence supporting ring annuloplasty over conventional De Vega's suture annuloplasty in severe TR [49]. Similarly, in an editorial, Alfieri and De Bonis summarized the results of six studies comparing the results of rigid ring annuloplasty and De Vega annuloplasty; TR recurrence was significantly greater with De Vega annuloplasty compared to rigid ring annuloplasty (6–30 % with rigid ring annuloplasty compared to 24–45 % for De Vega annuloplasty) [50].

References

1. Vassileva CM, Shabosky J, Boley T, Markwell S, Hazelrigg S. Tricuspid valve surgery: the past 10 years from the nationwide inpatient sample (nis) database. J Thorac Cardiovasc Surg. 2012;143:1043–9.
2. Dreyfus GD, Martin RP, Chan KMJ, Dulguerov F. Functional tricuspid regurgitation: a need to revise our understanding. J Am Coll Cardiol. 2015;65:2331–6.
3. Nishimura RA, Otto CM, Bonow RO, Carabello BA, Erwin JP, Guyton RA, O'Gara PT, Ruiz CE, Skubas NJ, Sorajja P, Sundt TM, Thomas JD. 2014 aha/acc guideline for the management of patients with valvular heart disease. J Am Coll Cardiol. 2014;63:e57–185.
4. Vahanian A, Alfieri O, Andreotti F, Antunes MJ, Baron-Esquivias G, Baumgartner H, Borger MA, Carrel TP, De Bonis M, Evangelista A, Falk V, Iung B, Lancellotti P, Pierard LA, Price S, Schafers H-J, Schuler G, Stepinska J, Swedberg K, Takkenberg J, Oppel UOV, Windecker S, Zamorano JL, Zembala M. ESC/EACTS guidelines on the management of valvular heart disease (version 2012). Eur Heart J. 2012;33:2451–96.
5. Colombo T, Russo C, Ciliberto GR, Lanfranconi M. Tricuspid regurgitation secondary to mitral valve disease: tricuspid annular function as guide to trcuspid valve repair. Cardiovasc Surg. 2001;9:369–77.
6. Ubago JL, Figueroa A, Ochoteco A, Colman T. Analysis of the amount of tricuspid valve annular dilatation required to produce functional tricuspid regurgitation. Am J Cardiol. 1983;52:155–8.
7. Kusajima K, Fujita T, Hata H, Shimahara Y, Miura S, Kobayashi J. Long term echocardiographic follow-up of untreated 2+ functional tricuspid regurgitation in patients undergoing mitral valve surgery. Inter Cardiovasc Thorac Surg. 2016;23(1):96–103.

8. Dreyfus J, Durand-Viel G, Raffoul R, Alkhoder S, Hvass U, Radu C, Al-Attar N, Ghodbhane W, Attias D, Nataf P, Vahanian A, Messika-Zeitoun D. Comparison of 2-dimensional, 3-dimensional, and surgical measurements of the tricuspid annular size: clinical implications. Circ Cardiovasc Imaging. 2015;8, e003241.
9. Filsoufi F, Chikwe J, Carpentier A. Rationale for remodelling annuloplasty to address functional tricuspid regurgitation during left-sided valve surgery. Eur J Cardiothorac Surg. 2015;47:1–3.
10. Goldstone AB, Howard JL, Cohen JE, MacArthur JW, Atluri P, Kirkpatrick JN, Woo YJ. Natural history of coexistent tricuspid regurgitation in patients with degenerative mitral valve disease: implications for future guidelines. J Thorac Cardiovasc Surg. 2014;148:2802–10.
11. Dreyfus GD, Corbi PJ, Chan KMJ, Bahrami TB. Secondary tricuspid regurgitation or dilatation: which should be the criteria for surgical repair? Ann Thorac Surg. 2005;79:127–32.
12. Yilmaz OG, Suri RMS, Dearani JA, Sundt TM, Daly RC, Burkhart HM, Enriquez-Sarano M, Schaff HV. Functional tricuspid regurgitation at the time of mitral valve repair for degenerative leaflet prolapse: the case for a selective approach. J Thorac Cardiovasc Surg. 2011;142:608–13.
13. Song H, Kim M-J, Chung CH, Choo SJ. Factors associated with development of late significant tricuspid regurgitation after successful left sided valve surgery. Heart. 2009;95:931–6.
14. Kwak J-J, Kim Y-J, Kim M-K, Kim H-K, Park JS, Kim HK, Kim K-B, Ahn H, Sohn D-W, Oh BH, Park Y-B. Development of tricuspid regurgitation late after left-sided valve surgery: a single center experience with long-term echocardiographic examinations. Am Heart J. 2008;155:732–7.
15. Benedetto U, Melina G, Angeloni E, Refice S, Roscitano A, Comito C, Sinatra R. Prophylactic tricuspid annuloplasty in patients with dilated tricuspid annulus undergoing mitral valve surgery. J Thorac Cardiovasc Surg. 2012;143:632–8.
16. Calafiore AM, Gallina S, Iaco AL, Contini M, Bivona A, Gagliardi M, Bosco P, Di Mauro M. Mitral valve surgery for functional mitral regurgitation: should moderate or more tricuspid regurgitation be treated? A propensity score analysis. Ann Thorac Surg. 2009;87:698–703.
17. De Bonis M, Lapenna E, Sorrentino F, La Canna G, Grimaldi A, Maisano F, Torracca L, Alfieri O. Evolution of tricuspid regurgitation after mitral valve repair for functional mitral regurgitation in dilated cardiomyopathy. Eur J Cardiothorac Surg. 2008;33:600–6.
18. Van de Veire NR, Braun J, Delgado V, Versteegh MIM, Dion RA, Klautz RJM, Bax JJ. Tricuspid annuloplasty prevents right ventricular dilatation and progression of tricuspid regurgitation in patients with tricuspid annular dilatation undergoing mitral valve repair. J Thorac Cardiovasc Surg. 2011;141:1431–9.
19. Navia JL, Brozzi NA, Klein AL, Ling LF, Kittayarak C, Nowicki ER, Batizy LH, Zhong J, Blackstone EH. Moderate tricuspid regurgitation with left sided degenerative heart valve disease: to repair or not to repair? Ann Thorac Surg. 2012;93:59–69.
20. Matsunaga A, Duran CMG. Progression of tricuspid regurgitation after repaired functional ischaemic mitral regurgitation. Circulation. 2005;112:I453–7.
21. Kim JB, Yoo DG, Kim GS, Song H, Jung S-H, Choo SJ, Chung CH, Lee JW. Mild-to-moderate functional tricuspid regurgitation in patients undergoing valve replacement for rheumatic mitral disease: the influence of tricuspid valve repair on clinical and echocardiographic outcomes. Heart. 2012;98:24–30.
22. Izumi C, Miyake M, Takahashi S, Matsutani H, Hashiwada S, Kuwano K, Hayashi H, Nakajima S, Nishiga M, Hanazawa K, Sakamoto J, Kondo H, Tamura T, Kaitani K, Yamanaka K, Nakagawa Y. Progression of isolated tricuspid regurgitation late after left-sided valve surgery. Circ J. 2011;75: 2902–7.
23. De Bonis M, Lapenna E, Pozzoli A, Nisi T, Giacomini A, Calabrese M, La Canna G, Pappalardo A, Miceli A, Glauber M, Barili F, Alfieri O. Mitral valve repair without repair of moderate tricuspid regurgitation. Ann Thorac Surg. 2015;100:2206–12.
24. Kara I, Koksal C, Erkin A, Sacli H, Demirtas M, Percin B, Diler MS, Kirali K. Outcomes of mild to moderate functional tricuspid regurgitation in patients undergoing mitral valve operations: a meta-analysis of 2,488 patients. Ann Thorac Surg. 2015;100: 2398–407.
25. Lee H, Sung K, Kim WS, Lee YT, Park S-J, Carriere KC, Park PW. Clinical and hemodynamic influences of prophylactic tricuspid annuloplasty in mechanical mitral valve replacement. J Thorac Cardiovasc Surg. 2016;151:788–95.
26. Zhu T-Y, Min X-P, Zhang H-B, Meng X. Preoperative risk factors for residual tricuspid regurgitation after isolated left sided valve surgery: a systematic review and meta-analysis. Cardiology. 2014;129:242–9.
27. Shiran A, Najjar R, Adawi S, Aronson D. Risk factors for progression of functional tricuspid regurgitation. Am J Cardiol. 2014;113:995–1000.
28. Chikwe J, Itagaki S, Anyanwu A, Adams DH. Impact of concomitant tricuspid annuloplasty on tricuspid regurgitation, right ventricular function, and pulmonary artery hypertension after repair of mitral valve prolapse. J Am Coll Cardiol. 2015;65:1931–8.
29. Di Mauro M, Bivona A, Iaco AL, Contini M, Gagliardi M, Varone E, Gallina S, Calafiore AM. Mitral valve surgery for functional mitral regurgitation: prognostic role of tricuspid regurgitation. Eur J Cardiothorac Surg. 2009;35:635–40.
30. Chen S-W, Tsai F-C, Tsai F-C, Chao Y K, Huang Y K, Chu J-J, Lin P-J. Surgical risk and outcome of repair versus replacement for late tricuspid regurgitation in redo operation. Ann Thorac Surg. 2012;93:770–5.
31. Bernal JM, Morales D, Revuelta C, Llorca J, Gutierrez-Morlote J, Revuelta JM. Reoperations after

tricuspid valve repair. J Thorac Cardiovasc Surg. 2005;130:498–503.

32. Teman NR, Huffman LC, Krajacic M, Pagani FD, Haft JW, Bolling SF. "Prophylactic" tricuspid valve repair for functional tricuspid regurgitation. Ann Thorac Surg. 2014;97:1520–5.
33. Mukherjee D, Nader S, Olano A, Garcia MJ, Griffin BP. Improvement in right ventricular systolic function after surgical correction of isolated tricuspid regurgitation. J Am Soc Echocardiogr. 2000;13:650–4.
34. Bertrand PB, Koppers G, Verbrugge FH, Mullens W, Vandervoort P, Dion RA, Verhaert D. Tricuspid annuloplasty concomitant with mitral valve surgery: effects on right ventricular remodelling. J Thorac Cardiovasc Surg. 2014;147:1256–64.
35. McCarthy PM, Bhudia SK, Rajeswaran J, Hoercher KJ. Tricuspid valve repair: durability and risk factors for failure. J Thorac Cardiovasc Surg. 2004;127: 674–85.
36. Tang GH, Tirone TE, Singh SK, Maganti MD. Tricuspid valve repair with an annuloplasty ring results in improved long-term outcomes. Circulation. 2006;114:I577.
37. Ghoreishi M, Brown JM, Stauffer CE, Young CA, Byron MJ, Griffith BP, Gammie JS. Undersized tricuspid annuloplasty rings optimally treat functional tricuspid regurgitation. Ann Thorac Surg. 2011;92:89–96.
38. Pfannmuller B, Doenst T, Eberhardt K, Seeburger J, Borger MA, Mohr FW. Increased risk of dehisence after tricuspid valve repair with rigid annuloplasty rings. J Thorac Cardiovasc Surg. 2012;143:1050–5.
39. Kilic A, Saha-Chaudhuri P, Rankin JS, Conte JV. Trends and outcomes of tricuspid valve surgery in north america: an analysis of more than 50,000 patients from the society of thoracic surgeons database. Ann Thorac Surg. 2013;96:1546–52.
40. LaPar DJ, Mulloy DP, Stone ML, Crosby IK, Lau CL, Kron IL, Ailawadi G. Concomitant tricuspid valve operations affect outcomes after mitral operations: a multi institutional, statewide analysis. Ann Thorac Surg. 2012;94:52–8.
41. Kim JB, Jung S-H, Choo SJ, Chung CH, Lee JW. Surgical outcomes of severe tricuspid regurgitation: predictors of adverse clinical outcomes. Heart. 2013;99:181–7.
42. Yiu K-H, Wong A, Pu L, Chiang M-F, Sit K-Y, Chan D, Lee H-Y, Lam Y-M, Chen Y, Siu C-W, Lau C-P, Au W-K, Tse H-F. Prognostic value of preoperative right ventricular geometry and tricuspid valve tethering area in patients undergoing tricuspid annuloplasty. Circulation. 2014;129:87–92.
43. Gonzalez-Santos JM, Arnaiz-Garcia ME, Sastre-Rincon JA, Bueno-Codoner ME, Dalmau-Sorli MJ, Arevalo-Abascal A, Lopez-Rodriguez J, Diego-Nieto A. Acute right coronary artery occlusion after tricuspid valve ring annuloplasty. Ann Thorac Surg. 2015; 99:2213–6.
44. Diez-Villanueva P, Gutierrez-Ibanes E, Cuerpo-Caballero GP, Sanz-Ruiz R, Abeytua M, Soriano J, Sarnago F, Elizaga J, Gonzalez-Pinto A, Fernandez-Aviles F. Direct injury to right coronary artery in patients undergoing tricuspid annuloplasty. Ann Thorac Surg. 2014;97:1300–5.
45. DeBonis M, Lapenna E, Taramasso M, Manca M, Calabrese MC, Buzzatti N, Rossodivita A, Pappalardo F, Dorigo E, Alfieri O. Mid-term results of tricuspid annuloplasty with a three-dimensional remodelling ring. J Cardiac Surg. 2012;27(3):288–94.
46. Fukuda S, Gillinov AM, McCarthy PM, Stewart WJ, Song JM, Kihara T, Daimon M, Shin MS, Thomas JD, Shiota T. Determinants of recurrent or residual functional tricuspid regurgitation after tricuspid annuloplasty. Circulation. 2006;114:I582.
47. Min S-Y, Song J-M, Kim J-H, Jang M-K, Kim Y-J, Song H, Kim D-H, Lee JW, Kang D-H, Song J-K. Geometric changes after tricuspid annuloplasty and predictors of residual tricuspid regurgitation: a real time three-dimensional echocardiography study. Eur Heart J. 2010;31:2871–80.
48. Gatti G, Dell'Angela L, Morosin M, Maschietto L, Pinamonti B, Benussi B, Forti G, Nicolosi GL, Sinagra G, Pappalardo A. Flexible band versus rigid ring annuloplasty for functional tricuspid regurgitation: two different patterns of right heart remodelling. Interact Cardiovasc Thorac Surg. 2016;23(1):79–89.
49. Khorsandi M, Banerjee A, Singh H, Srivastava AR. Is a tricuspid annuloplasty ring significantly better than a de vega's annuloplasty stitch when repairing severe tricuspid regurgitation? Interact Cardiovasc Thorac Surg. 2012;15(1):129–35.
50. Alfieri O, De Bonis M. Tricuspid valve surgery for severe tricuspid regurgitation. Heart. 2013;99: 149–50.
51. Carpentier A, Adams D, Filsoufi F. Carpentier's reconstructive valve surgery. 1st ed. Maryland Heights: Elsevier; 2010.

Suture Annuloplasty for Functional Tricuspid Regurgitation: Principles, Techniques and Results

22

Manuel J. Antunes

Abstract

The management of tricuspid regurgitation (TR) is a decision problem and is becoming increasingly controversial. The so-called functional TR, now more appropriately designated secondary TR, occurs in a significant proportion of patients, especially in association with acquired disease of the left heart valves of rheumatic origin. It is found more often in association with the mitral valve than with the aortic, and is rarer in degenerative disease. Although surgery is an obvious indication for severe TR, correction of less than severe but more than mild degrees of secondary TR is now recommended during surgery for left-sided heart valve disease. In our opinion, tricuspid valve replacement is only justified in cases of extensive destruction of the tricuspid valve, as in advanced infective endocarditis, or in patients with severe dysfunction of the right ventricle. In all other cases, tricuspid annuloplasty, with either suture or ring (or band), has been associated with excellent immediate and long term results. Suture annuloplasty is easy and quick to perform, efficient and inexpensive, and uses less foreign material. Although a degree of controversy remains, some comparative studies have shown similar outcomes of suture annuloplasty comparing to the use of rings or bands. Less favorable results may result from the fact that, although simpler, suture techniques may be more dependent on technical details. We have experienced excellent results in more than one thousand patients treated, for over 30 years, with our own modification of the De Vega annuloplasty.

Keywords

Tricuspid regurgitation • annuloplasty • suture annuloplasty • De Vega

M.J. Antunes
Cardiothoracic Surgery, Faculty of Medicine and University Hospital, Coimbra, Portugal
e-mail: antunes.cct.chuc@sapo.pt

K.M.J. Chan (ed.), *Functional Mitral and Tricuspid Regurgitation*,
DOI 10.1007/978-3-319-43510-7_22

Principles of Treatment

Management of tricuspid regurgitation (TR) is a decision problem and is becoming increasingly controversial. The so-called functional TR, now more appropriately designated secondary TR, occurs in 8–35 % of the patients, especially in association with acquired disease of the left heart valves of rheumatic origin. It is found more often in association with the mitral valve than with the aortic, and is rare in degenerative disease [1].

In his book "Perspectives on the Mitral Valve", published in 1987 [2], Professor John Barlow stated that "it is probable that this lesion (*tricuspid regurgitation*) is often partly or mainly organic", hence unable to regress after correction of the left-sided valve disease, thus hinting at the need for a "prophylactic annuloplasty".

In their much cited work published in 2005, Giles Dreyfus and co-workers analysed, intraoperatively, secondary tricuspid dilatation with or without regurgitation by measuring, in the cardioplegised heart, the largest diameter of the annulus between the two commissures bordering the anterior leaflet (Fig. 22.1). They came to a cut-off value of 70 mm, which would later be shown to correspond to 40 mm as measured by echocardiography in the diastole of a beating heart. The authors concluded that "secondary tricuspid dilatation is present in a significant number of patients with severe mitral regurgitation without tricuspid regurgitation. It is a progressive disease which does not resolve with correction of the primary lesion alone". Hence, "tricuspid anuloplasty at the time of mitral valve surgery in these patients results in improved functional capacity without any increase in perioperative morbidity or mortality" [3].

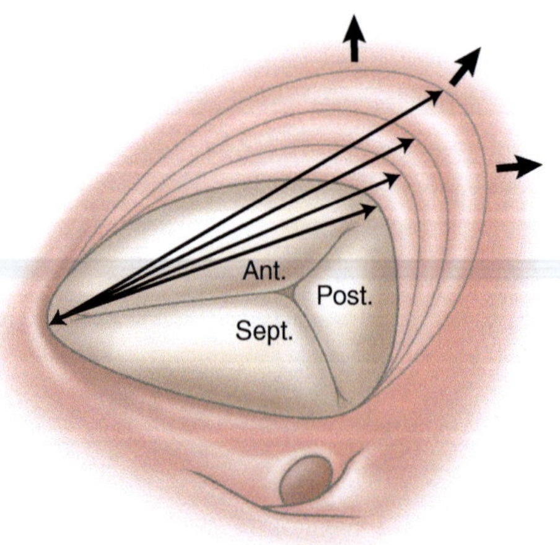

Fig. 22.1 Orientation and degree of the annular dilatation as assessed intraoperatively (Dreyfus et al. [3]. Permission granted by Elsevier)

Subsequently, the ESC/EACTS guidelines, published in 2012, recommended that "surgery of the tricuspid valve should be considered in patients with moderate primary TR undergoing left-sided valve surgery (IIa)" and that "surgery should be considered in patients with mild or moderate secondary TR with dilated annuli (≥40 mm or >21 mm/m^2 undergoing left-sided valve surgery (IIa)" [4]. On the other hand, the 2014 AHA/ACC guidelines suggest, as class IIa recommendation, that "tricuspid valve repair can be beneficial for patients with mild, moderate, or greater functional TR (stage B) at the time of left-sided valve surgery with either (1) tricuspid annular dilation or (2) prior evidence of right HF" [5].

Surgical Operative Techniques

In my opinion, only exceptionally will the TV need to be replaced as a first procedure, because the valve tolerates well a less-than-perfect repair (even in many cases of organic rheumatic disease, infective endocarditis, etc.). Hence, annuloplasty, when feasible, is the surgery of choice.

The first tricuspid annuloplasty was described in 1965 by Kay, as a modification of the mitral procedure he had described 2 years earlier. This pioneer used "three or four figure-of-eight sutures of 1-0 silk" to obliterate most, if not all, of the annulus of the anterior-inferior leaflet (currently denominated posterior leaflet) to "decrease the size of the annulus from an initial four or five finger breadths to two and one half finger breadths" [6], thus resulting in bicuspidization of the tricuspid valve (Fig. 22.2). The results then described were very encouraging and the procedure was quickly adopted by the surgical community.

In 1973, Alain Deloche and colleagues, from the Paris group, reported that 5/6 of the tricuspid

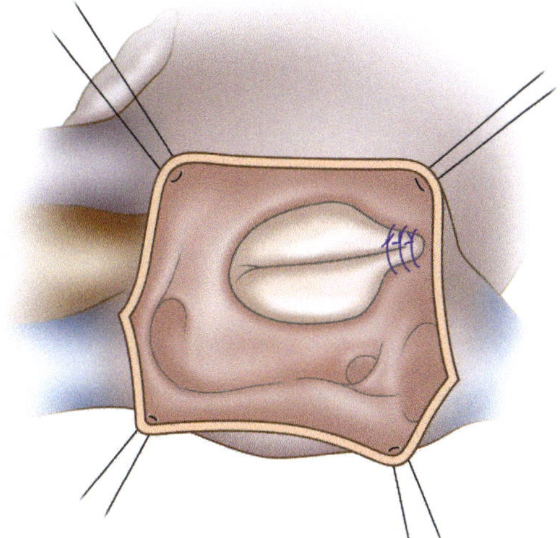

Fig. 22.2 The Kay procedure was the first tricuspid annuloplasty described. It consisted of 3 or 4 simple figure-of-eight sutures obliterating the posterior portion of the annulus, thus resulting in bicuspidization of the valve

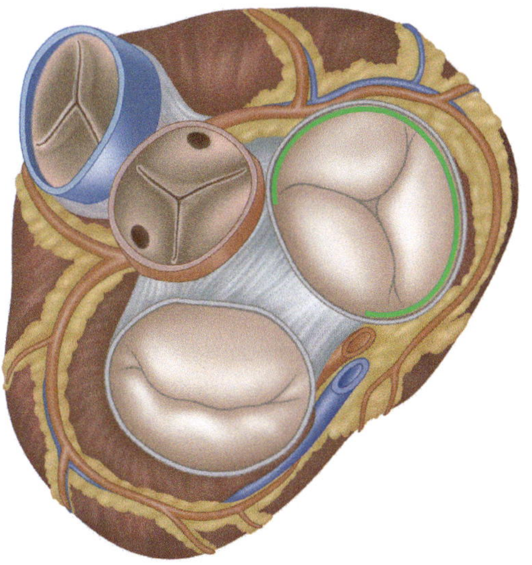

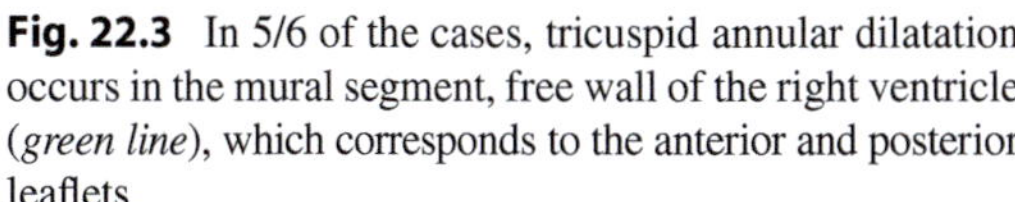

Fig. 22.3 In 5/6 of the cases, tricuspid annular dilatation occurs in the mural segment, free wall of the right ventricle (*green line*), which corresponds to the anterior and posterior leaflets

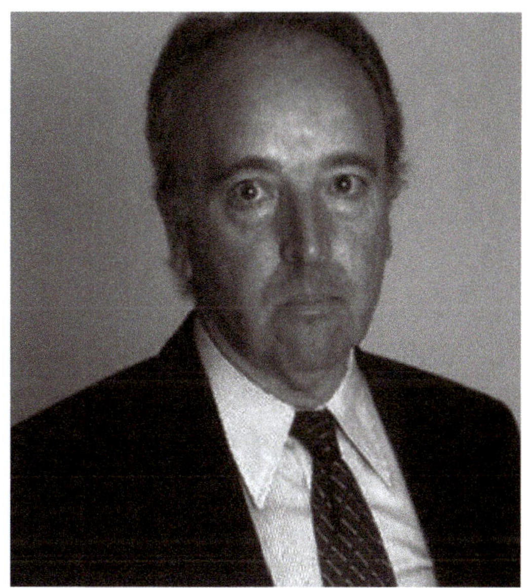

Fig. 22.4 Dr. Norberto De Vega

annular dilatation occurs in the mural segment, free wall of the right ventricle, which corresponds to the anterior and posterior leaflets (Fig. 22.3) [7]. Dr. Norberto de Vega, from Malaga, Spain, (Fig. 22.4) probably had the same intuition as, in 1972, he described that "the tricuspid regurgitation is usually caused by a selective expansion of the part of the tricuspid ring closely related to the free wall of the right ventricle (RV), area in which the anterior and posterior leaflets of the tricuspid apparatus are inserted" [8]. Hence, he devised the operation that carries his name and was then adopted by the majority of the surgeons. Classified as a selective, adjustable and permanent annuloplasty, it consists

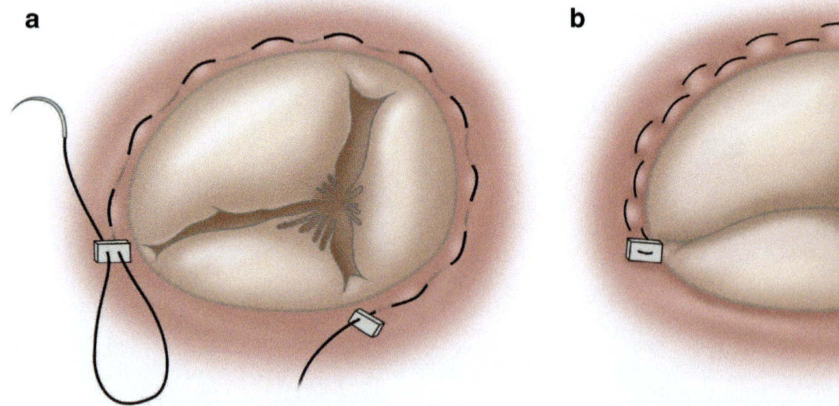

Fig. 22.5 De Vega suture annuloplasty. It consists of a double continuous suture extending from the antero-septal to the postero-septal commissures (Antunes and Barlow [1]). (**a**) A single row of suture (pledgeted at one end) is first placed along the annulus from the postero-septal commissure to the antero-septal commissure (where it is then passed through a pledget). (**b**) The same suture is then placed along the annulus again in the opposite direction forming a second row of sutures, and passing through the initial pledget, and tied after adjusting to the required length

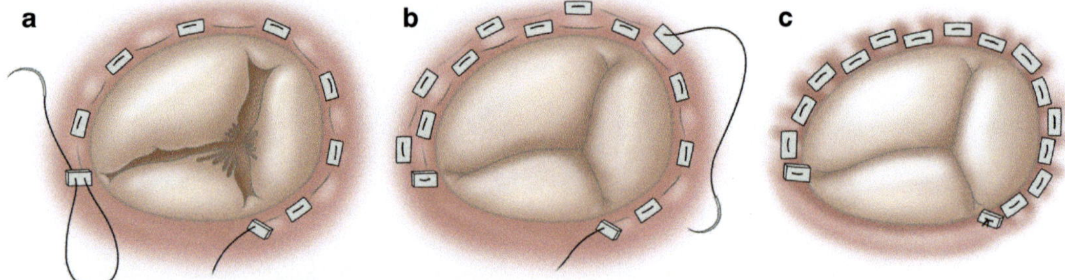

Fig. 22.6 Modified De Vega annuloplasty described by Antunes and Girdwood. It consists of the interposition of Teflon pledgets for each bite of the two-row suture (Antunes and Barlow [1]). (**a**) A single row of suture (pledgeted at one end) is first placed along the annulus from the postero-septal commissure to the antero-septal commissure; each bite of the suture through the annulus passes through a pledget. (**b**) The same suture is then placed along the annulus again in the opposite direction forming a second row of sutures; each bite through the annulus is again passed through a pledget. (**c**) The final result after tying the suture having determined the appropriate size

of a double continuous suture plication of the annulus, commenced anchored to the right fibrous trigone, at the level of the antero-septal commissure, and run along the annulus, ending at the level of the postero-septal commissure, both ends supported with Teflon pledgets (Fig. 22.5).

The procedure is simple and reproducible and only implies one important technical consideration, which consists of avoiding the right coronary artery which runs close to the anterior portion of the annulus. This requires somewhat superficial placement of the sutures and the procedure was often complicated by the 'guitar-string syndrome' which resulted of the suture tearing from the tissues.

To avoid this complication, in 1983 we described a simple modification of the De Vega technique which consists of the interposition of a small Teflon pledget in each bite in the annulus in both rows of the suture (Fig. 22.6) [9]. Since then, after more than one thousand procedures, we have not again seen a single case of that complication. A similar principle was used in 1989 by Revuelta et al. who used interrupted sutures supported by the Teflon pledgets along the annulus and termed it segmental tricuspid annuloplasty [10]. Another modification was described in 2007 by Sarraj and Duarte, who used a type of adjustable De Vega which consists of dividing it into two parts and using tourniquets to sequentially adjust the length

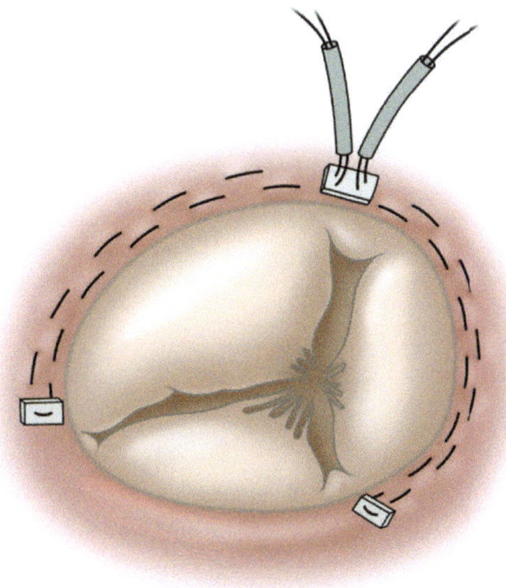

Fig. 22.7 Adjustable annuloplasty AS described by Saraj et al. (*Ann Thorac Surg*. 2007; 83: 698–9). This modification of the De Vega annuloplasty consists of two double-row sutures which can be tightened sequentially by tourniquets, thus selectively adjusting the size of the orifice (With permission from Elsevier)

of each part, hence the tightening of the orifice until competence is achieved (Fig. 22.7) [11].

Many other modifications were suggested but all were based on the concept idealised by De Vega and should all be named as modifications of the initial procedure. As initially described by De Vega, we use a monofilament propylene suture (size 3-0), but others use a 2-0 or 3-0 polyester suture [12].

Parallel to this evolution, Carpentier developed the ring concept in 1968, initially for treatment of the mitral valve regurgitation, followed by use in the tricuspid valve [13]. It consisted of a pre-shaped rigid flat ring which is almost complete but for the portion of the annulus where the bundle penetrates the ventricular septum. A possible downside of this concept is the fact that the ring fixes the annulus, thus preventing its natural dynamics during the cardiac cycle. Based on this, Duran and co-workers described the flexible ring in 1976 [14], which permits the dynamic alteration of the shape, but still prevents dilatation of the tricuspid orifice during diastole. Besides, the flexible ring becomes progressively stiff with time as a consequence of endothelial ingrowth, eventually even calcification. Many other types of rings and bands have been described and used clinically.

Results of Treatment

The techniques described are reproducible and easy to master, however requiring adherence to some important details, and can be performed rapidly, usually taking no longer than 10–15 additional minutes of operating time, hence with minor influence on morbidity or mortality. If necessary, the annuloplasty can be performed with the heart beating or fibrillating, after release of the aortic crossclamp. Apart from the suture material (and of pledgets), there is an absence of prosthetic material, which is an important consideration. And for those concerned about flexibility, it is fully preserved, although fibrosis around the sutures (and the pledgets) tends to transform it into a kind of band. Naturally, much cheaper than any commercially available devices, and this was a main consideration when Kay and De Vega devised their techniques. It may still be important today.

A few years ago, the group of Larry Cohn, from Boston, analysed 237 patients who underwent tricuspid annuloplasty for secondary tricuspid regurgitation as part of their cardiac surgical procedure, from 1999 to 2003. Bicuspidization was performed in 157 patients and ring annuloplasty in 80 patients. They found that both bicuspidization and ring annuloplasty were effective at eliminating tricuspid regurgitation at 3 years postoperatively. In fact, at that interval, both survival (75.3 % in the bicuspidization and 61.2 % in the ring annuloplasty group) and freedom from recurrence of moderate TR (75 % vs 69 %) tended to be better in bicuspidised patients than in those who received a ring. In the majority of the 44 patients (18.6 %) in whom moderate or greater recurrent TR developed, it happened within the first 6 months in both groups (Fig. 22.8). Hence, they concluded that "bicuspidization annuloplasty is a simple, inexpensive option for addressing functional tricuspid regurgitation" [15].

Shinn and colleagues, from the Mayo Clinic, analysed the outcomes of 479 patients (age 69.9 ± 11.1 years) who underwent tricuspid valve (TV) repair at the time of mitral valve (MV) surgery; (MV repair, n = 244). The etiologies were degenerative (n = 260, 54 %), rheumatic

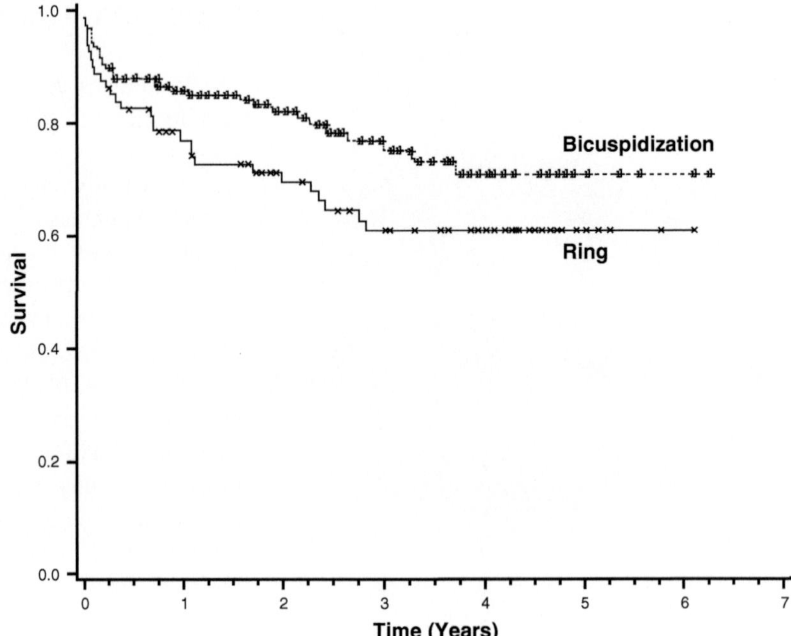

Fig. 22.8 Comparison of bicuspidization and ring annuloplasty for treatment of TR. There was a tendency for better survival in the bicuspidised patients (Ghanta et al. [15]. With permission from Elsevier)

(n = 150, 31 %), and ischemic (n = 69, 14 %). TV repair was performed using a flexible ring (n = 224, 47 %), rigid ring (n = 35, 7 %), Kay suture technique (n = 28, 6 %), or De Vega suture annuloplasty (n = 195, 41 %). They found that "freedom from TR ≥3+ was 98 % at dismissal, 83 % at 4 years, and 61 % at 8 years; which was similar between ring and suture methods, regardless of MV disease pathology" [16]. The single independent risk factor for late TR was preoperative TR ≥ 3+ (HR 2.21, p = 0.021) and TV reoperation was performed in only 5 patients, equally distributed among techniques.

Huang and co-workers studied the midterm clinical and echocardiographic results of a modified De Vega annuloplasty for repair of functional TR in 237 patients, with a mean follow-up time of 6.5 ± 3.2 years [17]. They found the De Vega suture annuloplasty to be effective at eliminating TR and producing right ventricular reverse remodeling at 5-year follow-up, although TR tended to increase with time.

In another study, the same group analysed a population of 448 patients in whom a modified De Vega annuloplasty (216 patients) or a ring annuloplasty (232 patients) were performed. They concluded that "the modified De Vega tricuspid annuloplasty is acceptable for repair of functional TR with improvements in clinical and echocardiographic status on a long-term basis, although the long-term recurrence-free survival appeared to be lower than that for ring annuloplasty" [18].

By contrast with these studies, Tang and co-workers, from the Toronto group, found that long-term survival, event-free survival and freedom from recurrent TR were significantly better in the ring group, and there was a trend toward fewer TV reoperations. Multivariable analysis demonstrated that the use of an annuloplasty ring was an independent predictor of long-term survival and event-free survival [19].

Therefore, there appear to be some discrepancies between the results of different reports. Trying to resolve this equation, Khorsandi and co-workers performed a meta-analysis on studies comparing suture and ring annuloplasty and found seven studies supporting the use of ring annuloplasty over De Vega's suture annuloplasty, while five studies found no significant difference in outcome between the two techniques. Conversely, two studies supported the

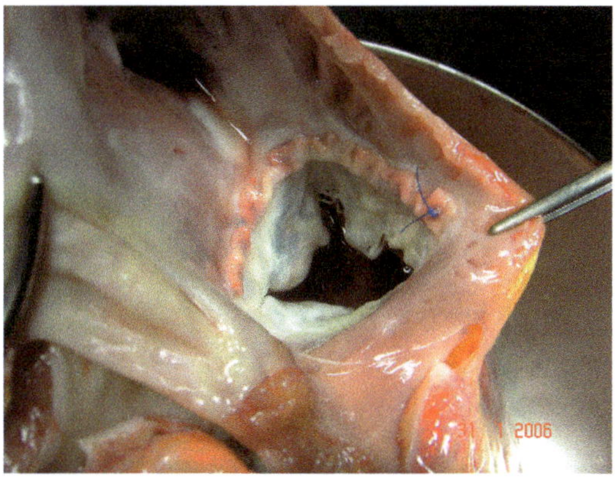

Fig. 22.9 Photograph of a heart retrieved during heart transplantation. Note that the modified de Vega annuloplasty, previously performed, did not extend to the posterior portion of the septal annulus (compare to Fig. 22.6)

use of De Vega's suture annuloplasty over ring annuloplasty [20].

There is, in my view, a plausible justification for these differences. While the technique of implantation of a prosthetic ring is very standardized, the performance of an annuloplasty is not, depending on small technical details and experience. For example, and contrary to what may be understood from most technical drawings, and from the initial description by De Vega, we have learnt a long time ago that the annuloplasty must be extended to the infero-posterior half of the septal portion of the tricuspid annulus, exactly in the same extent as the ring does (Fig. 22.9). A similar conclusion had been reached by Calafiore and colleagues [12].

In addition, the degree of narrowing of the tricuspid orifice is of extreme importance, and should be neither insufficient nor excessive. Kay and De Vega described the final size as equivalent to two and a half and two finger breaths, respectively. More recently, we have been tying the suture over a size 24 mm Hegar dilator or valve sizer. In fact, Hwang and co-workers, from Seoul, described the concept of tricuspid valve orifice index to optimize tricuspid valve annular reduction with the De Vega annuloplasty. These authors found that, after experience, "the De Vega annuloplasty for functional TR results in low rates of recurrence in the long-term. The tricuspid annulus should be reduced appropriately considering patients' body size (indexed tricuspid valve orifice diameter <22.5 mm/m^2) to prevent recurrent functional TR" [21].

In my view, the implantation of a ring is specifically indicated when there is organic involvement of the TV, usually with stenosis, where commissurotomy is also necessary, and in the case of significant dysfunction of the RV. However, in recent times, and following important studies on secondary mitral regurgitation, the importance of ventricular function has come into the equation, in the right as in the left ventricle. Kammerlander et al. recently concluded that "RV dysfunction, but not significant TR, is independently associated with survival late after left heart valve procedure" [22]. In the presence of significant right, as in left, ventricular dysfunction, the remodelling of the cavity results in malalignment of the subvalvular apparatus, with tethering, which, in turn, prevents correct apposition of the leaflets and causes regurgitation [23, 24]. But this occurs both in suture and ring annuloplasty, as they do not address the ventricular component of the disease [25], and may even be an indication for valve replacement.

However, even after adequate correction of the TR, reversal of the ventricular remodelling may not be complete or may not occur et al., especially if pulmonary hypertension does not regress adequately [26, 27]. Therefore, in my opinion, these patients should be maintained (for life) on anti-failure therapy (vasodilators and diuretics).

Conclusion

Correction of more than mild degrees of secondary TR is now recommended during surgery for left-sided heart valve disease. Tricuspid valve replacement is only justified in cases of extensive destruction of the tricuspid valve, as in advanced infective endocarditis, or in patients with severe dysfunction of the right ventricle. In all other cases, tricuspid annuloplasty, with either suture or ring (or band), has been associated with excellent immediate and longterm results. Suture annuloplasty is easy and quick to perform, efficient and inexpensive, and uses less foreign material. Results have generally been comparable with different types of annuloplasty.

Conflict of Interest None

References

1. Antunes MJ, Barlow JB. Management of tricuspid valve regurgitation. Heart. 2007;93:271–6.
2. Barlow JB. Perspectives on the mitral valve. Philadelphia: FA Davis Co; 1987. p. 338–59.
3. Dreyfus GD, Corbi PJ, Chan KM, Bahrami T. Secondary tricuspid regurgitation or dilatation: which should be the criteria for surgical repair? Ann Thorac Surg. 2005;79(1):127–32.
4. Vahanian A, Alfieri O, Andreotti F, Antunes MJ, Barón-Esquivias G, Baumgartner H, Borger MA, Carrel TP, De Bonis M, Evangelista A, Falk V, Lung B, Lancellotti P, Pierard L, Price S, Schäfers HJ, Schuler G, Stepinska J, Swedberg K, Takkenberg J, Von Oppell UO, Windecker S, Zamorano JL, Zembala M. Guidelines on the management of valvular heart disease (version 2012): the Joint Task Force on the Management of Valvular Heart Disease of the European Society of Cardiology (ESC) and the European Association for Cardio-Thoracic Surgery (EACTS). Eur J Cardiothorac Surg. 2012;42(4):S1–44.
5. Nishimura RA, Otto CM, Bonow RO, Carabello BA, Erwin JP 3rd, Guyton RA, O'Gara PT, Ruiz CE, Skubas NJ, Sorajja P, Sundt TM 3rd, Thomas JD, Anderson JL, Halperin JL, Albert NM, Bozkurt B, Brindis RG, Creager MA, Curtis LH, DeMets D, Guyton RA, Hochman JS, Kovacs RJ, Ohman EM, Pressler SJ, Sellke FW, Shen WK, Stevenson WG, Yancy CW; American College of Cardiology; American College of Cardiology/American Heart Association; American Heart Association.2014 AHA/ACC guideline for the management of patients with valvularheart disease: a report of the American College of Cardiology/American Heart Association Task Force on Practice Guidelines. J Thorac Cardiovasc Surg. 2014;148(1):e1–132.
6. Kay JH, Maselli-Campagna G, Tsuji HK. Surgical treatment of tricuspid insufficiency. Ann Surg. 1965;162(1):53–8.
7. Deloche A, Guerinon J, Fabiani JN, Morillo F, Caramanian M, Carpentier A, Maurice P, Dubost C. Anatomical study of rheumatic tricuspid valve diseases: application to the study of various valvuloplasties. Ann Chir Thorac Cardiovasc. 1973;12(4):343–9.
8. De Vega NG. La anuloplastia selectiva, regulable y permanente. Rev Esp Cardiol. 1972;25:555–6.
9. Antunes MJ, Girdwood RW. Tricuspid annuloplasty: a modified technique. Ann Thorac Surg. 1983;35:676–8.
10. Revuelta JM, Garcia-Rinaldi R. Segmental tricuspid annuloplasty: a new technique. J Thorac Cardiovasc Surg. 1989;97(5):799–801.
11. Sarraj A, Duarte J. Adjustable segmental tricuspid annuloplasty: a new modified technique. Ann Thorac Surg. 2007;83:698–9.
12. Calafiore AM, Di Mauro M. Tricuspid valve repair – indications and techniques: suture annuloplasty and band annuloplasty. Oper Tech Thorac Cardiovasc Surg. 2011;16:86–96.
13. Carpentier A. Reconstructive valvuloplasty. A new technique of mitral valvuloplasty. Presse Med. 1969; 77(7):251–3.
14. Duran CG, Ubago JL. Clinical and hemodynamic performance of a totally flexible prosthetic ring for atrioventricular valve reconstruction. Ann Thorac Surg. 1976;22(5):458–63.
15. Ghanta RK, Chen R, Narayanasamy N, McGurk S, Lipsitz S, Chen FY, Cohn LH. Suture bicuspidization of the tricuspid valve versus ring annuloplasty for repair of functional tricuspid regurgitation: midterm results of 237 consecutive patients. J Thorac Cardiovasc Surg. 2007;133(1):117–26.
16. Shinn SH, Schaff S, Park S; Dearani J, Joyce L, Greason K, Burkhart H, Stulak J, Daly D, Suri R. Outcomes of ring versus suture annuloplasty for tricuspid valve repair in patients undergoing mitral valve surgery: is there a difference? J Am Coll Cardiol. 2013;61(10_S). doi:10.1016/S0735-1097(13)62000-8.
17. Huang X, Gu C, Li B, Li J, Yang J, Wei H, Yu Y. Midterm clinical and echocardiographic results of a modified De Vega tricuspid annuloplasty for repair of functional tricuspid regurgitation. Can J Cardiol. 2013;29(12):1637–42.
18. Huang X, Gu C, Men X, Zhang J, You B, Zhang H, Wei H, Li J. Repair of functional tricuspid regurgitation: comparison between suture annuloplasty and rings annuloplasty. Ann Thorac Surg. 2014;97(4): 1286–92.
19. Tang GH, David TE, Singh SK, Maganti MD, Armstrong S, Borger MA. Tricuspid valve repair with an annuloplasty ring results in improved long-term outcomes. Circulation. 2006;114(1 Suppl): I577–81.
20. Khorsandi M, Banerjee A, Singh H, Srivastava AR. Is a tricuspid annuloplasty ring significantly better than a De Vega's annuloplasty stitch when repairing severe tricuspid regurgitation? Interact Cardiovasc Thorac Surg. 2012;15(1):129–35.
21. Hwang HY, Chang HW, Jeong DS, Ahn H. De Vega annuloplasty for functional tricupsid regurgitation: concept of tricuspid valve orifice index to optimize tricuspid valve annular reduction. J Korean Med Sci. 2013;28(12):1756–61.
22. Kammerlander AA, Marzluf BA, Graf A, Bachmann A, Kocher A, Bonderman D, Mascherbauer J. Right ventricular dysfunction, but not tricuspid regurgitation, is associated with outcome late after left heart valve procedure. J Am Coll Cardiol. 2014;64(24): 2633–42.

23. Dreyfus GD, Raja SG, John Chan KM. Tricuspid leaflet augmentation to address severe tethering in functional tricuspid regurgitation. Eur J Cardiothorac Surg. 2008;34:908–10.
24. Kim JH, Kim HK, Lee SP, Kim YJ, Cho GY, Kim KH, Kim KB, Ahn H, Sohn DW. Right ventricular reverse remodeling, but not subjective clinical amelioration, predicts long-term outcome after surgery for isolated severe tricuspid regurgitation. Circ J. 2014;78(2):385–92.
25. Bertrand PB, Koppers G, Verbrugge FH, Mullens W, Vandervoort P, Dion R, Verhaert D. Tricuspid annuloplasty concomitant with mitral valve surgery: effects on right ventricular remodeling. J Thorac Cardiovasc Surg. 2014;147(4):1256–64.
26. Dreyfus GD, Martin RP, Chan KM, Dulguerov F, Alexandrescu C. Functional tricuspid regurgitation: a need to revise our understanding. J Am Coll Cardiol. 2015;65(21):2331–6.
27. Navia JL, Novicki ER, Blackstone E, Brozzi NA, Nento DE, Atik FA, Rajeswaran J, Gillinov AM, Svensson LG, Lytle BW. Surgical management of secondary tricuspid valve regurgitation: annulus, commissure, or leaflet procedure? J Thorac Cardiovasc Surg. 2010;139:1473–82.

Addressing Severe Leaflet Tethering in Functional Tricuspid Regurgitation

23

K.M. John Chan

Abstract

Leaflet tethering occurs in functional tricuspid regurgitation due to remodeling of the right ventricle. It is distinct from tricuspid annular dilatation although the two pathologies may coexist. When present, it needs to be addressed during tricuspid valve repair to achieve long term durability of the repair. It is one of the risk factors for recurrent tricuspid regurgitation following tricuspid annuloplasty. Tricuspid valve replacement is a reasonable option in severe tricuspid regurgitation with severe leaflet tethering if valve repair is not possible.

Keywords

Tricuspid regurgitation • Tricuspid leaflet tethering • Tricuspid leaflet augmentation • Tricuspid valve replacement • Tricuspid valve

Leaflet tethering in functional tricuspid regurgitation (FTR) occurs in the more advanced stages of the disease due to remodeling and dilatation of the right ventricle with papillary muscle displacement [1–4]. It can occur in the absence of significant tricuspid annular dilatation and is reported to be more common in FTR associated with pulmonary hypertension, linked to right ventricular elongation and elliptical/spherical deformation [5]. This results in the tricuspid valve leaflets coapting or attempting to coapt below the plane of the tricuspid annulus [6]. Leaflet tethering is considered significant when the tethering height, i.e., the distance between the plane of the annulus and the leaflet coaptation point or theoretical leaflet coaptation point, is 8 mm or more at mid-systole in an apical four chamber echocardiographic view (Fig. 23.1) [2]. Leaflet coaptation, if present, is typically only occurring between the edges of the leaflets rather than between the body of the leaflets as is normal [6]. More often, the leaflets fail to coapt at all in these cases.

The tricuspid regurgitation (TR) is always severe in these cases and intervention on the tricuspid valve at the time of left sided heart valve surgery is usually indicated. However, adequate

K.M.J. Chan, BM BS, MSc, PhD, FRCS CTh
Department of Cardiothoracic Surgery,
Gleneagles Hospital, Jalan Ampang,
Kuala Lumpur 50450, Malaysia
e-mail: KMJohnChan@yahoo.com

K.M.J. Chan (ed.), *Functional Mitral and Tricuspid Regurgitation*,
DOI 10.1007/978-3-319-43510-7_23

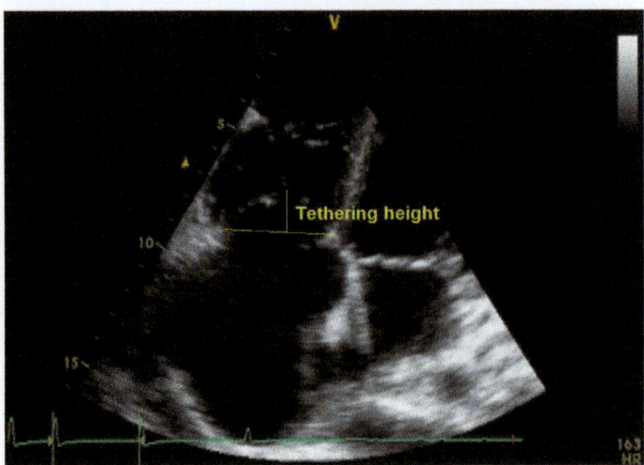

Fig. 23.1 Echocardiographic apical four chamber view demonstrating measurement of the tethering height at mid-systole. This is the distance between the plane of the tricuspid annulus and the coaptation point or theoretical coaptation point of the leaflets at mid systole

assessment of right ventricular function is advised prior to surgery to ensure that there is enough right ventricular function and reserve to cope with a competent repaired tricuspid valve. This is discussed in greater detail in a separate chapter.

Severe leaflet tethering, when present, cannot be addressed by tricuspid annuloplasty alone, which only addresses the tricuspid annular dilatation, as the recurrence rate of TR in such cases of 15–30% is significant [7–13]. In some cases of severe leaflet tethering, the annulus is not dilated, and doing an annuloplasty would not address the problem (Fig. 23.2). Leaflet tethering has been shown to be a predictor of residual TR at the time of hospital discharge following tricuspid annuloplasty, and of recurrent TR following tricuspid annuloplasty [11, 13, 14]. Re-operations in these patients carry a very high hospital mortality and these patients also have a reduced survival [10].

The leaflet tethering has to be adequately addressed surgically to ensure long term durability of the tricuspid valve repair. The most common technique used to address significant tricuspid leaflet tethering is to augment the tricuspid valve leaflet [15, 16]. Other techniques which have been described include the clover technique, whereby the central part of the free edges of the leaflets are sutured together [17]. Tricuspid valve replacement is an option if significant TR persists despite the use of these repair techniques.

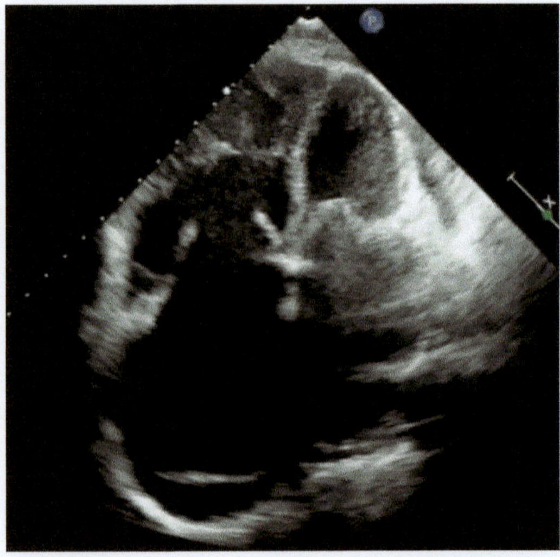

Fig. 23.2 Example of a patient with severe leaflet tethering but without annular dilatation. The tricuspid annular diameter was 38 mm

Tricuspid Leaflet Augmentation

Augmentation of the tricuspid valve leaflet was first described by Dreyfus, et al. in 2008 [15]. The principle of the operation is to increase the surface area of coaptation of the leaflets by increasing the size of the anterior leaflet using autologous pericardium. The autologous pericardial patch becomes the new body of the leaflet, and the whole of the native leaflet is the new coaptation surface which is brought towards the other leaflets allowing a generous surface area of coaptation and restoring valve competency (Fig. 23.3). The level of leaflet coaptation may still be occurring below the annulus but a generous surface of coaptation is present ensuring durability of the repair. The anterior leaflet is normally augmented as this is the leaflet most easily enlarged, and it is also usually the most significantly tethered, together with the posterior leaflet, due to their attachments to the anterior papillary muscle and hence to the free wall of the right ventricle [15]. The posterior leaflet can also be augmented if needed in addition to the anterior leaflet [16]. The septal leaflet is often small and redundant and not easily augmented although it is also possible to do so in selected cases with persistent TR after augmentation of the

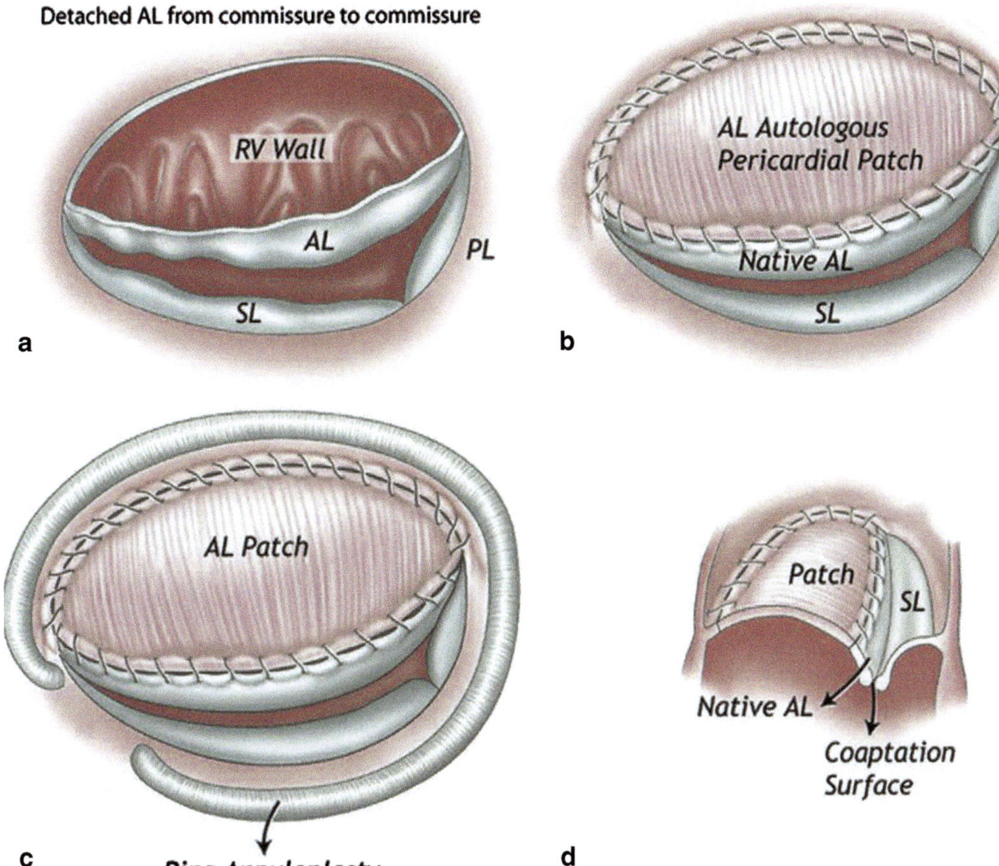

Fig. 23.3 Operative technique for anterior leaflet augmentation (From Dreyfus et al. [15]). (**a**) The anterior leaflet is detached from the annulus from commissure to commissure. (**b**) An autologous pericardial patch is sutured to the defect created. (**c**) An annuloplasty ring is implanted. (**d**) The autologous pericardial patch forms the new body of the leaflet, the native anterior leaflet forms the coaptation surface

anterior and posterior leaflets. Tricuspid leaflet augmentation has also been used with good results in severe TR secondary to rheumatic valve disease, in these cases, to address the loss of leaflet surface area due to the severely fibrotic and retracted leaflets [18].

Operative Technique

A patch of autologous pericardium is harvested, cleared of fatty tissue and treated in glutaraldehyde for 10 min and then washed in normal saline for a further 10 min. Treatment of the autologous pericardium in glutaraldehyde prevents calcification and retraction of the tissue in later years. The tricuspid valve is detached from its annular attachment along its entire length from the anteroseptal commissure to the anteroposterior commissure (Figs. 23.3 and 23.4). The secondary chordae are inspected and any chords significantly restricting the leaflet are divided. The previously harvested piece of autologous pericardium is cut into an oval shape to fit the size of the defect created. A generous patch is used with the diameter slightly greater than the distance between the anteroseptal and anteroposterior commissures and the height slightly greater than the distance between the annulus and the detached anterior leaflet. Care should be taken during the shaping and suturing of the patch to avoid distorting the normal geometry of the anterior leaflet, particularly its coaptation

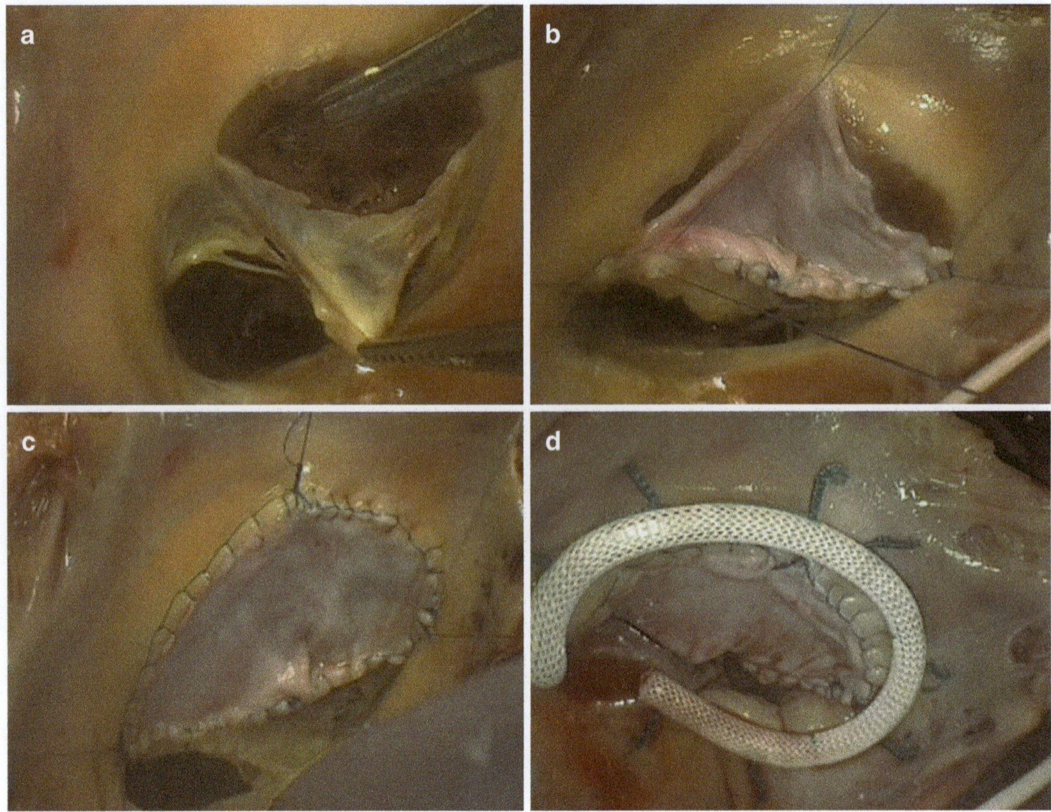

Fig. 23.4 Operative photographs for anterior leaflet augmentation (From Dreyfus et al. [15]). (**a**) The anterior leaflet is detached from the annulus from commissure to commissure. (**b**) The autologous pericardium is sutured to the detached anterior leaflet. (**c**) The autologous pericardial patch is then sutured to the annulus. (**d**) An annuloplasty ring is implanted

line. 5/0 Cardionyl suture (Peters Surgical, Bobigny, Cedex, France) or equivalent is used to suture the patch to the annulus on one side and the detached anterior leaflet on the other side. The suture is interlocked after each throw to ensure flat suturing and avoid the purse stringing effect. A tricuspid annuloplasty ring is then implanted sized by measurement of the autologous pericardial patch. A ring which is slightly smaller than the patch is selected (Fig. 23.2).

Augmentation of both anterior and posterior leaflets has also been described. In these cases, the anterior half of the posterior leaflet is also detached in addition to the anterior leaflet and a pericardial patch is used to close the defect [16]. The authors of this technique propose an alternative way to size the pericardial patch based on the size of the annuloplasty ring implanted, typically using a pericardial patch of 13–14 mm in height and 45–46 mm in length for a 28 mm or 30 mm rigid MC3 annuloplasty ring (Edwards Lifesciences, Irvine, CA, USA). In another variation of the technique, the entire anterior and posterior leaflets are detached from the annulus, from the anteroseptal commissure to the anteroposterior commissure. A patch the size of a 32 mm Carpentier Edwards ring is sutured in to fill the gap. At the anteroposterior commissure, the anterior and posterior leaflets are re-attached to the patch next to each other to reconstitute the commissure. The annuloplasty ring is then reimplanted [19].

Results

All the studies have reported good early results with tricuspid leaflet augmentation, with correction of the TR in all cases, reduction of leaflet tethering indices, and right ventricular reverse remodeling [15, 16, 19]. However, longer term follow up is necessary to determine the long term durability of the repair.

Clover (Edge-to-Edge) Technique

The clover technique of tricuspid valve repair was first described in 2004 and was used in patients with complex tricuspid valve lesions including leaflet prolapse from blunt trauma or myxomatous degeneration, and severe leaflet tethering due to ischemic dilated cardiomyopathy [17]. In this technique, the middle of the free edges of the tricuspid leaflets are sutured together using 5/0 polypropylene producing a clover shaped valve. An annuloplasty ring is then implanted to correct annular dilatation and stabilize the repair. At a mean follow-up of 12 months, TR was absent in five patients (38 %), mild in seven patients (53 %), and moderate in one patient (7 %), with no significant gradient across the tricuspid valve both at rest and exercise [17]. It should be noted that only one of the patients in this study had FTR with severely tethered leaflets; the lesion in all the other patients was leaflet prolapse secondary to blunt trauma or myxomatous degeneration. A potential limitation with the use of this technique in severely tethered leaflets is that although valve competency may be restored, this is achieved with increased leaflet tension which may limit the durability of the repair.

Tricuspid Valve Replacement

Replacement of the tricuspid valve is another option in severe FTR with severely tethered leaflets. It may be necessary if repair techniques with leaflet augmentation have failed to correct the TR and in cases of recurrent TR.

Choice of Prosthesis

Studies comparing mechanical and biological tricuspid valves have shown similar operative mortality, freedom from re-operation and survival between the two types of prosthesis [20–24]. Although patients receiving a mechanical tricuspid valve have a higher incidence of valve thrombosis, embolism and bleeding, patients receiving a bioprosthetic tricuspid valve have a higher incidence of structural valve deterioration, so that the valve-related event free survival and overall survival rates were not significantly different between the two groups [23, 24]. However, most studies do not extend beyond 10 years and the increased structural valve deterioration with bioprosthetic valves with time may outweigh the thrombosis, embolism and bleeding risk with mechanical valves over a longer time period particularly in younger patients. One meta-analysis comparing mechanical and biological prosthesis at a median follow-up of 7.3 years showed that the survival and freedom from re-operation was similar for both types of valves [21]. The thrombosis rate of mechanical valves in the tricuspid position was 0.87 % patient per year while the structural valve deterioration in biological valves in the tricuspid position was 1.02 % patient per year mainly due to pannus formation ($p=0.25$) [21]. The traditional belief that mechanical tricuspid valve prosthesis have a high incidence of valve thrombosis, and that biological tricuspid valve prosthesis have a very low incidence of structural valve deterioration therefore appears untrue. Interestingly, in this meta-analysis, 97 % of patients with a bioprosthetic tricuspid valve were receiving anticoagulation. Some authors recommend lifelong anticoagulation even for bioprosthetic tricuspid valves due to the possibility that thrombosis may be the mechanism involved in pannus formation [25, 26].

The choice of valve prosthesis should therefore be tailored according to the patient's characteristics and needs. Biological valves may be preferred over mechanical valves in older patients or in those in whom a limited life expectancy is expected due to the extent and severity of the cardiac disease, and in those unable to take lifelong anticoagulation. However, in younger patients and in those receiving a left sided mechanical valve prosthesis in whom a good life expectancy is predicted, a mechanical tricuspid valve replacement is reasonable. Mechanical valves may also be a better option in those with small annulus due to its better hemodynamics [27]. Nonetheless, in the United States, there has been an increased use of bioprosthesis in recent years from 34.9 % in 1999 to 53.8 % in 2008 [22].

Operative Technique

Typically, interrupted everting horizontal mattress pledgeted sutures are placed around the tricuspid annulus incorporating all of the tricuspid leaflets and therefore preserving all of the subvalvular apparatus. These are then passed around the prosthetic tricuspid valve before being lowered to the tricuspid annulus and tied down. Around the region of the conduction tissues at the septal annulus, it is best to pass the sutures through the septal leaflet adjacent to its attachment to the annulus, rather than through the annulus to avoid conduction problems.

Results

The operative mortality of tricuspid valve replacement ranges from 6.7 to 26 %, with lower mortality reported in more recent studies [22, 23, 27–32]. This may be related to improvements in myocardial protection, cardiopulmonary bypass, operative techniques with preservation of the subvalvular apparatus, post-operative care and better patient selection. Operative mortality and late survival is dependent on the patient's condition pre-operatively, particularly on the presence of heart failure, liver and kidney dysfunction. Patients with pre-operative icterus, hepatomegaly, raised pulmonary artery pressures, advanced heart failure, renal failure, cerebrovascular disease, chronic lung disease, or who are in NYHA class III or IV have increased mortality [28, 30, 32, 33]. In one study, the presence of liver disease increased operative mortality from 13.1 to 27 % [22]. One propensity matched study reported similar operative and long term mortality in patients undergoing tricuspid valve replacement and in those undergoing tricuspid valve repair surgery [34]. The risk of requiring a permanent pacemaker is between 2.5 and 17.2 % [22, 23, 27, 33]. The long term survival is dependent on the baseline risk profile of the patient; the reported Kaplan-Meier survival in various studies is 65–86 % at 5 years, 37–80 % at 9–10 years and 25–30 % at 14–15 years [28–30].

References

1. Park YH, Song JM, Lee EY, Kim YJ, Kang DH, Song JK. Geometric and haemodynamic determinant of functional tricuspid regurgitation: a real time three dimensional echocardiographic study. Int J Cardiol. 2008;124:160–5.
2. Kim HK, Kim YJ, Park JS, Kim KH, Kim KB, Ahn H, Sohn DW, Oh BH, Park YB, Choi YS. Determinants of the severity of functional tricuspid regurgitation. Am J Cardiol. 2006;98:236–42.
3. Spinner EM, Shannon P, Buice D, Jimenez JH, Veledar E, del Nido PJ, Adams DH, Yoganathan AP. In vitro characterization of the mechanisms responsible for functional tricuspid regurgitation. Circulation. 2011;124:920–9.
4. Spinner EM, Lerakis S, Higginson J, Pernetz M, Howell S, Veledar E, Yoganathan AP. Correlates of tricuspid regurgitation as determined by 3D echocardiography: pulmonary arterial pressure, ventricle geometry, annular dilatation, and papillary muscle displacement. Circ Cardiovasc Imaging. 2012;5:43–50.
5. Topilsky Y, Khanna A, Le Tourneau T, Park S, Michelena H, Suri R, Mahoney DW, Enriquez-Sarano M. Clinical context and mechanism of functional tricuspid regurgitation in patients with and without pulmonary hypertension. Circ Cardiovasc Imaging. 2012;5:314–23.
6. Dreyfus GD, Martin RP, Chan KMJ, Dulguerov F. Functional tricuspid regurgitation: a need to revise our understanding. J Am Coll Cardiol. 2015;65:2331–6.
7. Fukuda S, Gillinov AM, McCarthy PM, Stewart WJ, Song JM, Kihara T, Daimon M, Shin MS, Thomas JD, Shiota T. Determinants of recurrent or residual functional tricuspid regurgitation after tricuspid annuloplasty. Circulation. 2006;114:I582.
8. McCarthy PM, Bhudia SK, Rajeswaran J, Hoercher KJ. Tricuspid valve repair: durability and risk factors for failure. J Thorac Cardiovasc Surg. 2004;127:674–85.
9. Kwak J-J, Kim Y-J, Kim M-K, Kim H-K, Park JS, Kim HK, Kim K-B, Ahn H, Sohn D-W, Oh BH, Park Y-B. Development of tricuspid regurgitation late after left-sided valve surgery: a single center experience with long-term echocardiographic examinations. Am Heart J. 2008;155:732–7.
10. Bernal JM, Morales D, Revuelta C, Llorca J, Gutierrez-Morlote J, Revuelta JM. Reoperations after tricuspid valve repair. J Thorac Cardiovasc Surg. 2005;130:498–503.
11. Min S-Y, Song J-M, Kim J-H, Jang M-K, Kim Y-J, Song H, Kim D-H, Lee JW, Kang D-H, Song J-K. Geometric changes after tricuspid annuloplasty and predictors of residual tricuspid regurgitation: a real time three-dimensional echocardiography study. Eur Heart J. 2010;31:2871–80.

12. De Bonis M, Lapenna E, Sorrentino F, La Canna G, Grimaldi A, Maisano F, Torracca L, Alfieri O. Evolution of tricuspid regurgitation after mitral valve repair for functional mitral regurgitation in dilated cardiomyopathy. Eur J Cardiothorac Surg. 2008;33:600–6.
13. Fukuda S, Song JM, Gillinov AM. Tricuspid valve tethering predicts residual tricuspid regurgitation after tricuspid annuloplasty. Circulation. 2005;111:975–9.
14. De Bonis M, Lapenna E, Taramasso M, Manca M, Calabrese MC, Buzzatti N, Rossodivita A, Pappalardo F, Dorigo E, Alfieri O. Mid-term results of tricuspid annuloplasty with a three-dimensional remodelling ring. J Card Surg. 2012;27(3):288–94.
15. Dreyfus GD, Raja SG, Chan KMJ. Tricuspid leaflet augmentation to address severe tethering in functional tricuspid regurgitation. Eur J Cardiothorac Surg. 2008;34:908–10.
16. Choi JB, Kim NY, Kim KH, Kim MH, Jo KJ. Tricuspid leaflet augmentation to eliminate residual regurgitation in severe functional tricuspid regurgitation. Ann Thorac Surg. 2011;92:e131–3.
17. De Bonis M, Lapenna E, La Canna G. A novel technique for correction of severe tricuspid valve regurgitation due to complex lesions. Eur J Cardiothorac Surg. 2004;25:760–5.
18. Tang H, Xu Z, Zou L, Han L, Lu F, Lang X, Song Z. Valve repair with autologous pericardium for organic lesions in rheumatic tricuspid valve disease. Ann Thorac Surg. 2009;87:726–30.
19. Quarti A, Iezzi F, Soura E, Colaneri M, Pozzi M. Anterior and posterior leaflets augmentation to treat tricuspid valve regurgitation. J Card Surg. 2015;30:421–3.
20. Ratnatunga CP, Edwards M-B, Dore CJ, Taylor KM. Tricuspid valve replacement: UK heart valve registry mid-term results comparing mechanical and biological prostheses. Ann Thorac Surg. 1998;66:1940–7.
21. Rizzoli G, Vendramin I, Nesseris G, Bottio T, Guglielmi C, Schiavon D. Biological or mechanical prostheses in tricuspid position? A meta-analysis of intra-institutional results. Ann Thorac Surg. 2004;77:1607–14.
22. Vassileva CM, Shabosky J, Boley T, Markwell S, Hazelrigg S. Tricuspid valve surgery: the past 10 years from the Nationwide Inpatient Sample (NIS) database. J Thorac Cardiovasc Surg. 2012;143:1043–9.
23. Hwang HY, Kim K-H, Kim K-B, Ahn H. Mechanical tricuspid valve replacement is not superior in patients younger than 65 years who need long term anticoagulation. Ann Thorac Surg. 2012;93:1154–61.
24. Hwang HY, Kim K-H, Kim K-B, Ahn H. Propensity score matching analysis of mechanical versus bioprosthetic tricuspid valve replacements. Ann Thorac Surg. 2014;97:1294–9.
25. Solomon NA, Lim RC, Nand P, Graham KJ. Tricuspid valve replacement: bioprosthetic or mechanical valve? Asian Cardiovasc Thorac Ann. 2004;12:143–8.
26. De Brabandere K, Amsel BJ, Rodrigus I. The forgotten (tricuspid) valve: third time, right time. J Heart Valve Dis. 2015;24:331–4.
27. Said SM, Burkhart HM, Schaff HV, Johnson JN, Connolly HM, Dearani JA. When should a mechanical tricuspid valve replacement be considered? J Thorac Cardiovasc Surg. 2014;148:603–8.
28. Iscan ZH, Vural KM, Bahar I, Mavioglu L, Saritas A. What to expect after tricuspid valve replacement? Long term results. Eur J Cardiothroac Surg. 2007;32:296–300.
29. Nakano K, Eishi K, Kosakai Y, Isobe F, Sasako Y, Nagata S, Ueda H, Kito Y, Kawashima Y. Ten year experience with the Carpentier-Edwards pericardial xenograft in the tricuspid position. J Thorac Cardiovasc Surg. 1996;111:605–12.
30. Nooten GJV, Caes FL, Francois KJ, Taeymans Y, Primo G, Wellens F, Leclerq JL, Deuvaert FE. The valve choice in tricuspid valve replacement: 25 years of experience. Eur J Cardiothorac Surg. 1995;9:441–7.
31. Filsoufi F, Anyanwu AC, Salzberg SP, Frankel T, Cohn LH, Adams DH. Long-term outcomes of tricuspid valve replacement in the current era. Ann Thorac Surg. 2005;80:845–50.
32. Topilsky Y, Khanna A, Oh JK, Nishimura RA, Enriquez-Sarano M, Jeon YB, Sundt TM, Schaff HV, Park JS. Preoperative factors associated with adverse outcome after tricuspid valve replacement. Circulation. 2011;123:1929–39.
33. Kilic A, Saha-Chaudhuri P, Rankin JS, Conte JV. Trends and outcomes of tricuspid valve surgery in north america: an analysis of more than 50,000 patients from the Society of Thoracic Surgeons Database. Ann Thorac Surg. 2013;96:1546–52.
34. Moraca RJ, Moon MR, Lawton JS, Guthrie TJ, Aubuchon KA, Moazami N, Pasque MK, Damiano RJ. Outcomes of tricuspid valve repair and replacement: a propensity analysis. Ann Thorac Surg. 2009;87:83–9.

Percutaneous Approaches to Functional Tricuspid Regurgitation

24

Paolo Denti, Alberto Pozzoli, Azeem Latib, Antonio Colombo, and Ottavio Alfieri

Abstract

Functional tricuspid regurgitation (TR) is the most frequent etiology of tricuspid valve pathology in Western countries. Surgical avoidance of tricuspid repair has been accepted for years, based on the misleading concept that TR would disappear once the primary left-sided problem is treated. The current prevalence of moderate-to-severe TR is about 1.6 million in the United States, with only a small proportion treated, resulting in a large number of untreated patients with functional TR. Furthermore, significant residual TR has been reported in 10–45 % of patients after tricuspid surgical repair with different techniques. As a result, the pathophysiology and treatment of functional TR has gained significant interest in recent years. Percutaneous procedures may be an attractive alternative to surgery for patients deemed to be high-risk surgical candidates. Some of the concepts that have been developed for the percutaneous treatment of aortic and mitral regurgitation are currently being adapted to percutaneous tricuspid valve procedures.

Keywords

Functional tricuspid regurgitation • High risk patients • Percutaneous treatment • Animal study

Principles of Treatment

Functional tricuspid regurgitation (TR) is the most frequent etiology of patients presenting with TR. It is a common finding in patients with left-sided heart disease (around 50 % of patients with mitral valve regurgitation have concomitant TR) and a consistent number of them will develop significant functional TR following left-sided

P. Denti (✉) • A. Pozzoli • O. Alfieri
Heart Surgery Department, San Raffaele University Hospital, Via Olgettina 60, Milan, Italy
e-mail: denti.paolo@hsr.it

A. Latib • A. Colombo
EMO-GVM Centro Cuore Columbus, Milan, Italy

San Raffaele Scientific Institute, Milan, Italy

K.M.J. Chan (ed.), *Functional Mitral and Tricuspid Regurgitation*,
DOI 10.1007/978-3-319-43510-7_24

valve surgery [1, 2]. It has been estimated that 1.6 million patients in the US have moderate-to-severe TR and only less than 8000 patients underwent surgery [3, 4]. According to European guidelines, the surgical treatment of TR is currently indicated for all patients with mild or moderate functional TR when the annulus is dilated (>40 mm or >21 mm/m^2) and they should be considered for treatment when they become symptomatic or when progressive right ventricular (RV) dysfunction or dilatation is documented [5]. The presence of significant TR has a negative prognostic impact on survival in heart failure patients and is independently associated with a 1.5–2 fold increased risk of cardiovascular events during follow-up. Similarly, the late development of functional TR after left-sided valve surgery is also associated with a lower survival [1, 2, 6]. In this subgroup with long-standing TR that are medically managed for a long time, surgical correction can be prohibitive due to the presence of variable degrees of RV dysfunction, pulmonary vascular disease, right heart failure and reduced functional capacity (Table 24.1). The preoperative condition of the RV and the severity of secondary renal and hepatic impairment are the main predictors of limited survival [7, 8]. Considering the high-risk profile of patients with co-morbidities, it would be extremely attractive to find new solutions for a less-invasive treatment of TR. Over the past few years, the development and clinical use of percutaneous approaches to the aortic and mitral valve have been widespread, but limited data are available about the feasibility and efficacy of percutaneous tricuspid valve therapies [9, 10]. Some of the concepts that have been developed for the percutaneous treatment of the mitral regurgitation have been adapted to percutaneous repair of the TV [11].

Table 24.1 Hospital mortality for late tricuspid valve surgery

	Year	Hospital mortality (%)
King	1984	25
Kaul	1991	23.5
Staab	1999	8.8
Izumi	2002	14.2
McCarthy	2004	37
Dong-A Kwon	2006	25
Kwak	2008	16.6

Technique

The clinical experience with percutaneous tricuspid valve technologies are all very preliminary. While different approaches have been evaluated in the preclinical setting, one of the most promising concepts in this field seems to be annular remodeling therapy, since it addresses annular dilatation by reducing the antero-septal distance. Several devices are currently under pre-clinical and clinical evaluation, targeting different anatomic structures of the right heart, mainly the valve itself (the annulus, the leaflets and subvalvular apparatus), the right ventricle and the superior and inferior caval veins (Fig. 24.1).

TriCinch System

The TriCinch System (4TECH Cardio Ltd, Galway, Ireland) is a percutaneous device designed for TV remodeling, by means of a transfemoral implantation of a stainless steel corkscrew into the TV annulus at the level of the antero-posterior commissure. The corkscrew is connected through a Dacron band to a self-expanding nitinol stent. By pulling the system towards the inferior vena cava (IVC), the anchoring corkscrew remodels the antero-posterior annulus, adjustments on a beating heart under live echo guidance are possible, and when the correct level of tension is achieved, the tension is maintained by implantation of the stent in the IVC (Fig. 24.2). The stent is available in different sizes (27–43 mm in diameter, 60 mm in length) to guarantee oversizing in the hepatic region of the IVC and prevent stent migration. Extensive preclinical testing was performed with the TriCinch System in animal models, to prove the safety, technical feasibility and performance. More than 60 adult swines (40 acute and 24 chronic up to 90-days) were treated with the device through a transfemoral venous access [12]. All animals survived the acute implant, showing

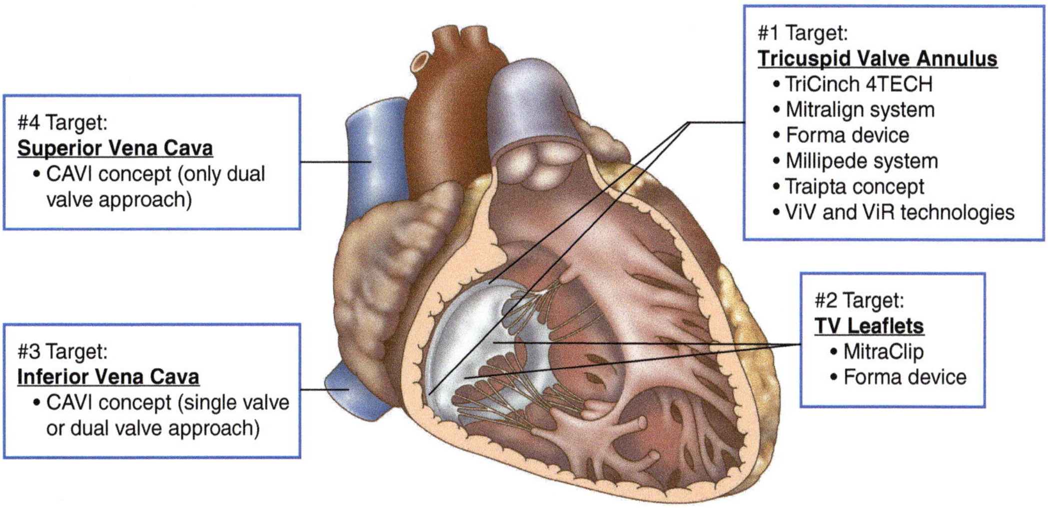

Fig. 24.1 Right heart anatomical targets to address for the treatment of functional TR with current devices under preclinical and clinical evaluation

the feasibility and the efficacy evaluation (30% reduction in septo-lateral TV annular dimension, significant increase in trans-tricuspid peak velocity and coaptation length). Furthermore, all the chronic animals correctly completed the follow-up period, demonstrating the safety of this type of technology in terms of stable implant into the TV annulus. The TriCinch System is currently under evaluation in the multicenter European First-in-Man PREVENT Study (Percutaneous Treatment of Tricuspid Valve Regurgitation With the TriCinch System; ClinicalTrials.gov identifier: NCT02098200), which is enrolling patients with functional TR that are suitable for transcatheter treatment. Preliminary results obtained in the first 3 successfully implanted patients showed reduction of the septolateral annular dimension that remained stable at 6-months after implantation, with sustained clinical and functional improvement [13, 14].

Mitralign System

The Mitralign device (Mitralign, Inc. Tewksbury, USA), which was originally designed for the treatment of functional mitral regurgitation [15], has recently been used to treat functional TR by performing a transcatheter bicuspidization of the TV though the transvenous jugular approach [16]. A steerable catheter is advanced in the right ventricle across the tricuspid valve and positioned under echocardiographic guidance. An insulated radiofrequency wire is then advanced from the base of the leaflet and within the annulus, toward the right atrium in the desired position, near the anteroposterior commissure. Once the wire is through the annulus, a pledget delivery catheter is advanced over the wire from the right atrium across the annulus to the right ventricle. The steps are then repeated on the opposite anatomic site of the posterior commissure (Fig. 24.3). A dedicated plication lock device brings the 2 pledgeted sutures together, plicating the annulus and bicuspidizing the TV. Preliminary results obtained in 7 high-risk patients with symptomatic FTR have been reported. Implantion was feasible in 5/7 patients with no reported adverse events, demonstrating its safety. Tricuspid annular dimension were acutely reduced in 4/5 patients [16, 17].

The FORMA Device

The FORMA Repair System (Edwards Lifescience, Irvine, US) is a valve spacer, which is positioned into the tricuspid regurgitant orifice in order to

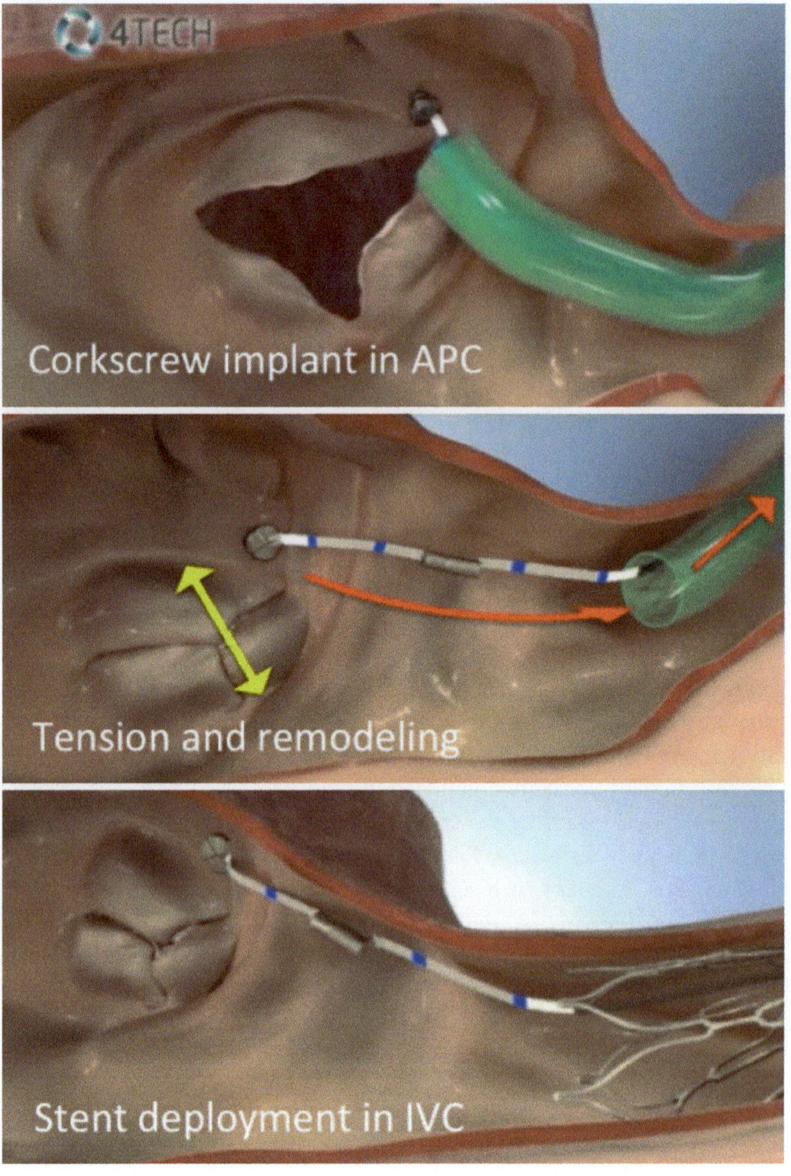

Fig. 24.2 Key phases of the implantation of the TriCinch device. *APC* antero-posterior commissure, *IVC* inferior vena cava (Courtesy of 4Tech Cardio Ltd)

create a platform for native leaflet coaptation. The device is delivered through subclavian venous access and is distally anchored to the RV apex. Proximal fixation is performed in a small surgically prepared pocket (as done for permanent pacemaker implantation). Preliminary results in 7 high-risk patients were recently reported. In all the patients, the device was successfully implanted without major complications, obtaining a mild-to-moderate acute reduction of TR grade. Thirty-day results, showed for 4 patients, reported clinical improvements and stable TR reduction [18].

The Millipede System

The Millipede system (Millipede, LLC, Ann Arbor, Michigan) involves the placement of a tricuspid annular ring with an attachment system via either minimally invasive surgical or percutaneous access to remodel the native tricuspid annular shape and diameter. It is repositionable and retrievable before deployment [10]. No updated preclinical feasibility or safety data are currently available and the company has changed its focus to concentrate on the mitral valve.

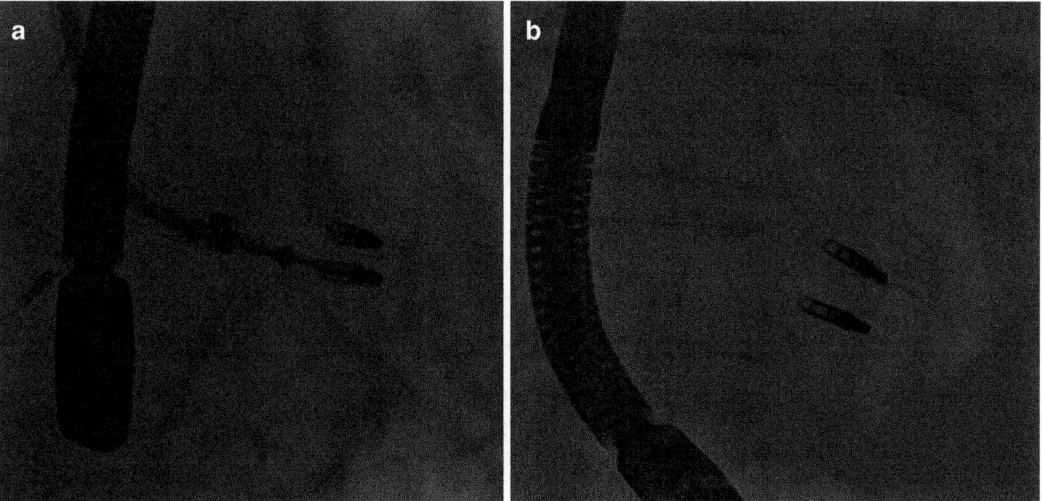

Fig. 24.3 Mitralign system. (**a**) Angiographic implantation of the second pledget in the antero-posterior commissure and (**b**) final fluoroscopic result of the procedure

MitraClip

Since the surgical edge-to-edge repair for the tricuspid valve, the clover technique, was associated with satisfactory results at mid-term follow-up [19], the implantation of the MitraClip device (Abbott, Abbott Park, Illinois) in the tricuspid position is currently under investigation. First-in-man use of MitraClip to treat TR was reported in a patient with congenitally corrected transposition of the great arteries [20]. Currently, MitraClip therapy for severe TR have been performed in 8 patients, of which 6 were done with the transjugular access and the other 2 cases transfemorally (Fig. 24.4). The numerous challenges of this approach include the three-leaflet configuration of the TV, the presence of huge annular dilatation and lack of coaptation, the different tissue properties of the tricuspid leaflets and also the use of reliable echo imaging to guide the procedure, which is actually not optimal for tricuspid interventional procedures.

Caval Valve Implantation (CAVI)

An alternative percutaneous approach to treat FTR was described by Corno et al. They reported the implantation of separate valves either in the inferior vena cava (single valve approach) alone or also in the superior vena cava (dual valve approach) to prevent damage to the liver and other organs [21–23]. The rationale of this procedure is to reduce hepatic, abdominal, and peripheral venous congestion leading to amelioration of right heart failure. Since the prostheses are implanted in a low-pressure venous system, lifelong anticoagulation would probably be required. In presence of advanced RV dysfunction, the single valve approach seems to be safer when RV dysfunction is severe, as it does not increase the RV preload. However, data are not yet available on whether the single or dual valve technique should be the optimal approach. Promising preliminary clinical results have been recently reported in 10 patients treated with the Sapien XT valve, preparing the landing zone in the inferior vena cava with a self-expandable stent. Acute hemodynamic as well as clinical improvements at follow-up have been reported in 5 patients, 3 treated with dual valve and 2 with single valve approach [24]. Two different clinical CAVI trials are enrolling high-risk patients with severe symptomatic TR: the TRICAVAL in Europe and the HOVER trial in US.

Transcatheter Tricuspid Valve Replacement

The feasibility of tricuspid valve-in-valve (Fig. 24.5) and valve-in-ring (Fig. 24.6) to treat

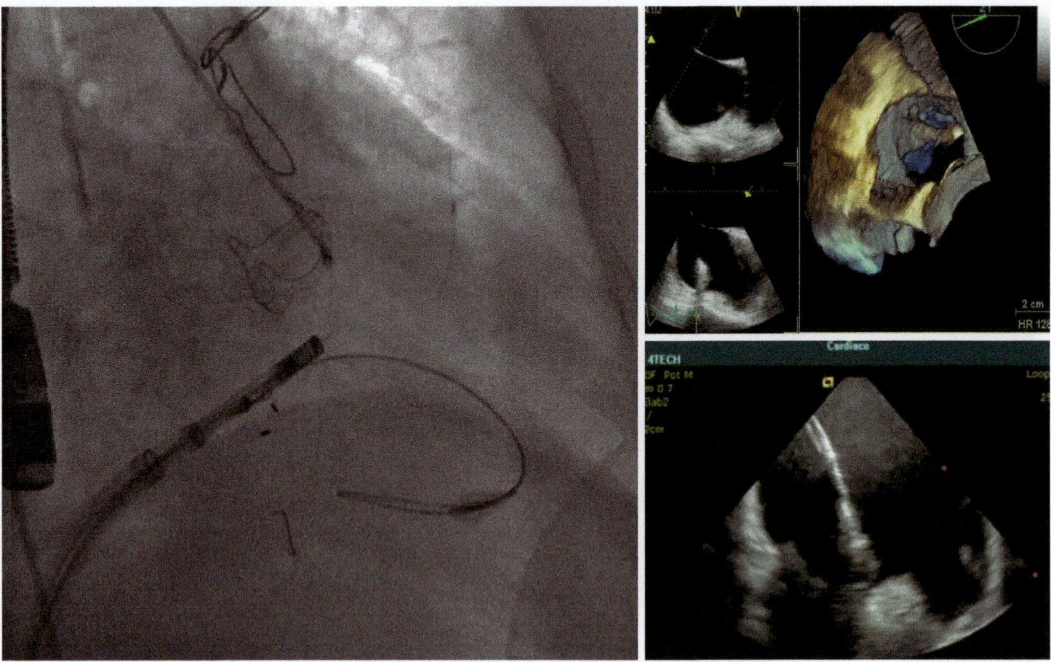

Fig. 24.4 The Mitraclip system grasping the tricuspidal leaflets through the right jugular vein, with intracardiac transfemoral echocardiographic guidance. Fluoroscopic implantation of two parallel devices to close the antero-septal commissure and the final echocardiographic result

degenerated surgical bioprostheses or after a failing surgical rigid ring annuloplasty was reported with different prostheses (Edwards Sapien, Sapien XT and Melody prosthesis) and approaches (mainly transfemoral and through the jugular vein) [25, 26]. The overall experience worldwide consists of 156 patients who underwent tricuspid valve-in-valve or valve-in-ring, they have been included in the Valve-in-Valve International Registry [27]. Acute satisfactory results were reported, but no data are available yet on the long-term outcomes. Currently, no reports exist on transcatheter tricuspid valve replacement in native tricuspid valves in human.

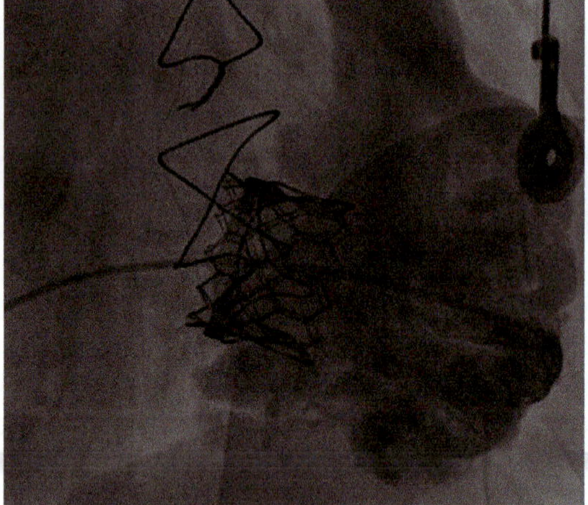

Fig. 24.5 Final angiographic result of a tricuspid Valve-in-Valve with a Edwards Sapien 3 (29 mm) implanted inside a degenerated surgical bioprosthesis (Carpentier-Edwards Perimount 29 mm)

Transatrial Intrapericardial Tricuspid Annuloplasty (TRAIPTA Concept)

A different approach is adopted by the TRAIPTA concept (Transatrial intrapericardial tricuspid annuloplasty) [28]. Pericardial access is obtained puncturing the right atrial appendage from within, after transfemoral venous access. A circumferential implant, which exerts compressive force over the tricuspid annulus, is delivered

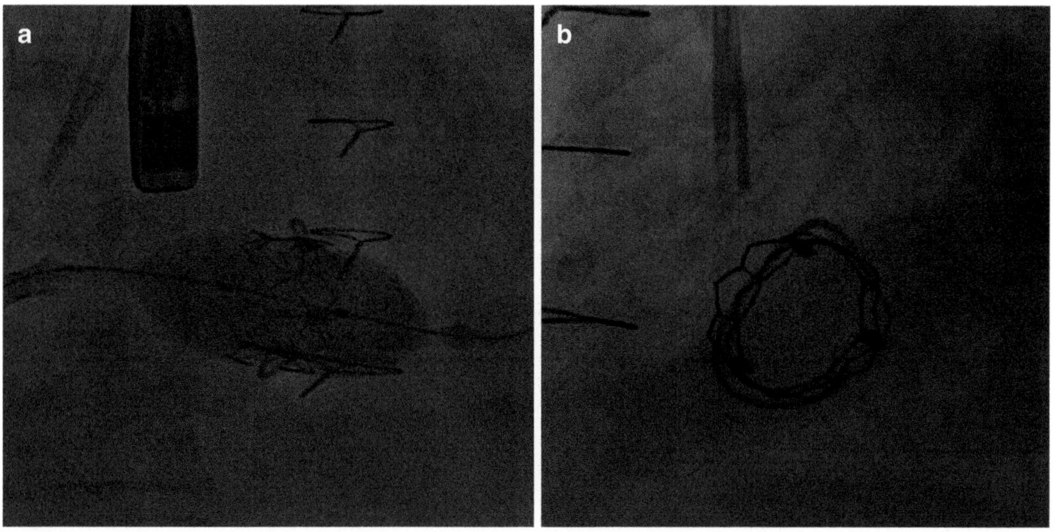

Fig. 24.6 Angiograms of a Valve-in-Ring procedure: implantation of an Edwards Sapien XT 26 mm (**a**) inside a Medtronic Contour 3D incomplete semi-rigid ring and final result after deployment (**b**)

along the atrioventricular groove within the pericardial space. Tension on the implant is then adjusted on a beating heart, to modify the tricuspid annulus thus lessening the regurgitation grade. The procedure is mainly guided by fluoroscopy. The right atrial puncture is finally sealed using nitinol closure devices. Preclinical experience showed safety of the implant. Significant improvement of leaflet coaptation and reduction of tricuspid valve area and diameters were also observed. The adoption of this technology could be limited by the fact that an essential requirement is the freedom of the intrapericardial space. Many of potential candidates will be surgical redo patients with FTR, in whom fibrotic adherences would represent a contraindication for this treatment. Also the risk of coronary compression requires further evaluation.

Early Results

Although only preliminary data are currently available, transcatheter-based techniques for the treatment of TR have been rapidly evolving over the last few years. Initial experiences showed that percutaneous tricuspid valve procedures, including repair and replacement, are feasible and seem to be safe. Some of these novel devices are based upon well-known surgical techniques that have subsequently progressed to less invasive approaches, while others are completely new concepts that should be validated in the clinical setting. It is not easily predictable as to how long it will take for transcatheter TV technology to become a routine therapeutic option in the clinical practice. The unmet clinical need is apparent, because of the huge number of patients with symptomatic severe TR who could benefit from an interventional treatment, currently deemed too high risk for conventional surgery. The consequence is that TR is an undertreated disease, leading to increased mortality and increased health costs. Less invasive percutaneous TV treatment could represent an emerging therapeutic option for this population. Imaging will play a central role in patient selection and procedural guidance.

References

1. Kwak JJ, Kim YJ, Kim MK, Kim HK, Park JS, Kim KH, Kim KB, Ahn H, Sohn DW, Oh BH, Park YB. Development of tricuspid regurgitation late after left-sided valve surgery: a single-center experience

with long-term echocardiographic examinations. Am Heart J. 2008;155(4):732–7.
2. Song H, Kim MJ, Chung CH, Choo SJ, Song MG, Song JM, Kang DH, Lee JW, Song JK. Factors associated with development of late significant tricuspid regurgitation after successful left-sided valve surgery. Heart. 2009;95(11):931–6.
3. Stuge O, Liddicoat J. Emerging opportunities for cardiac surgeons within structural heart disease. J Thorac Cardiovasc Surg. 2006;132(6):1258–61.
4. Health Research International Report. Report no. 057-1-US-0705-221) ES-5.
5. Vahanian A, Alfieri O, et al. Guidelines on the management of valvular heart disease (version 2012). Joint Task Force on the Management of Valvular Heart Disease of the European Society of Cardiology (ESC); European Association for Cardio-Thoracic Surgery (EACTS). Eur Heart J. 2012;33(19):2451–96.
6. Agarwal S, Tuzcu EM, Rodriguez ER, Tan CD, Rodriguez LL, Kapadia SR. Interventional cardiology perspective of functional tricuspid regurgitation. Circ Cardiovasc Interv. 2009;2:565–73.
7. Nath J, Foster E, Heidenreich PA. Impact of tricuspid regurgitation on long-term survival. J Am Coll Cardiol. 2004;43(3):405–9.
8. Shiran A, Sagie A. Tricuspid regurgitation in mitral valve disease incidence, prognostic implications, mechanism, and management. J Am Coll Cardiol. 2009;53:401–8.
9. McCarthy PM, Bhudia SK, Rajeswaran J, Hoercher KJ, Lytle BW, Cosgrove DM, Blackstone EH. Tricuspid valve repair: durability and risk factors for failure. J Thorac Cardiovasc Surg. 2004;127:674–85.
10. Taramasso M, Vanermen H, Maisano F, Guidotti A, La Canna G, Alfieri O. The growing clinical importance of secondary tricuspid regurgitation. J Am Coll Cardiol. 2012;59:703–10.
11. Rogers JH. Functional tricuspid regurgitation: percutaneous therapies needed. JACC Cardiovasc Interv. 2015;8(3):492–4. pii: S1936-8798(14)01756-7.
12. Taramasso M. Percutaneous remodeling of the tricuspid valve with a novel cinching device: acute and chronic experience in an in vivo animal model. Paris: EuroPCR; 2015.
13. Latib A, Agricola E, Pozzoli A, Denti P, Taramasso M, Spagnolo P, Juliard JM, Brochet E, Ou P, Sarano ME, Grigioni F, Alfieri O, Vahanian A, Colombo A, Maisano F. First-in-man implantation of a tricuspid annular remodeling device for functional tricuspid regurgitation. JACC Cardiovasc Interv. 2015;8(13):e211–4.
14. Maisano F. 4Tech percutaneous annuloplasty for tricuspid regurgitation. Chicago: TVT; 2015.
15. Siminiak T, Dankowski R, Baszko A, Lee C, Firek L, Kalmucki P, Szyszka A, Groothuis A. Percutaneous direct mitral annuloplasty using the Mitralign Bident system: description of the method and a case report. Kardiol Pol. 2013;71(12):1287–92.
16. Schofer J, Bijuklic K, Tiburtius C, Hansen L, Groothuis A, Hahn RT. First-in-human transcatheter tricuspid valve repair in a patient with severely regurgitant tricuspid valve. J Am Coll Cardiol. 2015; 65(12):1190–5.
17. Hahn RT. Mitralign for tricuspid regurgitation: case review and examples. Paris: EuroPCR; 2015.
18. Rodés-Cabau J. First-in-human experience: Edwards FORMA Repair System. Chicago: TVT; 2015.
19. Lapenna E, De Bonis M, Verzini A, La Canna G, Ferrara D, Calabrese MC, Taramasso M, Alfieri O. The clover technique for the treatment of complex tricuspid valve insufficiency: midterm clinical and echocardiographic results in 66 patients. Eur J Cardiothorac Surg Off J Eur Assoc Cardiothorac Surg. 2010;37(6):1297–303.
20. Franzen O, von Samson P, Dodge-Khatami A, Geffert G, Baldus S. Percutaneous edge-to-edge repair of tricuspid regurgitation in congenitally corrected transposition of the great arteries. Congenit Heart Dis. 2011;6(1):57–9.
21. Corno AF, Zhou J, Tozzi P, von Segesser LK. Offbypass implantation of a self-expandable valved stent between inferior vena cava and right atrium. Interact Cardiovasc Thorac Surg. 2003;2:166–9.
22. Lauten A, Doenst T, Hamadanchi A, Franz M, Figulla HR. Percutaneous bicaval valve implantation for transcatheter treatment of tricuspid regurgitation: clinical observations and 12-month follow-up. Circ Cardiovasc Interv. 2014;7(2):268–72.
23. Laule M, Stangl V, Sanad W, Lembcke A, Baumann G, Stangl K. Percutaneous transfemoral management of severe secondary tricuspid regurgitation with Edwards Sapien XT bioprosthesis: first-in-man experience. J Am Coll Cardiol. 2013;61(18): 1929–31.
24. Lauten A. Caval Valve Implantation (CAVI) for treatment of severe TR. San Francisco: TCT; 2014.
25. Godart F, Baruteau AE, Petit J, Riou JY, Sassolas F, Lusson JR, Fraisse A, Boudjemline Y. Transcatheter tricuspid valve implantation: a multicentre French study. Arch Cardiovasc Dis. 2014;107(11): 583–91.
26. Hoendermis ES, Douglas YL, van den Heuvel AF. Percutaneous Edwards SAPIEN valve implantation in the tricuspid position: case report and review of literature. EuroIntervention J EuroPCR Collaboration Working Group Interv Cardiol Eur Soc Cardiol. 2012;8(5):628–33.
27. Dvir D. Tricuspid valve-in-valve: update from VIVID registry and technical strategies to improve clinical outcomes. Chicago: TVT; 2015.
28. Rogers T, Ratnayaka K, Sonmez M, Franson DN, Schenke WH, Mazal JR, Kocaturk O, Chen MY, Faranesh AZ, Lederman RJ. Transatrial intrapericardial tricuspid annuloplasty. JACC Cardiovasc Interv. 2015;8(3):483–91.

Which Treatment Is Best for Which Patient in Functional Tricuspid Regurgitation?

25

K.M. John Chan

Abstract

A range of treatment options are available for functional tricuspid regurgitation. The type of treatment chosen needs to be tailored to each individual patient according to the stage of the disease.

Keywords

Functional tricuspid regurgitation • Tricuspid annuloplasty • Tricuspid leaflet augmentation • Tricuspid valve replacement • Tricuspid annular dilatation • Tricuspid leaflet tethering

The need for surgical intervention on the tricuspid valve and the most appropriate surgical intervention which should be performed is dependent on the severity of tricuspid regurgitation (TR) and the stage of tricuspid valve disease present. The stage of tricuspid valve disease is dependent on the tricuspid annular size, the mode of leaflet coaptation, and the severity of tricuspid leaflet tethering. As discussed earlier, three stages of functional TR can be recognized; this can be used to help guide treatment [1, 2]:

K.M.J. Chan, BM BS, MSc, PhD, FRCS CTh
Department of Cardiothoracic Surgery,
Gleneagles Hospital, Jalan Ampang,
Kuala Lumpur 50450, Malaysia
e-mail: kmjohnchan@yahoo.com

Stage 1: *The tricuspid annulus is not dilated, the leaflets coapt normally from body to body, there is no leaflet tethering.*

There is usually no TR or the TR is usually mild in this stage of disease. No surgical intervention is needed.

Stage 2: *The tricuspid annulus is dilated to more than 40 mm, the leaflets coapt abnormally from edge to edge only, there is no leaflet tethering or only mild leaflet tethering (less than 8 mm)*

TR is usually mild or moderate in this stage of disease but may increase in severity depending on right ventricular preload, afterload and contractility. Concomitant tricuspid annuloplasty should be performed at the time of left sided heart valve surgery. Annuloplasty using a rigid ring generally gives the best long term results. However, a flexible band annuloplasty or suture annuloplasty is acceptable if the

K.M.J. Chan (ed.), *Functional Mitral and Tricuspid Regurgitation*,
DOI 10.1007/978-3-319-43510-7_25

annulus is only mildly dilated and there is no more than moderate TR. A ring annuloplasty is recommended if the TR is severe or if there is severe dilatation of the tricuspid annulus.

Stage 3: *The tricuspid annulus is dilated to more than 40 mm, there is no leaflet coaptation, leaflet tethering is significant* (*greater than 8 mm*)

TR is usually severe under all physiological conditions in this stage of disease. In addition to concomitant tricuspid annuloplasty at the time of left sided heart valve surgery, the leaflet tethering needs to be addressed to ensure long term durability of the repair. The most appropriate procedure for this is augmentation of the anterior leaflet of the tricuspid valve. If necessary, augmentation of both the anterior and posterior leaflets can be performed. Tricuspid valve replacement is also an appropriate treatment in these patients if repair is not possible.

References

1. Dreyfus GD, Chan KMJ. Functional tricuspid regurgitation: a more complex entity than it appears. Heart. 2009;95:868–9.
2. Dreyfus GD, Martin RP, Chan KMJ, Dulguerov F. Functional tricuspid regurgitation: a need to revise our understanding. J Am Coll Cardiol. 2015;65:2331–6.

Future Directions in Functional Tricuspid Regurgitation

26

K.M. John Chan

Abstract

Much progress has been made in recent years on our understanding of functional tricuspid regurgitation, the indications for its treatment, and the best way to treat it depending on the stage of the disease. Much more needs to be done to better define some of the indications for surgical intervention and the type of surgery which should be performed. Longer term results are also needed for some of the newer techniques for tricuspid valve repair.

Keywords

Functional tricuspid regurgitation • Tricuspid valve repair • Tricuspid annuloplasty • Tricuspid leaflet augmentation • Tricuspid annular dilatation

Our understanding of functional tricuspid regurgitation (FTR) and the management of this condition has changed significantly over the last 10 years. Tricuspid annular dilatation is generally accepted as an indication for concomitant tricuspid valve intervention at the time of mitral or aortic valve surgery [1, 2]. However, the threshold size to indicate the need for surgical intervention on the tricuspid valve, although well established, continues to be challenged. A randomized controlled trial is needed to firmly address this.

An important point to note is that the benefits of doing concomitant tricuspid annuloplasty at the time of mitral or aortic valve surgery is not immediately apparent; these patients will survive the operation and be well enough to be discharged back home if the tricuspid valve is not operated on. However, the consequences of leaving the tricuspid valve alone in these patients will become apparent in future years when they develop recurrent TR and become symptomatic with a reduced survival [1]. At that stage, re-operative tricuspid valve surgery carries a high operative risk.

More recently, the concept of tricuspid leaflet tethering and the need to address this to ensure

K.M.J. Chan, BM BS, MSc, PhD, FRCS CTh
Department of Cardiothoracic Surgery,
Gleneagles Hospital, Jalan Ampang,
Kuala Lumpur 50450, Malaysia
e-mail: kmjohnchan@yahoo.com

K.M.J. Chan (ed.), *Functional Mitral and Tricuspid Regurgitation*,
DOI 10.1007/978-3-319-43510-7_26

long term durability of the tricuspid valve repair is also beginning to be appreciated [1, 2]. Surgical techniques have been developed to deal with this by augmenting the anterior leaflet. However, the long term results of this repair technique is needed and is still presently unknown.

Tricuspid valve replacement is still an accepted option in those with advanced disease in whom valve repair is not possible. Recent studies show a much improved operative risk with tricuspid valve replacement compared to earlier studies. A randomized trial is needed to compare the choice of prosthesis (biological versus mechanical) in younger patients.

Percutaneous approaches to functional TR have been developed and are being evaluated. This may be particularly useful in re-operative procedures.

Suggested Reading

1. Dreyfus GD, Chan KMJ. Functional tricuspid regurgitation: a more complex entity than it appears. Heart. 2009;95:868–9.
2. Dreyfus GD, Martin RP, Chan KMJ, Dulguerov F. Functional tricuspid regurgitation: a need to revise our understanding. J Am Coll Cardiol. 2015;65:2331–6.

Index

K.M.J. Chan (ed.), *Functional Mitral and Tricuspid Regurgitation*,
DOI 10.1007/978-3-319-43510-7

CPI Antony Rowe
Chippenham, UK
2017-02-24 22:39